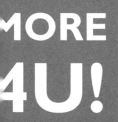
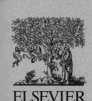

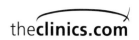

A. Simon Turner, BVSc, MS
CONSULTING EDITOR

VETERINARY CLINICS

OF NORTH AMERICA

Equine Practice

Neonatal Medicine and Surgery

GUEST EDITOR
L. Chris Sanchez, DVM, PhD

August 2005 • Volume 21 • Number 2

SAUNDERS

An Imprint of Elsevier, Inc.
PHILADELPHIA   LONDON   TORONTO   MONTREAL   SYDNEY   TOKYO

W.B. SAUNDERS COMPANY
A Division of Elsevier Inc.

Elsevier, Inc., 1600 John F. Kennedy Blvd., Suite 1800, Philadelphia, PA 19103-2899

http://www.vetequine.theclinics.com

VETERINARY CLINICS OF NORTH AMERICA: Volume 21, Number 2
EQUINE PRACTICE   ISSN 0749-0739
August 2005   ISBN 1-4160-2837-4
Editor: John Vassallo

The ideas and opinions expressed in *Veterinary Clinics of North America: Equine Practice* do not necessarily reflect those of the Publisher. The Publisher does not assume any responsibility for any injury and/or damage to persons or property arising out of or related to any use of the material contained in this periodical. The reader is advised to check the appropriate medical literature and the product information currently provided by the manufacturer of each drug to be administered to verify the dosage, the method and duration of administration, or contraindications. It is the responsibility of the treating physician or other health care professional, relying on independent experience and knowledge of the patient, to determine drug dosages and the best treatment for the patient. Mention of any product in this issue should not be construed as endorsement by the contributors, editors, or the Publisher of the product or manufacturers' claims.

Veterinary Clinics of North America: Equine Practice (ISSN 0749-0739) is published in April, August, and December by Elsevier, Inc. Corporate and editorial offices: Elsevier, Inc., 1600 John F. Kennedy Blvd., Suite 1800, Philadelphia, PA 19103-2899. Accounting and circulation offices: 6277 Sea Harbor Drive, Orlando, FL 32887-4800. Subscription prices are $145.00 per year for US individuals, $230.00 per year for US institutions, $73.00 per year for US students and residents, $169.00 per year for Canadian individuals, $285.00 per year for Canadian institutions, $185.00 per year for international individuals, $285.00 per year for international institutions and $93.00 per year for Canadian and foreign students/residents. To receive student/resident rate, orders must be accompanied by name of affiliated institution, date of term, and the *signature* of program/residency coordinator on institution letterhead. Orders will be billed at individual rate until proof of status is received. Foreign air speed delivery is included in all *Clinics* subscription prices. All prices are subject to change without notice. POSTMASTER: Send address changes to *Veterinary Clinics of North America: Equine Practice*, Elsevier, Customer Service Department, 6277 Sea Harbor Drive, Orlando, FL 32887-4800, USA; phone: (+1) (877) 8397126 [toll free number for US customers], or (+1) (407) 3454020 [customers outside US]; fax: (+1) (407) 3631354; e-mail: usjcs@elsevier.com

Reprints. For copies of 100 or more, of articles in this publication, please contact the Commercial Reprints Department, Elsevier Inc., 360 Park Avenue South, New York, New York 10010-1710. Tel. (212) 633-3813, Fax: (212) 462-1935 email: reprints@elsevier.com

Veterinary Clinics of North America: Equine Practice is covered in *Index Medicus, Excerpta Medica, Current Contents/Agriculture, Biology and Environmental Sciences, and ISI.*

Printed in the United States of America.

CONSULTING EDITOR

A. SIMON TURNER, BVSc, MS, Diplomate, American College of Veterinary Surgeons; Professor, Department of Clinical Sciences, College of Veterinary Medicine and Biomedical Sciences, Colorado State University, Fort Collins, Colorado

GUEST EDITOR

L. CHRIS SANCHEZ, DVM, PhD, Assistant Professor, Department of Large Animal Clinical Sciences, College of Veterinary Medicine, University of Florida, Gainesville, Florida

CONTRIBUTORS

JANE E. AXON, BVSc, MACVSc, Diplomate, American College of Veterinary Internal Medicine; Director, Clovelly Intensive Care Unit, Scone Veterinary Hospital, Scone, Australia

JAMES E. BRYANT, DVM, Partner and Surgeon, Pilchuck Veterinary Hospital, Snohomish, Washington

VIRGINIA A. BUECHNER-MAXWELL, DVM, MS, Diplomate, American College of Veterinary Internal Medicine; Associate Professor and Section Chief, Department of Large Animal Clinical Sciences, Virginia-Maryland Regional College of Veterinary Medicine, Virginia Tech, Blacksburg, Virginia

KEVIN T.T. CORLEY, BVM&S, PhD, MRCVS, Diplomate, American College of Veterinary Internal Medicine; Diplomate, American College of Veterinary Emergency and Critical Care; Head of Neonatal Foal Intensive Care Unit, Equine Referral Hospital, Royal Veterinary College, North Mymms, Hertfordshire, United Kingdom

EARL M. GAUGHAN, DVM, Professor, Large Animal Teaching Hospital, Auburn University College of Veterinary Medicine, Auburn University, Alabama

STEEVE GIGUÈRE, DVM, PhD, Diplomate, American College of Veterinary Internal Medicine; Associate Professor and Director of the Hofmann Equine Neonatal Intensive Care Unit, College of Veterinary Medicine, University of Florida, Gainesville, Florida

GUY D. LESTER, BVMS, PhD, Diplomate, American College of Veterinary Internal Medicine; Associate Professor of Equine Medicine, Department of Veterinary Clinical Sciences, School of Veterinary and Biomedical Sciences, Murdoch University, Murdoch, Western Australia

ROBERT J. MACKAY, BVSc, PhD, Professor and Chief, Department of Large Animal Clinical Sciences, University of Florida, Gainesville, Florida

K. GARY MAGDESIAN, DVM, Diplomate, American College of Veterinary Internal Medicine; Diplomate, American College of Veterinary Emergency and Critical Care; Diplomate, American College of Veterinary Clinical Pharmacology; Assistant Professor of Equine Critical Care Medicine, Department of Medicine and Epidemiology, University of California School of Veterinary Medicine, Davis, California

JONATHAN E. PALMER, VMD, Diplomate, American College of Veterinary Internal Medicine–Large Animal; Associate Professor of Medicine; Director of Neonatal/Perinatal Programs and Chief, Neonatal Intensive Care Service, Graham French Neonatal Section, Connelly Intensive Care Unit, The George D. Widener Hospital, New Bolton Center, School of Veterinary Medicine, University of Pennsylvania, Kennett Square, Pennsylvania

AMY C. POLKES, DVM, Diplomate, American College of Veterinary Internal Medicine; Damascus Equine Associates, Germantown, Maryland

MICHAEL B. PORTER, DVM, PhD, Diplomate, American College of Veterinary Internal Medicine; Department of Large Animal Clinical Sciences, College of Veterinary Medicine, University of Florida, Gainesville, Florida

SAMMY RAMIREZ, DVM, MS, Diplomate, American College of Veterinary Internal Medicine; Diplomate, American College of Veterinary Radiologists; College of Veterinary Medicine, Louisiana State University, Baton, Rouge, Louisiana

CLARE A. RYAN, DVM, Resident, Large Animal Internal Medicine, College of Veterinary Medicine, University of Florida, Gainesville, Florida

L. CHRIS SANCHEZ, DVM, PhD, Assistant Professor, Department of Large Animal Clinical Sciences, College of Veterinary Medicine, University of Florida, Gainesville, Florida

TROY N. TRUMBLE, DVM, PhD, Diplomate, American College of Veterinary Surgeons; Assistant Professor, Department of Large Animal Clinical Sciences, College of Veterinary Medicine, University of Florida, Gainesville, Florida

CONTENTS

Preface   xi
L. Chris Sanchez

Immunologic Disorders in Neonatal Foals   241
Steeve Giguère and Amy C. Polkes

Foals live in an environment heavily populated by bacteria, many
of which are capable of causing disease. Development of infection,
however, is the exception rather than the rule. The ability of the foal
to prevent infection by most pathogens is the result of a sophisticated set of defense mechanisms. These defense mechanisms can
be divided into adaptive and innate immunity. Innate immunity
encompasses defense mechanisms that preexist or are rapidly
induced within hours of exposure to a pathogen. Conversely, adaptive or acquired immunity represents host defenses mediated by
T and B lymphocytes, each expressing a highly specific antigen
receptor and exhibiting memory during a second encounter
with a given antigen. Immunologic disorders are relatively common in foals compared with their occurrence in adult horses. This
article summarizes the current understanding of the equine fetal
and neonatal immune system and reviews common immunodeficiency disorders as well as disorders resulting from allogenic
incompatibilities.

Equine Neonatal Sepsis   273
L. Chris Sanchez

Neonatal infection remains a leading cause of morbidity and mortality in the equine industry, despite advances in prevention and
treatment. Many factors can influence a foal's risk for the development of sepsis in the peripartum period. This article discusses those
factors, causative organisms, and therapeutic options. Factors that
influence prognosis and potential preventative strategies also are
addressed.

Neonatal Foal Diarrhea   295

K. Gary Magdesian

> Diarrhea is a significant cause of morbidity and mortality in the
> neonatal foal. Numerous noninfectious and infectious agents are
> responsible for enterocolitis and enteritis. This article provides an
> overview of the differential diagnoses for neonatal diarrhea and
> general and specific guidelines for therapy.

**Nondiarrheal Disorders of the Gastrointestinal Tract in
Neonatal Foals**   313

Clare A. Ryan and L. Chris Sanchez

> Neonates can have a variety of gastrointestinal disorders, primary
> and secondary in nature. Important primary disorders include con-
> genital abnormalities and meconium retention. One of the most
> important secondary lesions is generalized ileus. Gastric ulceration
> can occur as a primary or secondary event. This article addresses
> the pathophysiology, diagnosis, and treatment of gastrointestinal
> problems commonly observed in neonatal foals.

Maturity of the Neonatal Foal   333

Guy D. Lester

> The immature foal frequently represents a significant management
> challenge to even the most experienced clinician. The clinical
> course typically involves complications to a range of body systems,
> including the musculoskeletal, respiratory, and gastrointestinal sys-
> tems. Before the commencement of treatment, it is important to
> provide the owner with an estimation of short-term and long-term
> survival, expected costs, and possible complications. Formulation
> of an accurate prognosis can be a difficult task but is aided by
> knowledge not only of normal maturation but of the factors that
> affect this process.

Orthopedic Disorders in Neonatal Foals   357

Troy N. Trumble

> The first month of life is a vulnerable time for foals. They must
> adjust to their environment while they are still compromised
> immunologically, and their musculoskeletal system is rapidly
> growing and adjusting to stresses from an increasing amount of
> exercise. Therefore, if a foal is born with or acquires an abnormality
> or disease related to the musculoskeletal system, rapid adjustments
> must be made to allow the foal to grow and respond so that fut-
> ure athletic performance will not be compromised. Problems must
> be identified early, which requires thorough examinations. This
> article summarizes treatment options for orthopedic disorders that
> present or become clinically evident within the first month of life.

Neurologic Disorders of Neonatal Foals 387

Robert J. MacKay

Neurologic examination of the neonatal foal is quite different from the process used to examine older foals and adult horses. Abnormal neurologic signs are best appreciated in the context of a detailed knowledge of general neonatal medicine and awareness of normal foal behavior and milestones of development. A systematic approach to neurologic examination is provided. The results of such examination are used to localize a lesion or lesions in the nervous system. Descriptions and treatment strategies are given for most common and important neonatal neurologic diseases.

Equine Neonatal Thoracic and Abdominal Ultrasonography 407

Michael B. Porter and Sammy Ramirez

Pathologic disorders of the equine neonate often develop shortly after foaling as a result of prematurity, dystocia, trauma, or septicemia. Recognition of these disorders requires routine patient assessment along with diagnostic aids, including abdominal and thoracic ultrasonography. Fortunately, modern technology affords today's equine practitioners the opportunity to use ultrasonography to advance their practice, and it is the authors' hope that this article might help in those efforts.

Resuscitation and Emergency Management for Neonatal Foals 431

Kevin T.T. Corley and Jane E. Axon

Early intervention can dramatically alter outcome in foals. Cardiopulmonary cerebral resuscitation can be successful and clinically worthwhile when applied to foals that arrest as part of the birthing process. Readily available equipment and an ordered plan starting with addressing the respiratory system (airway and breathing) followed by the circulatory system (circulation and drugs) are the keys to success. Hypoglycemia is common in foals that are not nursing and in septic foals. Support of serum glucose can be an important emergency treatment. Respiratory support with oxygen therapy should be considered in all foals following resuscitation and dystocia. Other foals that are likely to benefit from oxygen are those that are dyspneic, cyanotic, meconium-stained after birth, or recumbent. Emergency therapies, applied correctly, are expected to result in decreased mortality and morbidity.

Ventilatory Support of the Critically Ill Foal 457

Jonathan E. Palmer

Critically ill foals often have respiratory failure and benefit from respiratory support. Conventional mechanical ventilation using modern mechanical ventilators is easily adapted to foals. Establishing ventilator settings is a dynamic process aided by constant monitoring of blood gas values, end-tidal carbon dioxide, airway pressures, respiratory volumes, airway resistance, and respiratory compliance. Early weaning is as important as timely initiation of ventilation.

Nutritional Support for Neonatal Foals 487
Virginia A. Buechner-Maxwell

In recent years, equine neonatal medicine has made significant advances. The importance of nutritional support for the sick neonatal foal has been recognized, and methods of providing that support have been developed. Today, the clinician has many options when designing a nutritional plan for the neonatal foal. When the foal's gut permits, enteral diets are an inexpensive source of nutrients. Under conditions where the gut requires rest, methods for delivering nutrients by the parenteral route have also been developed. In this article, the nutrition of the normal and sick foal is described. Guidelines for designing a nutritional plan are also reviewed.

Abdominal Surgery in Neonatal Foals 511
James E. Bryant and Earl M. Gaughan

Abdominal surgery in foals under 30 days old has become more common with improved neonatal care. Early recognition of a foal at risk and better nursing care have increased the survival rates of foals that require neonatal care. The success of improved neonatal care also has increased the need for accurate diagnosis and treatment of gastrointestinal, umbilical, and bladder disorders in these foals. This chapter focuses on the early and accurate diagnosis of specific disorders that require abdominal exploratory surgery and the specific treatment considerations and prognosis for these disorders.

Index 537

GOAL STATEMENT

The goal of the *Veterinary Clinics of North America: Equine Practice* is to keep practicing veterinarians up to date with current clinical practice in equine medicine by providing timely articles reviewing the state of the art in equine care.

ACCREDITATION

The *Veterinary Clinics of North America: Equine Practice* offers continuing education credits, awarded by Cummings School of Veterinary Medicine at Tufts University, Office of Continuing Education.

Cummings School of Veterinary Medicine at Tufts University is a designated provider of continuing veterinary medical education. Veterinarians participating in this learning activity may earn up to 6 credits per issue up to a maximum of 18 credits per year. Credits awarded may not apply toward license renewal in all states. It is the responsibility of each participant to verify the requirements of their state licensing board.

Credit can be earned by reading the text material, taking the examination online at *http://www.theclinics.com/home/cme*, and completing the program evaluation. Following your completion of the test and program evaluation, and review of any and all incorrect answers, you may print your certificate.

TO ENROLL

To enroll in the *Veterinary Clinics of North America: Equine Practice* Continuing Veterinary Medical Education Program, call customer service at 1-800-654-2452 or sign up online at *http://www.theclinics.com/home/cme*. The CVME program is now available at a special introductory rate of $49.95 for a year's subscription.

FORTHCOMING ISSUES

December 2005
New Therapies in Joint Disease
Troy N. Trumble, DVM, PhD, *Guest Editor*

April 2006
Case Studies
Jennifer MacLeay, DVM, PhD, *Guest Editor*

August 2006
Advances in Diagnosis and Management of Infection
Louise Southwood, BVSc, PhD, *Guest Editor*

RECENT ISSUES

April 2005
Wound Management
Christine L. Theoret, DMV, PhD, *Guest Editor*

December 2004
Infection Control
Fairfield T. Bain, DVM,
J. Scott Weese, DVM, DVSc, *Guest Editors*

August 2004
Updates in Ophthalmology
Tim J. Cutler, MVB, MS, *Guest Editor*

VETERINARY
CLINICS
Equine Practice

Vet Clin Equine 21 (2005) xi–xii

Preface

Neonatal Medicine and Surgery

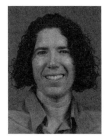

L. Chris Sanchez, DVM, PhD
Guest Editor

In most ways, the field of equine neonatology has advanced significantly since the topic was first broached by this series just over 20 years ago. In other ways, we seem to be fighting the same battles. Thus, the goal of this edition of *Veterinary Clinics of North America: Equine Practice* was to address many of the topics commonly encountered in neonatal practice and to provide the reader with the most up-to-date information possible. We have tried to bring forth a mixture of theoretical and practical information to each subject. Hopefully, we have succeeded.

Readers may notice that several important areas appear to be missing from this issue. Recent editions of this series ("Critical Care for All Ages," April 2004; "Respiratory Disease," April 2003; "Updates in Ophthalmology," August 2004; and "Modern Diagnostic Imaging," April 2001) have covered many important issues in the health care and management of foals; thus, the reader is directed elsewhere for additional information. Exclusion of these topics allowed for inclusion of others, thereby providing a broader base of knowledge in the field of neonatology. Even with these omissions, many questions remain, and this edition is simply one more piece of a very large puzzle.

Serving as the guest editor for this issue has been both an honor and a pleasure, but it has most certainly not been a solo effort. I would first like to thank the authors, without whom this issue clearly would not have been possible. These authors comprise both recognized experts in the field and new faces that you will likely see frequently in the future. I also thank John Vassallo, at Elsevier, for his patience and assistance. Most importantly, I am

doi:10.1016/j.cveq.2005.04.012   *vetequine.theclinics.com*

grateful to the many foals that, through their misfortune, have allowed all of us to become better clinicians over the years.

L. Chris Sanchez, DVM, PhD
Department of Large Animal Clinical Sciences
College of Veterinary Medicine
University of Florida
PO Box 100136
2015 SW 16th Avenue
Gainesville, FL 32610-0136

E-mail address: sanchezl@mail.vetmed.ufl.edu

ELSEVIER
SAUNDERS

VETERINARY
CLINICS
Equine Practice

Vet Clin Equine 21 (2005) 241–272

Immunologic Disorders
in Neonatal Foals

Steeve Giguère, DVM, PhD[a],*, Amy C. Polkes, DVM[b]

[a]*Department of Large Animal Clinical Sciences, College of Veterinary Medicine,*
University of Florida, PO Box 100136, Southwest 16th Avenue,
Gainesville, FL 32610, USA
[b]*Damascus Equine Associates, 19123 Highstream Drive, Germantown,*
MD 20874, USA

Foals live in an environment heavily populated by bacteria, many of which are capable of causing disease. Development of infection, however, is the exception rather than the rule. The ability of the foal to prevent infection by most pathogens is the result of a sophisticated set of defense mechanisms. These defense mechanisms can be divided into adaptive and innate immunity. Innate immunity encompasses defense mechanisms that preexist or are rapidly induced within hours of exposure to a pathogen. Conversely, adaptive or acquired immunity represents host defenses mediated by T and B lymphocytes, each expressing a highly specific antigen receptor and exhibiting memory during a second encounter with a given antigen. Immunologic disorders are relatively common in foals compared with their occurrence in adult horses. This article summarizes the current understanding of the equine fetal and neonatal immune system and reviews common immunodeficiency disorders as well as disorders resulting from allogenic incompatibilities.

Equine neonatal immunology

Development of the immune system in the fetus

Development of the equine immune system happens during fetal life, and the foal is practically immunocompetent at birth. Few studies have characterized fetal development of the equine immune system. The thymus

---

* Corresponding author.
E-mail address: gigueres@mail.vetmed.ufl.edu (S. Giguère).

is the first lymphoid organ to develop. Thymic corticomedullary organization of lymphocytes and antigen-responsive lymphocytes is present by day 80 of gestation [1,2]. Lymphocytes are present in the peripheral blood by day 120, and they proliferate in response to mitogens by day 140 [2]. Well-populated periarteriolar lymphocytic sheets, well-developed germinal centers, and significant responses to mitogens are present in the fetal spleen by day 200 [2]. Peripheral lymph nodes and intestinal lamina propria are populated with lymphocytes around day 90, and response to mitogens can be detected in the mesenteric lymph node by day 200 [1,2].

Immunoglobulin production is detectable in the serum of fetuses older than 185 days, and presuckle newborn foals have IgM concentrations of approximately 16 mg/dL [2]. Concentration of IgG is typically low and likely reflects the degree of in utero antigenic stimulation. In one study, serum IgG concentrations of presuckle foals at birth ranged from 0.2 to 17 mg/dL [2]. Specific antibody responses to in utero vaccination with coliphage T2 have been detected in equine fetuses as early as day 200 of gestation [3]. In other studies, administration of a Venezuelan equine encephalomyelitis antigen to equine fetuses from 232 to 283 days of gestational age resulted in higher serum neutralization titers than elicited by the same preparation in adult horses [4,5]. Collectively, the results of these studies indicate that functional T lymphocytes are present in the equine fetus by day 100 of gestation and functional B lymphocytes are present by day 200.

Transfer of passive immunity

The epitheliochorial placentation of mares does not allow transfer of maternal immunoglobulins to the fetus. As a result, foals are born with detectable but low concentrations of immunoglobulins. Although newborn foals are immunocompetent at birth, a primary immune response requires approximately 2 weeks to confer protection. Passive immunity acquired from the dam's colostrum is essential for preventing infection during this lag time between exposure to pathogens and development of a protective immune response. Colostrum is produced during the last 2 to 3 weeks of pregnancy under the influence of estrogen and progesterone [6]. Colostrum contains many soluble and cellular components that likely play a role in neonatal immunity and intestinal maturation. Soluble components include, among others, immunoglobulins, hormones, growth factors, cytokines, lactoferrin, CD14, and various enzymes (eg, lysozyme) [7,8]. Cellular components include lymphocytes, macrophages, neutrophils, and epithelial cells [9]. Only immunoglobulins have been studied comprehensively in horses. Immunoglobulins are transferred from the mare's blood to the mammary secretions through selective Fcγ receptors on the surface of epithelial cells. There is no correlation between serum and colostrum immunoglobulin concentrations in mares, suggesting that local production of immunoglobulins within the mammary gland may also occur [10]. Most mares produce between 1.8 to 2.8 L of colostrum. The predominant immunoglobulin in equine colostrum is IgG, with lesser quantities of IgA and IgM (Table 1) [10]. The predominant IgG subclass in colostrum is IgGb, followed by IgGa and IgG(T) [11]. IgA concentrations decrease rapidly in the first 8 hours after parturition and become negligible within 12 to 24 hours when the mare is actively suckled [12]. Colostral IgG concentrations are influenced by other factors, such as breed and age, with higher concentrations in mares from 3 to 10 years of age [12,13].

Normal foals consume colostrum within 2 hours of birth, and antibodies are detectable in the foal's serum within 4 to 6 hours [6]. In many domestic animal species, colostral immunoglobulin binds to a specialized Fc receptor on intestinal epithelial cells. Such receptors have not been identified in foals. Absorption of macromolecules in foals is nonselective and occurs by pinocytosis. Absorption of macromolecules is at its peak shortly after birth and decreases rapidly, with approximately 22% efficiency 3 hours after birth and less than 1% efficiency by 20 hours [14]. This rapid decrease in immunoglobulin absorption is caused by the replacement of specialized enterocytes capable of pinocytosis by mature enterocytes. Withholding the administration of macromolecules does not delay closure of the equine neonatal small intestine to immunoglobulin absorption [15]. The predominant IgG subclass in foal serum after ingestion of colostrum is IgGb [11,16]. Maternal IgG concentrations in foals peak 18 to 24 hours after birth and decline rapidly during the first 4 weeks of life, with a half-life for disappearance of approximately 18 days for IgGa, 32 days for IgGb, and 21

Table 1
Concentrations (mean ± SD) of IgG, IgM, and IgA in the colostrum, milk, and serum of horses

| Sample | n | Immunoglobulin (mg/dL) | | | Reference |
		IgG	IgA	IgM	
Colostrum	36	8912 ± 6200	957 ± 1098	123 ± 77	[10]
	6	16,583 ± 3618	NM	104 ± 35	[135]
	5	26,800 ± 5814	900 ± 300	NM	[11]
Milk[a]	5	50 ± 22	70 ± 20	NM	[11]
Serum: birth	35	5 ± 5	NM	16 ± 6	[2]
	5	3 ± 0.3	ND	NM	[11]
Serum: 24 h	36	1953 ± 1635	58 ± 42	34 ± 30	[10]
	10[b]	1600 ± 280	NM	50 ± 6	[30]
	5	3900 ± 412	40 ± 10	NM	[11]
Serum: 30 days	10[b]	1180 ± 280	NM	41 ± 8	[30]
	5	1770 ± 454	6 ± 4	NM	[11]
Serum: 120 days	10[b]	1360 ± 320	NM	46 ± 8	[30]
Serum: adults	35	2464 ± 1337	305 ± 337	136 ± 218	[10]
	6	2233 ± 262		104 ± 25	[136]
	25	1955 ± 413	NM	103 ± 40	[92]

Abbreviations: ND, none detected; NM, not measured.
[a] 28 Days postpartum.
[b] Only foals with adequate transfer of maternal immunoglobulins were included.

days for IgG(T) [11]. The time of disappearance of maternal IgG depends on the initial concentration absorbed, but concentrations are generally low by 6 months of age [17]. Serum concentrations of maternally derived IgA and IgM decrease more rapidly with half-lives of 3 to 5 days and are undetectable in most foals by 3 to 4 weeks of age [11,17].

Immune system during the neonatal period

Complement

The complement system is important for host defense against infection. Complement activation through the classic pathway requires antigen-antibody interaction. In contrast, the alternative pathway of complement activation is initiated by various cell surface constituents that are foreign to the host, such as the cell wall of bacteria or fungi. The activation of either pathway results in many important biologic consequences, such as lysis of some microorganisms, inflammation, viral neutralization, and opsonization of antigen. The two major opsonins in plasma are C3b and IgG. They enhance phagocytosis by binding to CD11b/CD18 (C3b) and Fcγ (IgG) receptors on the surface of phagocytes. Inactivation of complement results in a 60% to 80% decrease in the uptake of yeasts or *Streptococcus equi* subspecies *zooepidemicus* by equine neutrophils, demonstrating the importance of the complement system in uptake of pathogens by phagocytic cells [18–20]. Complement activity in newborn foals is approximately 13% of that of adult horses and increases with age, with approximately 64% of adult activity at 1 month and 85% at 5 months [21]. In contrast to IgG, complement activity does not increase significantly after ingestion of colostrum [21]. In the same study, complement activity in colostrum-deprived foals was significantly greater than postsuckle values in control foals [21].

Neutrophils

Chemotaxis and phagocytosis by foal neutrophils are low at birth and increase significantly after ingestion of colostrum [22,23]. Phagocytosis and killing of yeasts by neutrophils are lower in neonatal foals and increase with age, reaching adult levels by 3 to 4 weeks of age [23–25]. In contrast, phagocytosis of *Escherichia coli*, *Actinobacillus equuli*, and *Staphylococcus aureus* and killing of *Rhodococcus equi* by neonatal foal neutrophils are similar to those of adult horses [22,26–30]. The transient decrease in yeast uptake by neutrophils in some studies is attributable to the lower concentrations of opsonins in foal serum rather than functional immaturity of the neutrophils. This is evidenced by the fact that newborn foal neutrophils have similar or greater activity than neutrophils of adult horses when pooled adult sera are used for opsonization [24]. Similarly, deficiencies in chemotactic and phagocytic activity are also seen in adult horses when tested with neonatal foal serum [23]. Expression of CD18 on the neutrophils of foals is significantly higher than that of adult horses up to approximately 3 weeks of age, which may contribute to the greater phagocytic activity of foals' neutrophils [24]. Collectively, the results of these studies suggest that phagocytic cells of the newborn foal are functionally mature but that their chemotactic and phagocytic functions are limited by the reduced concentrations of opsonins in the foal's serum.

Adaptive immunity

Foals are born with circulating lymphocyte counts similar to those of adult horses. The number of circulating lymphocytes increases linearly, however, reaching counts approximately 2.5 times that of adult horses from 3 to 6 months of age [31,32]. This age-related increase in peripheral blood lymphocytes is caused by an increase in the numbers of CD4+ and CD8+ T lymphocytes and B lymphocytes [31,32]. This period coincides with an increase in serum IgG and IgM concentrations, suggesting activation of the humoral immune system. In contrast to the total number of cells, the percentage of CD4+ and CD8+ T lymphocytes and B lymphocytes remains fairly constant from birth to 6 months of age [31]. The absolute count and percentage of B lymphocytes in peripheral blood are higher in foals than in adult horses [31].

Proliferation of peripheral blood lymphocytes in response to mitogens is slightly reduced at birth but rapidly increases to adult levels [30,33]. Foals also have normal lymphokine-activated killing (LAK) cell activity of peripheral blood lymphocytes at birth and during early life [30]. Expression of mRNA for interferon-γ (IFNγ), interleukin (IL)-1α, and transforming growth factor-β (TGFβ) in blood lymphocytes stimulated with concanavalin A (ConA) increases with age during the first month of life [34]. In contrast, expression of other cytokines or chemokines, such as IL-1β, IL-2, IL-4, IL-6, IL-8, IL-10, IL-12, and TNFα did not change with increasing age [34]. The relatively low IFNγ expression at birth may suggest a reduced T helper 1 (Th1) response in the neonatal period. Several studies have shown that foals can mount cell-mediated immune responses to a variety of pathogens, including *Strongylus vulgaris*, *R equi*, and equine herpesvirus type 1 [35–38]. The age of development of protective cell-mediated immune responses to significant pathogens of foals and comparison of the magnitude of these responses with those of adult horses require further studies, however. Neonatal foals have significantly fewer T lymphocytes expressing major histocompatibility (MHC) class II antigens on their surface. Expression of MHC class II molecules increases progressively, reaching adult levels by approximately 4 months of age [30]. This suggests progressive development of antigen-activated memory T lymphocytes. Collectively, the results of these studies suggest that neonatal foals are immunocompetent but immunologically naive at birth.

Although foals can respond to foreign antigens from the day of birth, passively transferred maternal antibodies exert a considerable suppressive effect on antibody production. This is evidenced by the fact that the onset of antibody production is advanced in colostrum-deprived foals compared with foals with adequate transfer of passive immunity [6,21]. In the presence of transfer of passive immunity, IgGa, IgG(T), and IgA production peaks to levels comparable to those of adults by 8 to 12 weeks of age. In contrast, IgGb production is delayed and is still markedly below adult levels at 1 year of age [16]. The rate of decline of maternal antibodies varies, depending on the individual animal and the nature of the antigen. For many important pathogens, the concentration of maternal antibody in foals falls to nonprotective levels by 2 to 3 months of age. For equine influenza and tetanus, maternal antibodies in foals born from mares vaccinated in the last 2 months of pregnancy can persist until approximately 6 months of age and prevent adequate immune responses in foals vaccinated before reaching that age [17].

Host defense mechanisms of the respiratory system

Foals do not have organized lymphoid tissue in their lungs at birth, and lymphocytes and plasma cells are virtually absent in the first week of life. Plasma cells producing IgG, IgA, or IgM are present by 8 weeks of age, and foals exhibit well-developed bronchus- and bronchiole-associated lymphoid tissue by 12 weeks of age [39,40]. Foals are born without any detectable immunoglobulins in nasal mucosal secretions. After adequate transfer of passive immunity, concentrations of IgGa, IgGb, and IgG(T) in nasal secretions increase to values higher than what is found in adult horses [11]. Despite being the most abundant immunoglobulin in nasal secretions of adult horses, maternal IgA is not present on nasal mucosal surfaces in foals until they reach approximately 1 month of age, and IgA concentrations in nasal secretions reach adult values by approximately 6 weeks of age [11].

Total bronchoalveolar lavage (BAL) leukocyte count is low in foals and progressively increases until reaching adult values around 3 to 6 weeks of age [41,42]. In neonatal foals, the percentage of macrophages is 85% to 90%, whereas the percentage of lymphocytes is considerably lower (5%–20%) [41,42]. In adult horses, macrophages comprise 40% to 65% and lymphocytes comprise 30% to 70% of the BAL cell population [43,44]. The percentage of lymphocytes gradually increases, and the percentage of macrophages decreases, reaching adult values by approximately 3 months of age [30,41]. The increase in BAL fluid lymphocytes coincides with an increase in lymphocytes in peripheral blood. As in peripheral blood, the number of CD4+ and CD8+ T lymphocytes in BAL fluid is low for the first 2 months of life and then increases by 3 months of age [30,41]. In addition, there is lower expression of MHC class II antigens and CD44 (marker of lymphocyte activation) on foal BAL lymphocytes up to approximately 6 weeks of age [30,41].

Although the number of alveolar macrophages and lymphocyte populations in BAL fluid of foals has been studied, the function of pulmonary macrophages and lymphocytes has not been systematically investigated. In one study, the migrational activity of alveolar macrophages was significantly impaired in foals 2 to 3 days of age compared with 2-week-old foals and adult horses [45]. In another study, newborn foal alveolar macrophages had a lesser ability to phagocytize and kill *S aureus* than peripheral blood neutrophils from the same animals [46]. Phagocytosis and killing of *S aureus* by alveolar macrophages of 2- to 3-month-old foals are similar to what is found in adult horses [47]. In vitro phagocytosis and killing of *R equi* by alveolar macrophages from nonexposed foals are significantly lower what is found in adult horses, whereas phagocytosis and killing by alveolar macrophages from foals previously nebulized with *R equi* are similar to those of adults [47]. In the same study, opsonization of *R equi* significantly increased uptake and killing of *R equi* [47].

These results suggest an age-related maturation of the immune system in the respiratory tract of foals. Development of the immune system of the lung seems to occur at a slightly slower pace than what is seen in peripheral blood. Total immune cell number rather than function and lack of prior sensitization to antigen may be the limiting factors. Similar to what has been reported with peripheral blood neutrophils, chemotactic and phagocytic functions of alveolar macrophages may be limited by the lower concentration of opsonins in the neonatal period.

Assessment of the immune system

There are many clinical situations when a more thorough evaluation of the immune system is warranted. For example, any foal with an infection in the first month of life should be evaluated for failure of transfer of passive immunity (FPT). Other clinical situations that may indicate immunodeficiency in foals include recurrent infections, infections that are poorly responsive to appropriate therapy, infections caused by microorganisms of low pathogenicity, disease resulting from administration of a modified live vaccine, a family history of primary immunodeficiency, and failure to gain weight or grow normally. A complete review of immunodiagnostic tests available is beyond the scope of this article and can be found elsewhere [48,49]. The ability of the equine practitioner to perform a comprehensive evaluation of the immune system is limited by the fact that many immuno-diagnostic tests are only performed in specialized research laboratories and are not commercially available.

A complete blood cell count and blood cytology are often used as a starting point to assess the number of neutrophils, lymphocytes, and monocytes. B lymphocytes represent less than 30% of peripheral blood lymphocytes in foals and less than 10% to 20% in adult horses [31]. As a result, an animal with no B lymphocytes may have a normal total lymphocyte count. More specific tests readily available and useful to assess humoral immunity include measurement of serum IgG, IgM, and IgA concentrations by radial immunodiffusion or enzyme-linked immunosorbent assay (ELISA) and measurement of circulating B lymphocytes by flow cytometry (immunophenotyping). Interpretation of serum immunoglobulin concentrations in foals is confounded by antibody of maternal origin. IgA and IgM of maternal origin are virtually gone by 1 month of age, whereas maternal IgG may persist for 3 to 6 months. As a result, a foal less than 3 to 4 months of age may have normal serum IgG concentrations despite being unable to synthesize immunoglobulins. When the results of immunoglobulin concentrations or immunophenotyping indicate possible immunodeficiency, the ultimate approach for evaluating in vivo function of the humoral immune system is measurement of specific IgG before and 3 weeks after vaccination. Response to tetanus vaccination has been recommended for that purpose in adult horses [49]. Response to tetanus vaccination would not be suitable in foals less than 6 months of age born from vaccinated mares, however, because maternal antibody has been shown to inhibit response to vaccination almost completely until that age [17].

Evaluation of cell-mediated immunity is more difficult in a clinical setting. Lymphocyte phenotyping is commercially available and provides useful information on the number and percentage of T lymphocytes (eg, CD4, CD8). The only test of cell-mediated immunity that would be feasible in clinical practice is response to intradermal injection of phytohemagglutinin (PHA), which assesses delayed-type hypersensitivity T-lymphocyte responses [50]. In vitro tests of cell-mediated immune function require collaboration with a research laboratory performing these assays. In vitro lymphocyte proliferation responses to mitogens, such as ConA (T lymphocytes), PHA (T lymphocytes), pokeweed (T and B lymphocytes), and lipopolysaccharide (B lymphocytes) are commonly used.

Neutrophil and macrophage migration, phagocytic function, oxidative burst activity, and bactericidal activity in the horse have been measured using various approaches [24,25,51,52]. Evaluation of complement activity has also been reported [21,22,53]. Currently, these tests have limited availability.

The Coombs' test is useful when immune-mediated anemia is suspected because it detects immunoglobulin or complement on the surface of erythrocytes. Flow cytometry may also be used to detect immunoglobulins on the surface of erythrocytes or platelets [54]. This assay is more sensitive than the Coombs' test for the diagnosis of immune-mediated hemolytic anemia. Immunophenotyping and detection of surface immunoglobulins on the surface of equine platelets and erythrocytes are currently available commercially (Clinical Immunology Laboratory, Kansas State University, Manhattan, Kansas).

Immunodeficiencies

Immunodeficiency disorders are often classified as primary or secondary. Primary disorders have a presumed or established genetic basis, whereas secondary disorders are those resulting from failure of transfer of passive immunity, malnutrition, infection by immunosuppressive microorganisms, neoplasia, and treatment with immunosuppressive drugs. Immunodeficiencies may also be classified by the component of the immune system that is primarily affected. The most common immunodeficiency disorders of foals and the component(s) of the immune system they affect are presented in Table 2.

Failure of passive transfer of immunoglobulins

FPT is the most common immunodeficiency disorder of foals. There has been some controversy regarding the definition of FPT, but the most widely recognized classification defines FPT as serum IgG concentrations less than 400 mg/dL after 24 hours of age. Partial FPT is often defined as serum IgG concentrations from 400 to 800 mg/dL, whereas foals with adequate transfer of IgG have serum concentrations greater than 800 mg/dL. The incidence of FPT (IgG < 400 mg/dL) in foals has ranged between 3% and 20% [10,13,55–61].

Sepsis is the leading cause of morbidity and mortality in newborn foals [62]. Several studies have documented a positive correlation between FPT and bacterial sepsis [56–58,60,62]. In a prospective study, seven of eight colostrum-deprived foals developed clinical signs of infection and bacterial sepsis was confirmed by culture in five foals [63]. It is important to recognize that many foals with FPT remain healthy [55]. This suggests that, in addition to adequate immunoglobulin, other factors, such as environmental and management conditions, stress, concurrent disease, and virulence of the pathogen, may contribute to the development of sepsis.

Table 2
Clinical and laboratory features of characterized immunodeficiency disorders of horses

Disease	Breed	Age	IgG	IgA	IgM	T cells	B cells
FPT	All	<1 month	↓	↓	↓	N	N
SCID	Arabian	<5 months	↓[b]	↓	↓[c]	↓	↓
Agammaglobulinemia	Any[a]	<2 years	↓[b]	↓	↓[c]	N	↓
Transient hypogammaglobulinemia	Any	2–4 months	↓	N to ↓	N to ↓[c]	N	N
Selective IgM deficiency	Any	Any	N	N	↓[c]	N	N
Anemia, immunodeficiency, and peripheral ganglionopathy	Fell ponies	<3 months	↓[b]	N	↓[c]	N	↓

Abbreviations: N, normal concentrations; SCID, severe combined immunodeficiency; ↓, decreased concentrations.

[a] The disease has been recognized in Thoroughbreds, Standardbreds, and Quarter Horses, but the possibility that other breeds may be affected cannot be excluded. Only male horses have been affected.

[b] Serum IgG concentrations may be normal while antibodies of maternal origin are still circulating.

[c] Before 1 month of age, IgM of maternal origin may still be present.

Causes of failure of passive transfer of immunoglobulins

The three potential causes of FPT are production failure, ingestion failure, and absorption failure. Failure of the mare to provide sufficient colostrum for the foal may occur for a variety of reasons. Insufficient production of colostrum can occur with a premature birth, where the mare has not yet produced colostrum at the time of foaling. Serious illness in the mare during gestation can also contribute to a lack of colostrum production. A well-recognized problem leading to insufficient production of colostrum is ingestion of endophyte-infected fescue during the third trimester of gestation. This may cause a thickened placenta, premature placental separation, and a decrease in colostrum and milk production [64]. Finally, the mare may produce an ample volume of colostrum that is of poor quality with inadequate IgG concentrations. Colostral immunoglobulin concentration can vary widely between mares [10]. Subjectively, good-quality colostrum should be thick and sticky with a yellow appearance. Good-quality colostrum has IgG concentrations in excess of 3000 mg/dL. Immunoglobulin concentration can be directly measured by single radial immunodiffusion. Alternatively, fairly accurate stall-side estimation of colostral immunoglobulin concentrations can be achieved by refractometry, specific gravity, or glutaraldehyde coagulation. The equine colostrometer (Jorgensen Laboratories, Loveland, Colorado) is a modified hydrometer that measures the specific gravity of colostrum. A specific gravity of greater than 1.060 corresponds to an IgG concentration of greater than 3000 mg/dL [65]. A handheld refractometer (Bellingham & Stanley, Lawrenceville, Georgia) used to measure alcohol and sugar content of wine can also be used. A reading of greater than 23% on the sugar scale or greater than 16° on the alcohol scale corresponds to IgG concentrations greater than 6000 mg/dL [66]. Finally, the ability of glutaraldehyde to form a solid clot in the presence of gamma globulins can be used to estimate IgG content of colostrum. Formation of a solid clot in 10 minutes or less corresponds to IgG concentrations greater than 3800 mg/dL [67]. Mares with premature lactation before foaling often leak colostrum, leading to low IgG concentrations at the time of foaling. Twinning, placentitis, and premature placental separation can cause premature lactation in the mare.

The second cause of FPT is failure to ingest colostrum. A foal that is ill or weak at birth may not be capable of nursing the mare sufficiently. Congenital musculoskeletal abnormalities, such as contracted tendons or injury to the foal during birth, may also prevent the foal from nursing the mare after birth. The mare may reject the foal and prevent the foal from nursing. This usually requires intervention to ensure the safety of the foal and provide for ingestion of colostrum.

Finally, the foal may ingest an adequate volume of good-quality colostrum but fail to absorb sufficient immunoglobulins if vigorous nursing does not occur during the first 6 to 12 hours of life. Malabsorption has been postulated as a possible cause of FPT in foals that ingest adequate quantities of high-quality colostrum in the first 12 hours of life. In rats, glucocorticoids enhance maturation of enterocytes, resulting in loss of their ability to absorb immunoglobulins [68]. This has led to the hypothesis that stress with release of endogenous corticosteroids may decrease IgG absorption in foals. Administration of corticotropin to increase endogenous cortisol concentrations in foals does not have a negative impact on immunoglobulin absorption, however [69]. Finally, foals with concurrent illness may also have differences in metabolism and catabolism of ingested immunoglobulins, resulting in low serum concentrations despite adequate initial absorption.

Diagnosis

Assessment of passive transfer is important to accomplish within the first 24 hours. This is the period when the foal is most vulnerable to infectious organisms if transfer of immunoglobulins has not been achieved. Serum immunoglobulin status can be determined as early as 6 hours after birth if the foal has nursed sufficiently. Generally, immunoglobulin concentration is measured at 18 to 24 hours; at that time, serum IgG concentration has reached its peak. If there is concern or uncertainty regarding adequate ingestion of colostrum, however, the foal should be evaluated before 12 hours so that oral supplementation of colostrum or an oral immunoglobulin preparation can be given. Foals that develop clinical signs of illness should have their immunoglobulin concentration assessed to determine the need for therapeutic intervention even if IgG was adequate during an earlier routine check.

Single radial immunodiffusion is the most quantitatively accurate test available but requires an 18- to 24-hour incubation period. This long delay before test results are available is the major disadvantage of this test, because rapid identification of FPT is imperative for timely therapeutic intervention. Several stall-side tests or kits are available to estimate immunoglobulin concentration in whole blood, serum, or plasma [70–74]. Criteria for selection of a screening kit for FPT in foals include overall accuracy, time necessary to perform the assay, and cost. The zinc sulfate turbidity (Equi Z; VMRD, Pullman, Washington) and glutaraldehyde coagulation (Gamma-Check-E; Veterinary Dynamics, Templeton, California) tests are good initial screening tests because they are relatively inexpensive and results can be obtained in 5 minutes (glutaraldehyde coagulation) to 1 hour (zinc sulfate turbidity). These tests are fairly sensitive for the diagnosis of FPT, but they lack specificity. As a result, the predictive value of a negative test is good, indicating that the foal likely has adequate transfer of maternal immunoglobulin. In contrast, a positive test does not necessarily indicate that the foal has FPT, and additional testing is warranted. Many practitioners prefer the convenience and ease of use of immunoassays. Quantitative (DVM Stat; CAA, WestBand, Wisconsin) and semiquantitative (Snap; Idexx Laboratories, Westbrooke, Maine or Foal

IgG Midland Quick Test; Midland Bioproducts Corp., Boone, Iowa) immunoassays are commercially available.

Prevention and treatment

If FPT is likely in a foal because of premature lactation, poor colostrum quality, or reduced colostral intake, colostrum or an alternative source of immunoglobulin should be administered orally or by nasogastric tube preferably within 2 to 6 hours of birth. Good-quality equine colostrum is the preferable approach. The quantity of colostrum required depends on its IgG concentration, the size of the foal, and the efficiency of IgG absorption by the foal's gastrointestinal tract. Administration of 1 to 2 L of good-quality colostrum is typically recommended for a 45-kg foal. Feedings should begin approximately 2 hours after birth in volumes of 200 to 400 mL per feeding. Bovine colostrum may be used when equine colostrum is not available. Bovine colostrum is not ideal, because bovine immunoglobulins have a short serum half-life of 7 to 10 days in foals and are not specifically directed against equine pathogens [75,76]. Concentrated equine IgG is commercially available (Seramune; Sera, Shawnee Mission, Kansas). Administration of the recommended dose (two doses of 150 mL administered 1–2 hours apart) to foals by nasogastric tube within 4 hours of birth resulted in detectable IgG concentrations (average of 105 $\pm$ 2.6 mg/dL) but failed to raise IgG concentrations above 800 mg/dL [77]. Equine serum or plasma may also be given orally; however, oral administration of plasma or serum is not cost-effective because of the low concentration and limited oral absorption of immunoglobulins. Regardless of the type of oral product administered, IgG concentration should always be rechecked at 18 to 24 hours of age to ensure that adequate transfer of immunoglobulins has been achieved.

Therapy with intravenous plasma is indicated in foals with IgG concentrations below 400 mg/dL at 18 to 24 hours after birth. Clinically healthy foals with no apparent risk factors for sepsis and IgG concentrations between 400 and 800 mg/dL may not require plasma therapy if they are kept in a relatively clean environment. Foals with an IgG concentration between 400 and 800 mg/dL should be administered plasma intravenously if they are not perfectly normal on physical or laboratory evaluation, however. Plasma should be administered intravenously in a sufficient quantity to raise IgG above 800 mg/dL.

There are many US Department of Agriculture (USDA)–licensed equine plasma products commercially available. These products are convenient and relatively safe, because donors are screened for major alloantigens, alloantibodies, and infectious agents. Donors are vaccinated against common equine pathogens, and the minimum IgG concentration is indicated on the bag. An alternative to commercial sources is plasma obtained from a local donor. This has the theoretic advantage of providing antibodies against pathogens unique to the foal's environment. The donor should be blood typed, void of alloantibodies, and ideally negative for the

Aa and Qa erythrocyte alloantigens that are frequently associated with neonatal isoerythrolysis (NI). The IgG concentration of the donor plasma should be greater than 1200 mg/dL to provide sufficient immunoglobulins. The last alternative for therapy is administration of a concentrated serum product. The advantage of concentrated serum over plasma is a refrigerated shelf life of 3 years. Two to three units of concentrated serum administered intravenously is required to match the increase in the foal's IgG concentrations that is achieved with one unit of plasma, however, eliminating the cost benefit of serum product over plasma [78].

Immunoglobulin concentrations in commercially available plasma range between 1500 and 2500 mg/dL or greater depending on the product. One unit (950 mL) of plasma containing 1500 to 1700 mg/dL of IgG typically increases serum IgG concentrations in the average 45-kg foal by 200 to 300 mg/dL, whereas plasma containing 2500 mg/dL of IgG or greater may increase IgG concentrations by 400 to 800 mg/dL. As a result, 1 to 3 L may be necessary to achieve a final serum concentration of greater than 800 mg/dL in a foal with complete FPT. In addition to the severity of FPT, the size of the foal, IgG concentration of the plasma, and severity of concomitant disease may influence the increase in IgG attained after plasma transfusion. Foals with sepsis may differ in catabolism and distribution of immunoglobulins and thus require additional volumes of plasma to achieve adequate serum IgG concentrations. Therefore, the serum IgG should be reassessed after administration to determine if additional plasma is needed. Septic foals may also require repeated plasma transfusions throughout the course of their disease to maintain adequate circulating immunoglobulins.

Plasma should be thawed and warmed to body temperature before administration. A whole-blood filter should always be used when administering plasma or serum products. Recommendations for the rate of administration are empiric. Generally, the first 50 mL is given at a slow rate to observe for potential adverse reactions, such as tachypnea, tachycardia, hyperthermia, urticaria, or changes in behavior. If there are no reactions noted, the remainder of the transfusion can be administered at 20 to 30 mL/kg/h, although some manufacturers recommend much faster administration. Slower flow rates are generally safer, because adverse reactions can be identified before administration of a large volume. Rapid flow rates are especially discouraged when several units must be administered to normovolemic foals because of the potential for volume overload. If minor adverse reactions are observed, the rate of infusion should be decreased until the signs subside. If an adverse reaction does not diminish after slowing the rate or if a severe reaction occurs, the transfusion should be discontinued.

Severe combined immunodeficiency

Severe combined immunodeficiency (SCID) is a genetic disorder affecting human beings, dogs, mice, and Arabian foals. Affected individuals lack

GIGUÈRE & POLKES

functional B and T lymphocytes and are incapable of producing antigen-specific immune responses. SCID has been identified in Arabian foals from Australia, Canada, the United Kingdom, and the United States [79]. The disease is inherited in Arabian horses as an autosomal recessive trait [80]. The SCID trait results from a 5–base pair deletion in the gene encoding the catalytic subunit of DNA-dependent protein kinase (DNA-PK) [81]. The lack of activity of DNA-PK leads to a failure of T and B lymphocytes to cut, rearrange, and anneal the genes that encode their surface-expressed antigen-specific receptors [81]. Failure to complete these gene rearrangement events results in elimination of lymphocyte precursors; as a consequence, affected foals are born without mature functional B and T lymphocytes.

Clinical presentation

Foals with SCID seem normal at birth and may not show clinical signs until 1 to 3 months of age. The time of onset of clinical signs is determined by the extent of transfer of passive immunity and level of exposure to pathogens. The inability to mount specific humoral and cell-mediated immune responses allows affected foals to become susceptible to multiple infections as maternal immunity wanes.

Most affected foals present with infections of the respiratory tract from bacterial, viral, or fungal agents. Common specific causative agents include adenovirus, *R equi*, and *Pneumocystis carinii* [82]. Gastrointestinal disease from protozoal organisms, such as *Cryptosporidium*, is also not uncommon [82].

Adenovirus is probably the most significant of the pathogens isolated, because it has been found in up to two thirds of affected foals [82]. Although adenovirus begins in the respiratory tract, it can extend to the gastrointestinal tract, leading to endocrine and exocrine pancreatic disease with subsequent weight loss and impaired growth [82].

Diagnosis

The definitive diagnosis of SCID in an Arabian foals relies on genetic testing (VetGen, Ann Arbor, Michigan). DNA from blood or cheek swabs is amplified by polymerase chain reaction and hybridized with probes specific for the normal and mutant alleles of the catalytic subunit of DNA-PK [83].

Arabian foals with SCID are persistently and severely lymphopenic (<1000 lymphocytes per microliter). T- and B-lymphocyte counts are severely decreased. Persistent lymphopenia in an Arabian foal is an indication for genetic testing even if the foal is apparently healthy. Immunoglobulin concentrations of affected foals may be normal at birth if transfer of passive immunity was adequate. Affected foals fail to produce their own immunoglobulins, however. Because the half-life of IgM is much shorter than that of IgG, foals with SCID have undetectable IgM concentrations by 3 to 4 weeks of age [79].

Management and prognosis

Medical management of foals with SCID is unrewarding. Foals may initially respond to medical therapy; however, the infections tend to recur, and affected foals generally do not survive beyond 5 months of age. In one foal, the disease could be corrected by bone marrow transplantation from a histocompatible full-sibling donor [84]. In contrast, complete correction of immunologic defects could not be achieved by engraftment of fetal cells or equine leukocyte antigen haploidentical bone marrow cells [85].

Prevention of the disease relies on responsible breeding practices that incorporate genetic testing into the breeding program. Mares and stallions intended for breeding use should be tested to determine if they are free of or heterozygous for the SCID gene. Ideally, only horses exempt from the SCID gene (homozygous normal) should be bred. Under no circumstances should two heterozygous horses be selected for breeding. If an owner elects to breed a mare or stallion heterozygous for the gene, he or she should ensure that the breeding partner is homozygous normal. In addition, foals resulting from such matings should be tested before use for breeding purposes because they have 50% chance of being heterozygous.

Selective IgM deficiency

Selective IgM deficiency has been reported in foals and adult horses. The molecular mechanism for disease development is unknown, and a genetic basis is unproven at this time. The association of some cases of IgM deficiency with neoplasia and spontaneous recovery in others suggest that at least some cases represent a secondary rather than a primary immunodeficiency disorder.

Clinical presentation

Two clinical presentations have been recognized. The first and most common clinical presentation involves foals between 2 and 8 months of age. Affected foals are often small for their age, and they experience repeated episodes of bacterial infections [86]. The respiratory tract is commonly involved. The disorder most often affects Quarter Horses and Arabians, but the disease has been recognized in other breeds as well [61,87].

The second clinical presentation involves adult horses. Early reports suggested a strong association between IgM deficiency in adult horses and lymphoma [88–91]. More recently, it has been recognized that IgM deficiency may also be found in horses diagnosed with a variety of medical conditions other than lymphoma [92]. The sensitivity and specificity of a serum IgM concentration of less than 60 mg/dL for detecting equine lymphoma were low at 50% and 35%, respectively [92]. At a cutoff of less than 23 mg/dL, the sensitivity was low at 28% but specificity improved at 88% [92]. These results indicate that IgM concentrations should not be used as a screening test for equine lymphoma.

Diagnosis

The diagnosis of selective IgM deficiency is made by measuring serum immunoglobulin concentrations. Affected horses have a significant reduction or complete absence of IgM and normal concentrations of IgA, IgG, and IgG(T). Serum IgM concentrations more than 2 SDs below that of age-matched controls have been considered diagnostic [61,79]. Initial studies reported normal IgM concentrations in adult horses to be 120 ± 30 mg/dL, indicating that horses with IgM concentrations less than 60 mg/dL would be considered IgM deficient. In a recent study, 5 (20%) of 24 normal fit horses were found to have IgM concentrations consistently below 60 mg/dL [92]. Based on these results, a cutoff for IgM concentration of less than 23 mg/dL has been proposed for the diagnosis of IgM deficiency in adult horses [92]. Blood lymphocyte counts and lymphocyte phenotyping are normal in foals or adult horses with selective IgM deficiency unless they are influenced by underlying diseases, such as lymphoma. Other laboratory findings may reflect concurrent or underlying diseases.

Management and prognosis

There is no specific treatment for selective IgM deficiency. Plasma transfusions are generally not beneficial because of the short half-life of IgM. Antimicrobial therapy and supportive care may at least temporarily control bacterial infections. In a retrospective study, 7 of 11 foals with selective IgM deficiency died from infections before they were 8 months of age [61]. Three additional foals survived beyond 1 year of age but had recurrent respiratory tract infections and exhibited delayed growth [61]. One foal had recurrent infection until 1 year of age and then completely recovered [61].

In a retrospective study of IgM deficiency (<60 mg/dL) in horses older than 1 year of age, 13 of 22 horses (59%) without lymphoma were apparently healthy 1 year after discharge from the hospital [92]. Serum IgM concentrations were greater than 60 mg/dL in only 2 of 10 horses in which it was rechecked, however [92].

Agammaglobulinemia

Agammaglobulinemia in people is a genetic disorder defined by the absence of mature B cells and plasma cells along with a functional T-lymphocyte population. Affected individuals lack the ability to produce immunoglobulins after immunization. The condition in human beings is inherited as an X-linked trait caused by a mutation in btk, a gene encoding a cytoplasmic tyrosine kinase [93]. As a result, only male patients are affected and female carriers seem to be clinically healthy. Five cases of agammaglobulinemia in male Thoroughbred, Quarter Horse, and Standardbred horses have been described [94–97]. The occurrence of cases only in male horses is compatible with but does not prove the fact that agammaglobulinemia may be an X-linked disorder as well. To the authors' knowledge, the btk gene has not been examined in affected horses to date.

Clinical presentation

Clinical signs of infectious disease involving the respiratory, digestive, and musculoskeletal systems become apparent as maternal immunoglobulins decrease. As with other primary immunologic disorders, affected individuals may initially respond to therapy but infections tend to recur.

Diagnosis

Horses with agammaglobulinemia have undetectable serum IgM and IgA concentrations, along with low serum concentrations of IgG and IgG(T). Serum IgG concentrations may be within normal limits if measured in young foals with adequate transfer of passive immunity, but these values decline as maternal immunity wanes. Blood lymphocyte counts are normal but lymphocyte phenotyping reveals an absence of B lymphocytes. T-lymphocyte numbers and function test results are normal. There is no serologic response to immunization.

Management and prognosis

Treatment of horses with agammaglobulinemia is generally unrewarding, because infections tend to recur. Aggressive antimicrobial therapy and periodic intravenous administration of plasma as a source of exogenous antibody may prolong the life of affected horses. Most horses do not survive past 2 years of age [79]. Because of the suspicion of a genetic disorder, affected horses should not be bred. A program for prevention is not possible until a specific genetic defect is identified and characterized.

Anemia, immunodeficiency, and peripheral ganglionopathy in Fell pony foals

A syndrome of severe anemia, immunodeficiency, and peripheral ganglionopathy has been described in Fell pony foals [98–102]. The molecular basis for the disorder is undefined.

Clinical presentation

Foals seem normal at birth, but clinical signs, including diarrhea, cough, and failure to suckle, become apparent in the first few weeks of life [102]. Frequent chewing movements and lingual hyperkeratosis are also commonly noted [102]. Severe anemia develops, characterized by pale mucous membranes and general ill-thrift. In some foals, cryptosporidial enteritis, adenoviral bronchopneumonia, or pancreatitis is found at necropsy, suggesting an immunodeficiency disorder [102].

Laboratory and pathologic findings

Severe anemia is a consistent clinicopathologic finding. The anemia is normocytic to macrocytic with small numbers of late erythroid precursors in the bone marrow. Total immunoglobulin concentrations are normal initially in affected foals with adequate transfer of passive immunity [102]. Affected foals lack the ability to synthesize IgGa, IgGb, and IgM, however [99]. Foals are often lymphopenic with normal to increased neutrophil counts [100]. There is a marked relative deficiency of B lymphocytes on immunohisto-chemistry analysis of the lymph nodes and thymus [102]. The mean population of B lymphocytes in peripheral blood is less than 10% of that present in normal foals, whereas circulating subpopulations of CD4+ and CD8+ T lymphocytes are unaffected [98]. Affected foals have reduced expression of MHC class II antigens and increased expression of CD11a/18 on their blood lymphocytes. The response of lymphocytes to mitogen stimulation (ConA, PHA, pokeweed mitogen [PWM]) is not significantly different from that of healthy foals [100].

Pathologic abnormalities include a small thymus with no secondary lymphoid follicles or plasma cells. *Cryptosporidium parvum* and adenovirus may be found at necropsy as the causative agents of diarrhea and bronchopneumonia, respectively [102]. Neuronal chromatolysis involving trigeminal, cranial mesenteric, and dorsal root ganglia are found at necropsy, although clinical neurologic abnormalities may not be apparent [102].

Diagnosis is made on the basis of clinical disease in a Fell pony foal along with histologic confirmation of bone marrow erythroid hypoplasia; absence of secondary lymphoid follicles and plasma cells; and neuronal chromatolysis involving the trigeminal, cranial mesenteric, and dorsal root ganglia.

Management and prognosis

Supportive care and antimicrobial therapy may be given for short-term survival. Blood transfusion is unsuccessful and does not affect outcome [102]. Most foals die by 3 months of age despite treatment [102].

Other immunodeficiency syndromes

Other rare immunodeficiency disorders have been reported in foals. The genetic basis and pathogenesis of these disorders are unknown. Transient hypogammaglobulinemia was reported in an Arabian foal [103]. The foal had low serum concentrations of IgG, IgG(T), IgM, and IgA at 3 months of age despite normal numbers and function of B and T lymphocytes in vitro. Spontaneous recovery occurred at 185 days of age [103]. An unusual selective immunoglobulin deficiency was described in a 10-month-old Arabian foal with normal serum concentrations of IgG but nondetectable concentrations of IgM, IgA, and IgG(T). In vitro testing showed normal responses to T-cell mitogens and weak responses to a B-cell mitogen. On postmortem examination, there was atrophy of the lymph nodes and lymphocyte depletion in the thymus and spleen [104]. Transient CD4 and CD8 T-cell lymphopenia has been reported in a foal [105]. This abnormality likely contributed to *P carinii* infection. Other heterogeneous immunodeficiency disorders of foals manifested by bacterial infections and oral candidiasis have been described [106].

Allogenic incompatibilities

Neonatal isoerythrolysis

NI is an important immunologic disease of newborn foals that results in hemolytic anemia. NI occurs after maternal alloantibodies present in the colostrum are ingested and absorbed by the foal. The alloantibodies are directed against surface antigen on the foal's erythrocytes, resulting in cell lysis, agglutination, or both. Several events must be present for NI to occur. First, the mare must be negative for the offending red blood cell (RBC) antigen. Second, the mare must be exposed to and produce antibody to the offending RBC antigen. Exposure may occur in previous pregnancies, through blood transfusion, or after transplacental contamination with fetal blood earlier during the current pregnancy. Finally, the foal from the current pregnancy must have inherited the offending RBC antigen from the stallion. Extravascular hemolysis is the primary mechanism for RBC removal, but complement-mediated intravascular hemolysis may also occur [107].

Pathogenesis

Population studies of blood types most frequently involved in NI show that approximately 14% of foals should have erythrocyte incompatibilities with the dam [108]. The true incidence of NI is much less than 14%, however, because alloimmunization does not occur during every incompatible pregnancy. Production of alloantibodies also varies by breed, with reports of 10% of Thoroughbred mares and 20% of Standardbred mares having detectable concentrations of anti-RBC antibodies in their serum [109]. Only a small percentage of these mares produce significant alloantibodies directed against specific antigenic factors on the foal erythrocytes to result in NI, however. The incidence of NI is 2% in Standardbreds and 1% in Thoroughbreds [109].

Seven RBC groups or systems have been recognized in the horse: A, C, D, K, P, Q, and U [110]. Each blood group produces surface molecules that contain antigenic sites known as factors. There are more than 30 factors that have been identified to date. The most common factors involved in NI are Aa and Qa, accounting for approximately 90% of cases of NI. Other factors that have been implicated in cases of NI include: Ab, Qrs, Qb, Qc, Dc, Da, Db, Ka, Pa, and Ua [111–113].

Mares without the Aa or Qa factor are at particular risk of producing NI-causing antibodies. Although 2% of Thoroughbred mares are actually

Aa-negative, only 50% of these mares make antibodies against Aa [109]. The probability of foals from an Aa-negative mare inheriting the Aa factor from the sire is 85% [112]. Therefore, the incidence of NI in the overall Thoroughbred population is low; however, among those mares that are negative for Aa and producing anti-Aa antibodies, the incidence is high. A larger percentage of Thoroughbred mares are negative for the Qa factor (16%), but there is only a 60% chance of the foal inheriting Qa from the sire and only 3% of Qa-negative mares actually produce anti-Qa antibody [112]. In Standardbred mares, 22% of pacers and 3% of trotters are negative for Aa. Although a high percentage of Standardbred pacers are Aa-negative, only 17% of these mares make anti-Aa antibodies [112]. The percentage of Standardbred foals that inherit Aa from the sire is only 44% as compared with 85% in Thoroughbreds [112]. Standardbreds and Morgans have such a low frequency of Qa factor that this blood group is not considered a risk factor for these breeds.

Antibodies to Ca factor are actually found in higher numbers than antibodies to Aa or Qa factor, but these antibodies generally do not cause significant hemolysis. In fact, mares that are Ca-negative as well as Aa-negative are less likely to produce antibodies to Aa than mares that are Ca-positive, suggesting that antibody to Ca antigens may protect against the production of anti-Aa antibodies [114].

Clinical presentation

Foals are normal at birth but typically show clinical signs between 6 hours and 5 days of age [115]. Clinical signs vary in severity depending on the amount of antibody absorbed and the affinity of the alloantibody. Clinical signs may include weakness, lethargy, tachypnea, tachycardia, pale mucous membranes, icterus, pigmenturia, cardiovascular collapse, and hemodynamic shock [107]. Many of the clinical signs observed are a result of the decrease in oxygen-carrying capacity of blood. Death may precede development of icterus in peracute cases. In contrast, the disease may be subclinical in some mildly affected foals.

Laboratory findings

Clinicopathologic abnormalities include decreases in packed cell volume (PCV), RBCs, and hemoglobin. Bilirubin (mainly unconjugated) concentrations are increased as a result of increased RBC destruction. Hemoglobinuria may be present. Increased lactate concentrations, increased anion gap (metabolic acidosis), and decreased mixed venous oxygen tension may be found in more severely affected foals with impaired tissue oxygenation [116]. When present, azotemia may be the result of renal tubular injury from tissue hypoxia or the nephrotoxic effects of hemoglobin. Uncommonly, toxic hepatopathy (from severe hemolysis) or hepatocellular necrosis (from anoxia) may result in an increase in concentrations of liver enzymes, ammonia, and bile acids [107,117].

Diagnosis

The diagnosis of NI is based on clinical signs consistent with the disease in conjunction with laboratory findings demonstrating maternal alloanti-bodies to the foal's RBCs. There are several laboratory tests available to identify the presence of alloantibodies using agglutination or hemolysis as the end point.

The most reliable test is a hemolytic cross-match test. Hemolytic assays use an exogenous source of complement (usually from rabbit serum) to show hemolysis. RBCs from the foal are mixed with serum from the mare in the presence of complement. If alloantibodies are present, hemolysis occurs as complement is activated. Mare serum is considered positive for alloantibodies when dilutions greater than 1:16 show complete hemolysis. A cross-match between the mare's serum and foal's RBCs can also be performed to demonstrate agglutination. Alloantibodies responsible for NI are stronger hemolysins than agglutinins, however [118,119]. In addition, rouleaux formation poses a problem in interpretation of minor agglutina-tion. As a result, demonstration of hemolysis is simpler, quicker, and more accurate [119]. A Coombs' test can be used to demonstrate the presence of antibodies or complement bound to the foal's RBCs, but this test is not as reliable and not specific for NI.

The jaundiced foal agglutination (JFA) assay is easy to perform and has been shown to correlate well with the standard hemolytic test described previously [112]. In the JFA test, serial dilutions of the mare's colostrum are centrifuged in the presence of the foal's RBCs. Positive reactions characterized by formation of clumps of RBCs at the bottom of the tube at dilutions of 1:16 or greater are considered significant [112]. Additionally, the blood type of the mare and the presence of anti-RBC alloantibodies should be determined for future breeding management when there is a confirmed case of NI.

Treatment

Treatment of NI is based on the severity of disease and how early the problem is recognized. If the disease is recognized when the foal is less than 24 hours of age, the mare's colostrum should be withheld. After 24 hours of age, most of the colostral antibody has been depleted and the absorptive ability of the foal's intestine is negligible. In some cases, hemolysis may be so mild that no treatment is necessary. These foals should be monitored closely, and exercise and stress should be minimized. Severely affected individuals require a blood transfusion. Determining which foals require a blood transfusion is based on clinical and laboratory findings. Weakness, tachypnea, or tachycardia may be the result of decreased oxygen-carrying capacity of blood and suggests the need for a transfusion. Transfusion has traditionally been recommended when the PCV is 10% to 15% [107,120,121]. Simple reliance on PCV, RBC counts, or hemoglobin concentrations may be misleading because these parameters are also influenced by plasma volume and may not necessarily reflect a change in the oxygen-carrying capacity of blood. Physiologic markers of impaired tissue oxygenation are likely superior to PCV or hemoglobin concentrations as transfusion triggers. The most practical marker of impaired tissue oxygenation in foals is measurement of lactate concentrations. Anaerobic metabolism is not the only cause of hyperlactatemia, however. The oxygen extraction ratio (O_2ER) has been shown to be an accurate transfusion trigger in laboratory animals and people [122–124]. A normal O_2ER in conscious healthy foals is approximately 20% [125]. As the hematocrit decreases, there is a progressive decrease in oxygen delivery. This decrease in oxygen delivery is compensated for by an increase in O_2ER up to 50% to 60% in an attempt to maintain constant oxygen uptake by tissues. When the hematocrit falls below a critical level, however, the increase in O_2ER is no longer sufficient to maintain constant oxygen uptake and tissue oxygenation begins to fall. Measurement of O_2ER requires placement of a central venous catheter to obtain mixed venous blood. The O_2ER is calculated as $(SaO_2 - SvO_2/SaO_2) \times 100$, where SaO_2 and SvO_2 represent arterial and mixed or central venous oxygen saturation, respectively. An O_2ER of 50% or greater has been shown to be a good indicator of the need for blood transfusion [122–124]. The use of O_2ER as a transfusion trigger in general equine practice is limited by the placement of a central venous catheter and availability of blood gas analyzers.

Washed RBCs from the dam are the ideal choice when a transfusion is needed. Because the mare's plasma contains the offending antibodies, RBCs should be washed a minimum of two times before administering the packed RBCs to the foal. Alternatively, cross-matching with particular attention to the reaction of the foal's serum with the donor's RBCs may be used to select an appropriate donor. If cross-matching is not available, a donor previously identified to be Aa-negative and Qa-negative and free of alloantibody would be a good choice based on the fact that these two antigens account for most cases of NI. The odds of randomly selecting an Aa-negative and Qa-negative donor vary with breed. If a donor must be used without first performing a cross-match, the best choice would be a Standardbred, Morgan, or Quarter Horse gelding that has no prior history of a blood transfusion.

The volume of blood required to increase the PCV to a desired value can be calculated from the following equation: body weight (kg) × 150 mL/kg × (PCV desired − PCV observed)/PCV of the donor, where 150 mL/kg represents the approximate blood volume of a 2-day-old foal. Typically, 2 to 4 L of blood is collected from the donor. The half-life of transfused RBCs in foals is 3 to 9 days and is not significantly different whether the donor is the mare or a compatible unrelated donor [126]. This period of time is sufficient to maintain oxygen delivery until the bone marrow responds adequately in most foals.

Polymerized bovine hemoglobin (Oxyglobin; Biopure Corp., Cambridge, Massachusetts) has a long shelf life (36 months), and cross-matching is not necessary because of the lack of erythrocyte membranes. Oxyglobin (10–20 mL/kg) may be used in an emergency situation in foals with NI to improve the oxygen-carrying capacity of blood while cross-matching is performed or the mare's RBCs are washed [116]. Oxyglobin has been shown to improve hemodynamics and oxygen transport parameters in horses experiencing normovolemic anemia [116,127]. The short half-life of polymerized hemoglobin (18–43 hours) as compared with transfused RBCs prevents it from being the sole source of transfusion in most cases of NI in foals, however. Anaphylactoid reactions during administration of polymerized hemoglobin, albeit rare, have been reported in horses [127]. Additional therapy that may be indicated depending on the severity of the disease and concurrent problems includes broad-spectrum antibiotics for the prevention or treatment of sepsis, oxygen therapy, supplemental nutrition, and fluid therapy. Anticonvulsants may also be required for the more serious cases that develop seizures. Although corticosteroids may reduce the clearance of IgG-coated RBCs, their use is controversial, because many foals with NI may be septic or have concurrent infections.

Prognosis

The prognosis for NI depends on many factors, including the amount of antibody absorbed, the affinity of the antibody, the time before initiation of treatment, and secondary complications. The prognosis is favorable in most uncomplicated cases. In a recent retrospective study of 71 cases of NI, the survival rate was 73% [128]. The most common complication in foals with NI is sepsis attributable to many possible contributing factors, including stress, lack of nutrition (too weak to nurse), partial FTP, decreased immunologic defenses from an overwhelmed reticuloendothelial system, or bacterial translocation through the gut as a result of tissue hypoxia. In rare instances, renal failure, liver failure, or kernicterus may also occur. In the retrospective study mentioned previously [128], 12% of foals developed sepsis, 9% developed kernicterus, and 5% had moderate to severe hepatopathy.

Kernicterus is a well-recognized complication in human infants with excessive bilirubinemia (unconjugated) from severe or continued hemolysis. Kernicterus has also been recognized as a complication of NI in foals [117]. Not every foal with severe hyperbilirubinemia develops kernicterus, however. The clinical signs associated with kernicterus in foals include lethargy, depression, and decreased appetite progressing to rigidity, opisthotonus, convulsions, and death [117]. The diagnosis is made by histopathologic evaluation with deposition of unconjugated bilirubin and neuronal necrosis of specific areas of the cerebral gray matter, including the basal ganglia, hippocampal cortex, subthalamic nuclei, and cerebellum. Treatment of human infants with severe hyperbilirubinemia includes phototherapy, exchange transfusion, and administration of phenobarbital to increase bilirubin conjugation [129]. These therapies have not been critically investigated in foals.

Prevention

Prevention of NI requires proactive screening to determine if a foal may be at risk. Broodmares should be blood typed to determine if they are at risk. Mare negatives for Aa or Qa factor are particularly at risk. One strategy could be to breed these mares to an Aa/Qa-negative stallion, thus eliminating the possibility of the foal inheriting the offending antigen. This approach is impractical in breeds in which a large percentage of the population carries these antigens, however. In the case of incompatible mating or mating between horses of unknown blood groups, serum from the mare should be screened for anti-RBC antibodies within 30 days before foaling. If results of serum testing are equivocal (eg, positive but low titer), the test should be repeated closer to parturition. If results demonstrate anti-RBC antibodies, a hemolytic test or the JFA test should be performed before the foal nurses. Colostrum should be withheld from the foal and an alternative source provided pending test results. If the mare's colostrum is determined to contain alloantibodies, the foal should be held off the mare for a minimum of 24 hours and fed colostrum negative for alloantibodies. During this time, the mare's udder should be stripped every 2 hours to help maintain milk production. Serum IgG should be measured in the foal 12 to 24 hours after birth to ensure adequate transfer of immunoglobulins.

Mares negative for Ca often make anti-Ca antibody. Although these antibodies are not known to cause NI, they confuse the issue of screening because they cause false-positive reactions in most screening tests. As described previously, other blood group antigens have been associated with NI in horses. Approximately 1 in 2000 pregnancies may result in sensitization against antigens other than Aa or Qa [120]. As a result, it is not practical to consider all mares without these antigens to be at risk for NI.

Neonatal isoerythrolysis in mule foals

Mule foals are the result of a mating between a donkey sire and a horse dam. The occurrence of NI in mule foals has been reported to be higher than in horse foals because of a unique RBC antigen (donkey factor) that is found on all donkey RBCs [130,131]. This unique donkey factor antigen is not found on horse RBCs; thus, theoretically all mule pregnancies are incompatible with regard to this factor [131]. Although all mule pregnancies are at risk for NI, many mule foals remain clinically normal. The incidence of NI in mule foals is approximately 10% [131]. Although rare in horse foals, thrombocytopenia is a common feature in mule foals with NI [130].

Because horses do not have the donkey factor or have naturally occurring antibody to it, any horse would be a suitable donor of whole blood. If the dam's cells are used, however, they must be washed thoroughly.

Neonatal alloimmune thrombocytopenia with or without ulcerative dermatitis

Neonatal alloimmune thrombocytopenia occurs when maternal antibodies are produced against fetal platelet antigens inherited from the stallion. Neonatal alloimmune thrombocytopenia is not uncommon in mule foals with NI. The disease has also been reported in horse foals [132,133]. Most affected foals are less than 4 days of age at the time of presentation. Some but not all affected foals present with oral and lingual ulcers as well as crusting and erythema around the eyes; the muzzle; or the perineal, inguinal, axillary, trunk, or neck regions [133]. Histopathologic examination of the skin reveals multifocal dermoepidermal vesicles that may progress to dermoepidermal separation with fibrin, cellular debris, and RBCs filling the cleft [133]. Clinical signs on presentation in foals without skin lesions are often nonspecific and include weakness, lethargy, and decreased ability to nurse. Petechial hemorrhages and prolonged bleeding from venipuncture sites may be identified on physical examination. Spontaneous hemorrhage may be seen in severely affected foals, resulting in epistaxis, melena, or hyphema. The main laboratory finding is thrombocytopenia unless other disease processes are present concurrently. Affected foals often have moderate concurrent neutropenia [133]. The presence of severe thrombocytopenia combined with the absence of other clotting anomalies is suggestive of alloimmune thrombocytopenia.

The fact that mares bred from different sires have birthed affected foals in sequential years suggests an alloimmune process. A definitive diagnosis of immune-mediated thrombocytopenia is based on the detection of immunoglobulins on the surface of the foal's platelets by flow cytometry [54]. Indirect assays showing that antibodies from the mare's serum or milk (but not that from a control horse) bind to the foal's platelets are necessary to confirm that the disease is alloimmune [132]. A specific platelet or skin antigen associated with alloimmune thrombocytopenia and ulcerative dermatitis in foals has not been identified. Treatment of clinically affected foals consists of administration of platelet-rich plasma from a compatible donor identified on minor cross-match. Whole blood may be used when thrombocytopenia results in severe hemorrhage and clinically significant anemia. Whole blood or plasma must be collected in plastic bags to preserve platelets. In one report, the foal's platelets were negative for platelet-associated antibody by 9 days of age, presumably because platelet-reactive alloantibodies are rapidly removed by mononuclear phagocytes [132]. Platelet counts gradually increase in most foals within 7 to 10 days, and skin lesions typically resolve within 10 to 14 days. There is no evidence that corticosteroids improve the outcome of affected foals.

Other immune-mediated diseases

Neonatal neutropenia suspected to be alloimmune in origin has been described in a foal based on severe neutropenia and increased staining for IgG on the surface of the affected foal's neutrophils [134]. Administration of a single injection of granulocyte colony stimulating factor (6 μg/kg administered subcutaneously) resulted in a considerable increase in peripheral neutrophils, and the foal made an uneventful recovery [134]. Immune-mediated anemia and thrombocytopenia unrelated to maternally derived antibody have also been described in foals [135].

References

[1] Mackenzie CD. Histological development of the thymic and intestinal lymphoid tissue of the horse. J S Afr Vet Assoc 1975;46(1):47–55.
[2] Perryman LE, McGuire TC, Torbeck RL. Ontogeny of lymphocyte function in the equine fetus. Am J Vet Res 1980;41(8):1197–200.
[3] Martin BR, Larson KA. Immune response of equine fetus to coliphage T2. Am J Vet Res 1973;34(10):1363–4.
[4] Mock RE, Morgan DO, Jochim MM, et al. Antibody response of the fetus and adult equine to Venezuelan equine encephalomyelitis virus (VEE-TC-84): Immunoglobulins $G_{a\&b}$, M, and T. Equine Infect Dis 1978;IV:209–19.
[5] Morgan DO, Bryans JT, Mock RE. Immunoglobulins produced by the antigenized equine fetus. J Reprod Fertil Suppl 1975;23:735–8.
[6] Jeffcott LB. Studies on passive immunity in the foal. 1. Gamma-globulin and antibody variations associated with the maternal transfer of immunity and the onset of active immunity. J Comp Pathol 1974;84(1):93–101.
[7] Kelly GS. Bovine colostrums: a review of clinical uses. Altern Med Rev 2003;8(4):378–94.
[8] Zou E, Brady HA, Hurley WL. Protective factors in mammary gland secretions during the periparturient period in the mare. J Equine Vet Sci 1998;18:184–8.
[9] Le Jan C. Cellular components of mammary secretions and neonatal immunity: a review. Vet Res 1996;27(4–5):403–17.
[10] Kohn CW, Knight D, Hueston W, et al. Colostral and serum IgG, IgA, and IgM concentrations in Standardbred mares and their foals at parturition. J Am Vet Med Assoc 1989; 195(1):64–8.
[11] Sheoran AS, Timoney JF, Holmes MA, et al. Immunoglobulin isotypes in sera and nasal mucosal secretions and their neonatal transfer and distribution in horses. Am J Vet Res 2000;61(9):1099–105.
[12] Pearson RC, Hallowell AL, Bayly WM, et al. Times of appearance and disappearance of colostral IgG in the mare. Am J Vet Res 1984;45(1):186–90.
[13] LeBlanc MM, Tran T, Baldwin JL, et al. Factors that influence passive transfer of immunoglobulins in foals. J Am Vet Med Assoc 1992;200(2):179–83.
[14] Jeffcott LB. Studies on passive immunity in the foal. II. The absorption of 125I-labelled PVP (polyvinyl pyrrolidone) by the neonatal intestine. J Comp Pathol 1974;84(3):279–89.
[15] Raidal SL, McTaggart C, Yovich JV, et al. Effect of withholding macromolecules on the duration of intestinal permeability to colostral IgG in foals. Proc Am Assoc Equine Pract 2000;46:260–3.

[16] Holznagel DL, Hussey S, Mihalyi JE, et al. Onset of immunoglobulin production in foals. Equine Vet J 2003;35(6):620–2.

[17] Wilson WD, Mihalyi JE, Hussey S, et al. Passive transfer of maternal immunoglobulin isotype antibodies against tetanus and influenza and their effect on the response of foals to vaccination. Equine Vet J 2001;33(7):644–50.

[18] Reifenberg K, Stahl M, Losch U. Complement-dependence of polymorphonuclear yeast cell phagocytosis: a comparison between man and various domestic animals. Zentralbl Veterinarmed B 1990;37(8):561–9.

[19] Grondahl G, Johannisson A, Jensen-Waern M. Opsonic effect of equine plasma from different donors. Vet Microbiol 1997;56(3–4):227–35.

[20] Asbury AC, Gorman NT, Foster GW. Uterine defense mechanisms in the mare: serum opsonins affecting phagocytosis of *Streptococcus zooepidemicus* by equine neutrophils. Theriogenology 1984;21(2):375–85.

[21] Bernoco MM, Liu IK, Willits NH. Hemolytic complement activity and concentrations of its third component during maturation of the immune response in colostrum-deprived foals. Am J Vet Res 1994;55(7):928–33.

[22] Grondahl G, Sternberg S, Jensen-Waern M, et al. Opsonic capacity of foal serum for the two neonatal pathogens *Escherichia coli* and *Actinobacillus equuli*. Equine Vet J 2001;33(7): 670–5.

[23] Bernoco M, Liu IK, Wuest-Ehlert CJ, et al. Chemotactic and phagocytic function of peripheral blood polymorphonuclear leucocytes in newborn foals. J Reprod Fertil Suppl 1987;35:599–605.

[24] Grondahl G, Johannisson A, Demmers S, et al. Influence of age and plasma treatment on neutrophil phagocytosis and CD18 expression in foals. Vet Microbiol 1999;65(3):241–54.

[25] Demmers S, Johannisson A, Grondahl G, et al. Neutrophil functions and serum IgG in growing foals. Equine Vet J 2001;33(7):676–80.

[26] Hietala SK, Ardans AA. Neutrophil phagocytic and serum opsonic response of the foal to *Corynebacterium equi*. Vet Immunol Immunopathol 1987;14(3):279–94.

[27] Martens JG, Martens RJ, Renshaw HW. *Rhodococcus* (*Corynebacterium*) *equi*: bactericidal capacity of neutrophils from neonatal and adult horses. Am J Vet Res 1988;49(3):295–9.

[28] Takai S, Morozumi Y, Higashiyama S, et al. Nitroblue tetrazolium reduction by neutrophils of newborn foals, adult horses, and a foal infected with *Rhodococcus* (*Corynebacterium*) *equi*. Jpn J Vet Sci 1986;48:405–8.

[29] Yager JA, Duder CK, Prescott JF, et al. The interaction of *Rhodococcus equi* and foal neutrophils *in vitro*. Vet Microbiol 1987;14(3):287–94.

[30] Flaminio MJ, Rush BR, Davis EG, et al. Characterization of peripheral blood and pulmonary leukocyte function in healthy foals. Vet Immunol Immunopathol 2000;73(3–4): 267–85.

[31] Flaminio MJ, Rush BR, Shuman W. Peripheral blood lymphocyte subpopulations and immunoglobulin concentrations in healthy foals and foals with *Rhodococcus equi* pneumonia. J Vet Intern Med 1999;13(3):206–12.

[32] Smith R III, Chaffin MK, Cohen ND, et al. Age-related changes in lymphocyte subsets of Quarter horse foals. Am J Vet Res 2002;63(4):531–7.

[33] Sanada Y, Noda H, Nagahata H. Development of lymphocyte blastogenic response in the neonatal period of foals. Zentralbl Veterinarmed A 1992;39(1):69–75.

[34] Boyd NK, Cohen ND, Lim WS, et al. Temporal changes in cytokine expression of foals during the first month of life. Vet Immunol Immunopathol 2003;92(1–2):75–85.

[35] Prescott JF, Markham RJ, Johnson JA. Cellular and humoral immune response of foals to vaccination with *Corynebacterium equi*. Can J Comp Med 1979;43(4):356–64.

[36] Dennis VA, Klei TR, Miller MA, et al. Immune responses of pony foals during repeated infections of *Strongylus vulgaris* and regular ivermectin treatments. Vet Parasitol 1992; 42(1–2):83–99.

[37] Chong YC, Duffus WP. Immune responses of specific pathogen free foals to EHV-1 infection. Vet Microbiol 1992;32(3–4):215–28.

[38] Ellis JA, Steeves E, Wright AK, et al. Cell-mediated cytolysis of equine herpesvirus-infected cells by leukocytes from young vaccinated horses. Vet Immunol Immunopathol 1997; 57(3–4):201–14.

[39] Banks EM, Kyriakidou M, Little S, et al. Epithelial lymphocyte and macrophage distribution in the adult and fetal equine lung. J Comp Pathol 1999;120(1):1–13.

[40] Blunden AS, Gower SM. A histological and immunohistochemical study of the humoral immune system of the lungs in young Thoroughbred horses. J Comp Pathol 1999;120(4): 347–56.

[41] Balson GA, Smith GD, Yager JA. Immunophenotypic analysis of foal bronchoalveolar lavage lymphocytes. Vet Microbiol 1997;56(3–4):237–46.

[42] Zink MC, Johnson JA. Cellular constituents of clinically normal foal bronchoalveolar lavage fluid during postnatal maturation. Am J Vet Res 1984;45(5):893–7.

[43] Moore BR. Diagnostic use of bronchoalveolar lavage in horses. Equine Pract 1996;18(5): 7–15.

[44] Sweeney CR, Rossier Y, Ziemer EL, et al. Effects of lung site and fluid volume on results of bronchoalveolar lavage fluid analysis in horses. Am J Vet Res 1992;53(8):1376–9.

[45] Liu IK, Walsh EM, Bernoco M, et al. Bronchoalveolar lavage in the newborn foal. J Reprod Fertil Suppl 1987;35:587–92.

[46] Fogarty U, Leadon DP. Comparison of systemic and local respiratory tract cellular immunity in the neonatal foal. J Reprod Fertil Suppl 1987;35:593–8.

[47] Hietala SK, Ardans AA. Interaction of Rhodococcus equi with phagocytic cells from R. equi-exposed and non-exposed foals. Vet Microbiol 1987;14(3):307–20.

[48] Sandbulte MR, Roth JA. Methods for analysis of cell-mediated immunity in domestic animal species. J Am Vet Med Assoc 2004;225(4):522–30.

[49] Young KM, Lunn DP. Immunodiagnostic testing in horses. Vet Clin North Am Equine Pract 2000;16(1):79–103.

[50] Hodgin EC, McGuire TC, Perryman LE, et al. Evaluation of delayed hypersensitivity responses in normal horses and immunodeficient foals. Am J Vet Res 1978;39(7):1161–7.

[51] Flaminio MJ, Rush BR, Davis EG, et al. Simultaneous flow cytometric analysis of phagocytosis and oxidative burst activity in equine leukocytes. Vet Res Commun 2002; 26(2):85–92.

[52] Raidal SL, Bailey GD, Love DN. Flow cytometric determination of oxidative burst activity of equine peripheral blood and bronchoalveolar lavage-derived leucocytes. Vet J 1998; 156(2):117–26.

[53] Grondahl G, Johannisson A, Jensen-Waern M, et al. Opsonization of yeast cells with equine iC3b, C3b, and IgG. Vet Immunol Immunopathol 2001;80(3–4):209–23.

[54] Davis EG, Wilkerson MJ, Rush BR. Flow cytometry: clinical applications in equine medicine. J Vet Intern Med 2002;16(4):404–10.

[55] Baldwin JL, Cooper WL, Vanderwall DK, et al. Prevalence (treatment days) and severity of illness in hypogammaglobulinemic and normogammaglobulinemic foals. J Am Vet Med Assoc 1991;198(3):423–8.

[56] Clabough DL, Levine JF, Grant GL, et al. Factors associated with failure of passive transfer of colostral antibodies in Standardbred foals. J Vet Intern Med 1991;5(6): 335–40.

[57] Haas SD, Bristol F, Card CE. Risk factors associated with the incidence of foal mortality in an extensively managed mare herd. Can Vet J 1996;37(2):91–5.

[58] McGuire TC, Crawford TB, Hallowell AL, et al. Failure of colostral immunoglobulin transfer as an explanation for most infections and deaths of neonatal foals. J Am Vet Med Assoc 1977;170(11):1302–4.

[59] Morris DD, Meirs DA, Merryman GS. Passive transfer failure in horses: incidence and causative factors on a breeding farm. Am J Vet Res 1985;46(11):2294–9.

[60] Raidal SL. The incidence and consequences of failure of passive transfer of immunity on a Thoroughbred breeding farm. Aust Vet J 1996;73(6):201–6.

[61] Perryman LE, McGuire TC. Evaluation for immune system failures in horses and ponies. J Am Vet Med Assoc 1980;176(12):1374–7.

[62] Cohen ND. Causes of and farm management factors associated with disease and death in foals. J Am Vet Med Assoc 1994;204(10):1644–51.

[63] Robinson JA, Allen GK, Green EM, et al. A prospective study of septicaemia in colostrum-deprived foals. Equine Vet J 1993;25(3):214–9.

[64] Cross DL, Redmond LM, Strickland JR. Equine fescue toxicosis: signs and solutions. J Anim Sci 1995;73(3):899–908.

[65] LeBlanc MM, McLaurin BI, Boswell R. Relationships among serum immunoglobulin concentration in foals, colostral specific gravity, and colostral immunoglobulin concentration. J Am Vet Med Assoc 1986;189(1):57–60.

[66] Chavatte P, Clement F, Cash R, et al. Field determination of colostrum quality by using a novel, practical method. Proc Am Assoc Equine Pract 1998;44:206–9.

[67] Jones D, Brook D. Investigation of the Gamma-Check-C test as a means of evaluating the IgG levels in equine colostrum. J Equine Vet Sci 1995;15:269–71.

[68] Halliday R. The effect of steroid hormones on the absorption of antibody by the young rat. J Endocrinol 1959;18(1):56–66.

[69] Carrick JB, Pollitt CC, Thompson HL, et al. Failure of the administration of ACTH to affect the absorption of colostral immunoglobulin in neonatal foals. Equine Vet J 1987; 19(6):545–7.

[70] Rumbaugh GE, Ardans AA, Ginno D, et al. Measurement of neonatal equine immunoglobulins for assessment of colostral immunoglobulin transfer: comparison of single radial immunodiffusion with the zinc sulfate turbidity test, serum electrophoresis, refractometry for total serum protein, and the sodium sulfite precipitation test. J Am Vet Med Assoc 1978;172(3):321–5.

[71] Bauer JE, Brooks TP. Immunoturbidimetric quantification of serum immunoglobulin G concentration in foals. Am J Vet Res 1990;51(8):1211–4.

[72] Beetson SA, Hilbert BJ, Mills JN. The use of the glutaraldehyde coagulation test for detection of hypogammaglobulinaemia in neonatal foals. Aust Vet J 1985;62(8):279–81.

[73] Bertone JJ, Jones RL, Curtis CR. Evaluation of a test kit for determination of serum immunoglobulin G concentration in foals. J Vet Intern Med 1988;2(4):181–3.

[74] Pusterla N, Pusterla JB, Spier SJ, et al. Evaluation of the SNAP foal IgG test for the semiquantitative measurement of immunoglobulin G in foals. Vet Rec 2002;151(9):258–60.

[75] Lavoie JP, Spensley MS, Smith BP, et al. Absorption of bovine colostral immunoglobulins G and M in newborn foals. Am J Vet Res 1989;50(9):1598–603.

[76] Holmes MA, Lunn DP. A study of bovine and equine immunoglobulin levels in pony foals fed bovine colostrum. Equine Vet J 1991;23(2):116–8.

[77] Vivrette SL, Young K, Manning S, et al. Efficacy of Seramune in the treatment of failure of passive transfer in foals. Proc Am Assoc Equine Pract 1998;44:136–7.

[78] McClure JT, DeLuca JL, Lunn DP, et al. Evaluation of IgG concentration and IgG subisotypes in foals with complete or partial failure of passive transfer after administration of intravenous serum or plasma. Equine Vet J 2001;33(7):681–6.

[79] Perryman LE. Primary immunodeficiencies of horses. Vet Clin North Am Equine Pract 2000;16(1):105–16.

[80] Perryman LE, Torbeck RL. Combined immunodeficiency of Arabian horses: confirmation of autosomal recessive mode of inheritance. J Am Vet Med Assoc 1980;176(11):1250–1.

[81] Shin EK, Perryman LE, Meek K. A kinase-negative mutation of DNA-PK(CS) in equine SCID results in defective coding and signal joint formation. J Immunol 1997;158(8):3565–9.

[82] Perryman LE, McGuire TC, Crawford TB. Maintenance of foals with combined immunodeficiency: causes and control of secondary infections. Am J Vet Res 1978;39(6): 1043–7.

[83] Shin EK, Perryman LE, Meek K. Evaluation of a test for identification of Arabian horses heterozygous for the severe combined immunodeficiency trait. J Am Vet Med Assoc 1997; 211(10):1268–70.

[84] Bue CM, Davis WC, Magnuson NS, et al. Correction of equine severe combined immunodeficiency by bone marrow transplantation. Transplantation 1986;42(1):14–9.

[85] Perryman LE, Bue CM, Magnuson NS, et al. Immunologic reconstitution of foals with combined immunodeficiency. Vet Immunol Immunopathol 1987;7(1–4):495–508.

[86] Perryman LE, McGuire TC, Hilbert BJ. Selective immunoglobulin M deficiency in foals. J Am Vet Med Assoc 1977;170(2):212–5.

[87] Weldon AD, Zhang C, Antczak DF, et al. Selective IgM deficiency and abnormal B-cell response in a foal. J Am Vet Med Assoc 1992;201(9):1396–8.

[88] Ansar AS, Furr M, Chickering WR, et al. Immunologic studies of a horse with lymphosarcoma. Vet Immunol Immunopathol 1993;38(3–4):229–39.

[89] Perryman LE, Wyatt CR, Magnuson NS. Biochemical and functional characterization of lymphocytes from a horse with lymphosarcoma and IgM deficiency. Comp Immunol Microbiol Infect Dis 1984;7(1):53–62.

[90] Perryman LE, Wyatt CR. Suppressor lymphocyte activity in normal and immunodeficient horses. Thymus 1984;6(4):263–72.

[91] Furr MO, Crisman MV, Robertson J, et al. Immunodeficiency associated with lymphosarcoma in a horse. J Am Vet Med Assoc 1992;201(2):307–9.

[92] Perkins GA, Nydam DV, Flaminio MJ, et al. Serum IgM concentrations in normal, fit horses and horses with lymphoma or other medical conditions. J Vet Intern Med 2003; 17(3):337–42.

[93] Vetrie D, Vorechovsky I, Sideras P, et al. The gene involved in X-linked agammaglobulinaemia is a member of the src family of protein-tyrosine kinases. Nature 1993;361(6409): 226–33.

[94] Deem DA, Traver DS, Thacker HL, et al. Agammaglobulinemia in a horse. J Am Vet Med Assoc 1979;175(5):469–72.

[95] Banks KL, McGuire TC, Jerrells TR. Absence of B lymphocytes in a horse with primary agammaglobulinemia. Clin Immunol Immunopathol 1976;5(2):282–90.

[96] McGuire TC, Banks KL, Evans DR, et al. Agammaglobulinemia in a horse with evidence of functional T lymphocytes. Am J Vet Res 1976;37(1):41–6.

[97] Perryman LE, McGuire TC, Banks KL. Animal model of human disease. Infantile X-linked agammaglobulinemia. Agammaglobulinemia in horses. Am J Pathol 1983;111(1): 125–7.

[98] Thomas GW, Bell SC, Phythian C, et al. Aid to the antemortem diagnosis of Fell pony foal syndrome by the analysis of B lymphocytes. Vet Rec 2003;152(20):618–21.

[99] Thomas GW, Bell SC, Carter SD. Immunoglobulin and peripheral B-lymphocyte concentrations in Fell pony foal syndrome. Equine Vet J 2005;37(1):48–52.

[100] Bell SC, Savidge C, Taylor P, et al. An immunodeficiency in Fell ponies: a preliminary study into cellular responses. Equine Vet J 2001;33(7):687–92.

[101] Richards AJ, Kelly DF, Knottenbelt DC, et al. Anaemia, diarrhoea and opportunistic infections in Fell ponies. Equine Vet J 2000;32(5):386–91.

[102] Scholes SF, Holliman A, May PD, et al. A syndrome of anaemia, immunodeficiency and peripheral ganglionopathy in Fell pony foals. Vet Rec 1998;142(6):128–34.

[103] McGuire TC, Poppie MJ, Banks KL. Hypogammaglobulinemia predisposing to infection in foals. J Am Vet Med Assoc 1975;166(1):71–5.

[104] Boy MG, Zhang C, Antczak DF, et al. Unusual selective immunoglobulin deficiency in an Arabian foal. J Vet Intern Med 1992;6(4):201–5.

[105] Flaminio MJ, Rush BR, Cox JH, et al. CD4 + and CD8 + T-lymphocytopenia in a filly with Pneumocystis carinii pneumonia. Aust Vet J 1998;76(6):399–402.

[106] McClure JJ, Addison JD, Miller RI. Immunodeficiency manifested by oral candidiasis and bacterial septicemia in foals. J Am Vet Med Assoc 1985;186(11):1195–7.

[107] Whiting JL, David JB. Neonatal isoerythrolysis. Compend Contin Educ Pract Vet 2000;22: 968–75.

[108] Becht JL. Neonatal isoerythrolysis in the foal. I. Background, blood group antigens, and pathogenesis. Compend Contin Educ Pract Vet 1983;5(Suppl):S591–6.

[109] Bailey E. Prevalence of anti-red blood cell antibodies in the serum and colostrum of mares and its relationship to neonatal isoerythrolysis. Am J Vet Res 1982;43(11): 1917–21.

[110] Bowling AT, Clark RS. Blood-group and protein polymorphism gene-frequencies for 7 breeds of horses in the United States. Anim Blood Groups Biochem Genet 1985;16: 93–108.

[111] MacLeay JM. Neonatal isoerythrolysis involving the Qc and Db antigens in a foal. J Am Vet Med Assoc 2001;219(1) 50, 79–81.

[112] Bailey E, Conboy HS, McCarthy PF. Neonatal isoerythrolysis of foals: an update on testing. Proc Am Assoc Equine Pract 1987;33:341–55.

[113] Zaruby JF, Hearn P, Colling D. Neonatal isoerythrolysis in a foal, involving anti-Pa alloantibody. Equine Vet J 1992;24(1):71–3.

[114] Bailey E, Albright DG, Henney PJ. Equine neonatal isoerythrolysis: evidence for prevention by maternal antibodies to the Ca blood group antigen. Am J Vet Res 1988; 49(8):1218–22.

[115] Becht JL, Semrad SD. Hematology, blood typing, and immunology of the neonatal foal. Vet Clin North Am Equine Pract 1985;1(1):91–116.

[116] Perkins GA, Divers TJ. Polymerized hemoglobin therapy in a foal with neonatal isoerythrolysis. J Vet Emerg Crit Care 2001;11(2):141–6.

[117] David JB, Byars TD. Kernicterus in a foal with neonatal isoerythrolysis. Compend Contin Educ Pract Vet 1998;20:517–22.

[118] Becht JL, Page EH, Morter RL, et al. Experimental production of neonatal isoerythrolysis in the foal. Cornell Vet 1983;73(4):380–9.

[119] Becht JL, Page EH, Morter RL, et al. Evaluation of a series of testing procedures to predict neonatal isoerythrolysis in the foal. Cornell Vet 1983;73(4):390–402.

[120] McClure Blackmer JJ, Parish SM. Diseases caused by allogenic incompatibilities. In: Smith BP, editor. Large animal internal medicine. St. Louis, MO: Mosby; 2002. p. 1604–13.

[121] Vaala WE. Transfusion therapy. In: Koterba AM, Drummond WH, Kosch PC, editors. Equine clinical neonatology. Philadelphia: Lea & Febiger; 1990. p. 701–11.

[122] Levy PS, Chavez RP, Crystal GJ, et al. Oxygen extraction ratio: a valid indicator of transfusion need in limited coronary vascular reserve? J Trauma 1992;32(6):769–73.

[123] Sehgal LR, Zebala LP, Takagi I, et al. Evaluation of oxygen extraction ratio as a physiologic transfusion trigger in coronary artery bypass graft surgery patients. Transfusion 2001;41(5):591–5.

[124] Wilkerson DK, Rosen AL, Gould SA, et al. Oxygen extraction ratio: a valid indicator of myocardial metabolism in anemia. J Surg Res 1987;42(6):629–34.

[125] Corley KTT. Monitoring and treating haemodynamic disturbances in critically ill neonatal foals. Part 1: haemodynamic monitoring. Equine Vet Educ 2002;4:345–58.

[126] Smith JE, Dever M, Smith J, et al. Post-transfusion survival of 50Cr-labeled erythrocytes in neonatal foals. J Vet Intern Med 1992;6(3):183–5.

[127] Belgrave RL, Hines MT, Keegan RD, et al. Effects of a polymerized ultrapurified bovine hemoglobin blood substitute administered to ponies with normovolemic anemia. J Vet Intern Med 2002;16(4):396–403.

[128] Polkes AC. Neonatal isoerythrolysis: overview, management strategies and long-term outcome. ACVIM Forum Proceedings 2003;21:248–50.

[129] Dennery PA, Seidman DS, Stevenson DK. Neonatal hyperbilirubinemia. N Engl J Med 2001;344(8):581–90.

[130] Traub-Dargatz JL, McClure JJ, Koch C, et al. Neonatal isoerythrolysis in mule foals. J Am Vet Med Assoc 1995;206(1):67–70.

[131] McClure JJ, Koch C, Traub-Dargatz J. Characterization of a red blood cell antigen in donkeys and mules associated with neonatal isoerythrolysis. Anim Genet 1994;25(2):119–20.

[132] Buechner-Maxwell V, Scott MA, Godber L, et al. Neonatal alloimmune thrombocytopenia in a quarter horse foal. J Vet Intern Med 1997;11(5):304–8.

[133] Perkins GA, Miller WH, Divers TL, et al. Ulcerative dermatitis, thrombocytopenia, and neutropenia in neonatal foals. J Vet Intern Med 2005;19(2):211–5.

[134] Davis EG, Rush B, Bain F, et al. Neonatal neutropenia in an Arabian foal. Equine Vet J 2003;35(5):517–20.

[135] Sockett DC, Traub-Dargatz J, Weiser MG. Immune-mediated hemolytic anemia and thrombocytopenia in a foal. J Am Vet Med Assoc 1987;190(3):308–10.

[136] Lavoie JP, Spensley MS, Smith BP, Mihalyi J. Colostral volume and immunoglobulin G and M determinations in mares. Am J Vet Res 1989;50(4):466–70.

ELSEVIER
SAUNDERS

VETERINARY
CLINICS
Equine Practice

Vet Clin Equine 21 (2005) 273–293

Equine Neonatal Sepsis

L. Chris Sanchez, DVM, PhD

*Department of Large Animal Clinical Sciences, College of Veterinary Medicine, University of
Florida, PO Box 100136, 2015 S.W. 16th Avenue, Gainesville, FL 32610-0136, USA*

Sepsis represents a major disease process with clinical and economic importance worldwide. Sepsis has been implicated as the major cause of morbidity and mortality in the equine neonate [1,2]. Because the response of the body to microbial invasion of the bloodstream involves a systemic inflammatory response, foals can deteriorate rapidly despite aggressive treatment. This deterioration often leaves the equine practitioner in a difficult situation, and sepsis and its associated repercussions have prompted much of the advanced neonatal care to which this article is dedicated.

Pathophysiology and associated definitions

Much of the clinical syndrome classically associated with sepsis is caused by a nonspecific inflammatory response not necessarily the infectious organism itself. Many terms have been coined referring to this response and its associated syndromes and processes. A set of definitions were described in 1991 by the American College of Chest Physicians and the Society of Critical Care Medicine, and a summary of this consensus report follows [3]. The systemic inflammatory response syndrome (SIRS) refers to a systemic inflammatory response, regardless of the inciting cause, which results in at least two of the following four clinical manifestations: fever; tachycardia; tachypnea or hyperventilation; and leukocytosis, leukopenia, or a relative increase of circulating immature neutrophils. When SIRS occurs in response to a confirmed infectious process, the process is termed sepsis. Infection refers to the invasion of normally sterile host tissue by microorganisms or to the inflammatory response generated in response to those organisms. The presence of viable bacteria in the blood is termed bacteremia, and the presence of other viable pathogens in the blood is described similarly (ie, viremia, fungemia, and other conditions). When sepsis is associated with

---

E-mail address: sanchezl@mail.vetmed.ufl.edu

doi:10.1016/j.cveq.2005.04.007

organ dysfunction, hypoperfusion, or hypotension, the event is termed severe sepsis. Septic shock is defined as sepsis-induced hypotension that persists despite adequate fluid therapy and is accompanied by hypoperfusion abnormalities or organ dysfunction. Manifestations of organ dysfunction in the horse can include laminitis and coagulopathy in addition to classic examples of renal, gastrointestinal, hepatic cardiovascular, or pulmonary dysfunction [4]. The multiple organ dysfunction syndrome (MODS) describes the alteration of organ function in an acutely ill patient such that homeostasis cannot be maintained. MODS can occur either as a primary event (ie, as a direct result of trauma) or secondary to a host response. Recently, a syndrome of immunosuppression caused by an over-pronounced systemic anti-inflammatory response resulting in increased circulating levels of anti-inflammatory mediators, leukocyte anergy, or increased susceptibility to infection has been termed the compensatory anti-inflammatory response syndrome (CARS). If an individual fluctuates between episodes of SIRS and CARS, the term mixed anti-inflammatory response syndrome (MARS) applies [5].

Endotoxin plays a critical role in the pathophysiology of septic shock in gram-negative sepsis [6,7] and is particularly important in the foal, because the most frequently isolated organisms are gram-negative bacteria [2,8]. The pathophysiology of sepsis and the systemic inflammatory response have been reviewed extensively in both humans and horses [3,9–11]. This article focuses on aspects of these processes that pertain specifically to the neonatal foal; a detailed discussion of the cellular and systemic events associated with sepsis and SIRS has been described previously [4].

Predisposing factors and routes of infection

Many events can predispose an equine neonate to infection, such as maternal illness, alterations in gestational length, partial or complete failure of passive transfer, poor sanitary conditions, improper umbilical care, and other factors. These events can be summarized as prenatal (or maternal) and postnatal factors.

Maternal factors include dystocia, premature placental separation, placentitis, and various other forms of maternal illness such as colic. Such problems have been reported in 24% of bacteremic foals in a recent study [12]. Many of these factors can be interrelated, with placentitis as a primary event and other problems such as premature placental separation occurring secondarily. In utero infection of the fetus caused by placentitis occurs typically through ascending infection and often results in premature delivery [13]. Because chronic placentitis in the mare often results in precocious fetal maturation, a premature foal born to such a mare likely has a greater chance of being septic but a higher probability of survival than a foal born at a similar gestational age to a mare without placentitis or other chronic stimulation.

Most postnatal risk factors are intertwined with possible routes of infection. The main exception to this is the failure of passive transfer (FPT) of IgG. Because the foal is relatively immuno-naïve at the time of birth, reasonably an absence of this natural provision of protection would lead to an increased risk of postnatal infection. A number of studies have documented a close relationship between the concentration of foal serum IgG and incidence of disease [14–17]. Clearly, factors other than the magnitude of passive transfer also are involved in determining disease risk. The route and timing of transfer are likely relevant, along with the potential for bacterial challenge. Farm management is particularly important, including general cleanliness, stocking density, exposure to disease, maternal nutrition, and prepartum vaccination and deworming programs. One study [18] has demonstrated that foals with partial FPT were not at any greater risk of disease than those with adequate transfer on a well-managed Standardbred farm.

Postnatal routes of infection include the umbilicus, gastrointestinal tract, and respiratory tract. Although the umbilicus has been regarded tradition-ally as the most important site for bacterial pathogen entry into the foal, the role of the intestinal tract has been recently reevaluated [19]. It was suggested that too much emphasis was placed on the magnitude of colostral transfer, rather than the timing of transfer. This concept was raised 30 years ago, when it was demonstrated that noninvasive *Escherichia coli* could be taken up by the intestine of neonatal piglets before gut closure [20]. In the pig and the lamb, the ability to absorb macromolecules is regulated by luminal content, and closure could be delayed for up to 5 days by deprivation of milk or colostrum. Conversely, other investigators [21,22] have demonstrated that the period before closure could be shortened by feeding a large volume of colostrum or milk shortly after birth.

Less work has been performed in the foal, but several key details have been established. The foal does not fully discriminate between maternal IgG and other macromolecules, and absorption of macromolecules occurs through specialized cells through pinocytosis. The absorption of macro-molecules peaks shortly after birth and declines to less than 1% by 20 hours [23]. Unlike other species, absorption of IgG does not appear to be Fc receptor-mediated in the foal. The foal will selectively absorb IgG and IgM over IgA [24]. Unlike the piglet or the lamb, intestinal permeability to IgG cannot be delayed through withholding of macromolecules in the foal [25]. It is not known whether premature closure can be induced by the feeding of macromolecules immediately after birth.

Significant postnatal factors other than FPT include gestational age and environmental conditions. Foals with exceptionally short or long lengths of gestation are at risk for the development of sepsis [26]. Unsanitary environmental conditions can result in an increased bacterial load to the neonatal gastrointestinal tract, especially during the initial periods of udder seeking.

Clinical signs and diagnosis

Physical examination findings

The initial clinical signs can be vague and vary widely but frequently include depression, decreased or absent suckling from the mare, and lethargy, which may progress to recumbence. The flat-out foal presenting with septic shock used to be a common presentation, but, as awareness and the overall level of neonatal care has increased, fewer foals present in this state. For those foals considered normal at any point before onset of illness, depression and anorexia often are the first signs noted. The examination of the foal should always include an examination of the mare's udder for fill, and depressed foals will often stand with their head underneath the mare and can have dried streaming milk on their foreheads. Thus, dehydration and hypoglycemia become more significant problems as time progresses, because of lack of intake. Tachycardia and tachypnea are common but not always present. The mucous membranes often develop a bright or injected appearance, and the capillary refill time may be rapid. Rectal temperature may be normal or mildly increased, and sepsis should not be ruled out on the basis of a normal rectal temperature. Hypothermia can be associated with advanced sepsis or moderate to severe prematurity. Left untreated, these early signs will progress to septic shock, in which there is deterioration of the cardiovascular system (cyanosis, muddy mucous membranes, tachycardia, weak pulse, and peripheral shutdown) and often death.

In addition to the systemic parameters mentioned previously, septic foals also can have additional localizing signs associated with specific foci of infection. Diarrhea is one of the most common early localizing signs in foals with sepsis and no other evidence of enteric pathogens. Occasionally, diarrhea can be the first clinical sign noted. Other localizing signs of sepsis include uveitis, seizures, joint effusion with or without lameness, lameness alone or in association with edema and pain over a physis, respiratory disease or distress, subcutaneous abscesses, patent urachus, and omphalitis. Importantly, many foals with umbilical remnant infection or abscessation often have normal external umbilical structures. Thus, ultrasonographic examination is recommended in any presumed septic foal.

Clinicopathologic findings

Clinical signs and historical information alone often are sufficient for a suspicion of sepsis. However, in addition to the physical examination findings, laboratory data may be helpful in diagnosing early sepsis. Leukopenia, characterized by neutropenia, is the most common hematologic finding associated with acute sepsis. In one study [27], septic foals less than 1 week of age had a lower total white blood count (WBC), neutrophils and lymphocytes, and higher bands and monocytes than healthy age-matched controls. Premature or dysmature foals also will commonly have neutropenia in the absence of sepsis; however, septic foals typically have a degenerative left shift and evidence of toxicity (Doehle bodies, toxic granulation, and vacuolization), whereas these findings are not typical of uncomplicated prematurity. In older septic foals (8–14 days), the total WBC, neutrophils, and bands have been shown to be higher than in age-matched controls [27]. A high fibrinogen concentration at or shortly after birth should raise the suspicion of in utero infection [28].

Abnormal serum glucose concentrations are common in septic foals. Hypoglycemia is common initially, especially in foals less than 24 hours of age [28]. Although hypoglycemia is related predominantly to decreased intake, endotoxemia can contribute to hypoglycemia by decreasing hepatic gluconeogenesis and increasing peripheral glucose uptake. In the initial phase of treatment, the rate of supplementation should be monitored carefully because many foals subsequently develop hyperglycemia in response to dextrose infusion. Other biochemical abnormalities common in septic foals include azotemia and hyperbilirubinemia [2].

Common abnormalities found on arterial blood gas analysis include acidemia and increased lactate. One early report [28] has demonstrated a high incidence of metabolic, respiratory, or mixed acidosis. A recent report [29] has indicated significant differences in arterial lactate concentration between foals with a positive versus negative blood culture, those that met the criteria for SIRS versus those that did not, and those that met the criteria for septic shock versus those that did not. These differences were noted at admission and at 18 to 36 hours after admission for the blood culture and SIRS variables, but numbers precluded an analysis for the septic shock variable. Stewart and colleagues [12] have noted that foals with gram-negative enteric bacteremia were more likely to have an elevated $Paco_2$ than other foals with bacteremia.

The coagulation and fibrinolytic systems of the septic newborn often are abnormal, with clinically relevant decreases in antithrombin III and elevations in prothrombin time (PT), activated partial thromboplastin time (APTT), and fibrinogen and fibrin degradation products [27]. A detectable plasma endotoxin concentration but not a blood culture result has been significantly correlated with abnormal PT and APTT in this study; thus endotoxemia not bacteremia is likely associated with the development of coagulopathy in septic foals [27]. Some patients may develop active hemorrhage or thrombosis, which can include thrombosis of major arteries such the aorta, iliac, femoral, or brachial arteries.

Definitive diagnosis

A blood culture is the gold standard for the diagnosis of systemic bacterial infection. The identification of a causative organism allows for directed antimicrobial therapy as well as the determination of patterns in infection. Samples for culture should be collected from a large vein (usually the jugular or cephalic but other sites such as the saphenous vein can be used as well) after surgical clip and aseptic preparation. The sample should be collected in a sterile syringe without anticoagulant and placed immediately into an appropriate medium, such as thioglycolate and tryptic soy broth (BBL SEPTI-CHEK, Becton Dickinson, Sparks, MD). A fresh needle should be used for the instillation of blood into the culture medium. A sample collection from a venous catheter is acceptable, provided the procedure is performed directly from the catheter at the time of placement without compromising sterile technique. For foals that are receiving antimicrobial therapy before sample collection, an appropriate medium, for example tryptic soy broth with resins (BBL SEPTI-CHEK), also is also available and may improve microbial recovery. Regardless of the bottle used, care should be taken to infuse the recommended volume of blood to promote optimum recovery.

Two limitations hamper the usefulness of blood cultures from a diagnostic standpoint. First, positive results are not usually available for at least 48 hours. Second, a positive blood culture, although extremely specific, does not confer optimal sensitivity. Many foals with histologic evidence of sepsis at necropsy have historical evidence of a negative blood culture. This finding can result from a number of factors, including previous antimicrobial therapy and low circulating bacterial population. In one study [30], only 40% of *E coli* infections were successfully identified by blood culture, relative to those organisms obtained from a culture at necropsy. Thus, a means of identifying at-risk foals would be a valuable tool for the attending clinician.

The first scoring systems were adopted and modified in the 1980s, with a stated aim of predicting whether a foal would be septic before the return of blood culture results [31,32]. The modified "sepsis score" currently used in many hospitals is calculated based on a number of historical and physical findings and laboratory data and has a reported sensitivity and specificity of 92.8% and 85.9%, respectively [32]. The sepsis score has not been as accurate at other institutions. Recent data have shown a false-negative rate of 48% in blood culture-positive foals in Ohio [12]. In a study at the University of Georgia [33] that examined foals with a sepsis score greater than 11, a positive blood culture, or greater than 3 foci of infection, 43 of 247 foals had a sepsis score less than 11 but at least one of the other criteria, and 46 of 250 had a sepsis score greater than 11 without either of the other criteria. In a Virginia study [32], the modified and original sepsis scores [31] each produced a positive predictive values of 84%, with negative predictive values of 55 and 53%, respectively [34]. Results from these studies stress the importance of regional and institutional variability in the accuracy of scoring systems.

The modified sepsis score was reevaluated recently at the University of Florida, the same geographic population for which it was originally generated, and obtained a similar sensitivity (89%) but lower specificity

(67.5%) using positive blood culture alone as a gold standard, rather than including evidence of specific foci of infection at necropsy as well (Sanchez and Lester, unpublished observations, 2003). Because of the heavy weighting of historical information and related problems, moderately to severely premature foals often can have a positive sepsis score without a positive blood culture. However, because many of the maternal problems resulting in prematurity also can lead to systemic sepsis, this crossover is easily predictable. The problems with the clinical application of these scoring systems are their relatively low specificity and negative predictive value. Thus, although a "positive" score is supportive of sepsis in a suspected animal, a "negative" score alone should not be used to withhold antibiotic therapy from an at-risk foal. Similarly, the use of a positive score alone, without complimentary culture results or necropsy findings, should be used cautiously to confirm a diagnosis of sepsis for retrospective studies.

Causative organisms

Retrospective studies have evaluated the most common organisms isolated from both blood culture and necropsy specimens in septic foals over the years. A summary of the reported bacterial isolates is presented in Table 1. Although gram-positive organisms predominated in the 1940s to 1950, E coli has remained the predominant organism isolated from septic foals in recent studies, regardless of clinic location or methodology [8,12,28,30,33,35]. As far as the next most prominent isolate, however, era and geographic location appear to play a major role. In Pennsylvania in the late 1990s, gram-positive bacteria (Enterococcus spp, Streptococcus spp, and Staphylococcus spp) cumulatively played a major role in disease pathogenesis [8], whereas Actinobacillus spp accounted for approximately 30% of all isolates at Ohio State University in the late 1990s [12]. A Georgia study [33] has reported a dramatic decrease in the percentage of E coli isolates between 1986 and 1990 and later 5-year sampling periods (1991–1995 and 1996–2000). The predominant organisms with increased percentages over the same period were Enterococcus spp and Staphylococcus spp. A study [36] evaluating trends by decade (1980s and 1990s) in a Florida population, found that E coli remained the predominant isolate, percentages of gram-negative nonenteric and gram-positive organisms remained steady, the percentage of anaerobes increased, and the gram-negative nonenteric organisms decreased.

Systemic fungal infections also can occur in neonatal foals. The most commonly implicated organism is Candida albicans, a dimorphic fungus, although other organisms may play a similar role [37,38]. These infections have been associated typically with prolonged hospitalization and invasive monitoring techniques [38] or immunodeficiency [37]. Prolonged antimicrobial therapy and the administration of parental nutrition have been

Table 1
Summary of reported frequency of bacterial isolates

	Study							
	Wilson and Madigan [30]	Koterba et al [28]	Raisis et al [35]	Marsh and Palmer [8]	Stewart et al [12]	Henson and Barton [33]		
Years of study	1978–1987	1982–1983	1989–1992	1991–1998	1993–2000	1986–1990	1991–1995	1996–2000
Number of animals	47	27	24	155	101		250	
Blood cultures only?[a]	No	Yes	No	Yes	Yes		No	
Admission only?[b]	No	No	No	No	Yes		No	
Isolates (%)								
E. coli	30.6	56	50	18.7	39	59	29	26
Enterobacter spp	3.5	3.7	12.5	12.3	14	18	8	9
Klebsiella spp	12.9	7.4		3.9	11	16	15	7
Proteus spp		3.7	4		1			
Salmonella spp		3.7	12.5	2.9	5	17	1	3
Actinobacillus spp	18.8	7.4	12.5	8.9	30	11	8	7
Pasteurella spp		3.7		1.5				
Pseudomonas spp	4.7	3.7		4.9	2			
Enterococcus spp				9.4	14	0	2	19
Streptococcus spp	8.3		8	9.4	10	33	15	8
Staphylococcus spp	3.5	3.7		9.8	3	7	8	15
Clostridium spp	2.4	3.7						
Acinetobacter spp				4.9				
Citrobacter spp	4.7							
All anaerobes				4.5	6			
Other gram-negative bacteria	4.7			4.5				
Other gram-positive bacteria	5.9							

Data are expressed as a percentage of the total isolates from each study.

[a] Blood cultures only: whether samples analyzed were restricted to culture of blood only or if they included culture of blood or infected tissue collected at necropsy.

[b] Admission only: whether samples analyzed were restricted to those obtained on the date of a particular foal's admission to the hospital.

suggested as risk factors for the development of candidiasis. A common clinical sign is a fever unresponsive to antimicrobial therapy. Most foals with systemic infection also will develop thrush (white plaques on the lingual surface) either concurrently or before showing clinical signs of systemic infection; thus, a daily oral examination is recommended for all hospitalized foals. Antifungal therapy should be strongly considered in any presumed septic foal that develops thrush and is clearly indicated in any animal with a confirmed isolate.

Therapy

Important topics in the treatment of neonatal sepsis are provided below. Providing nutritional support is critical to the care of affected neonates but will not be discussed here because that topic is covered elsewhere in this issue.

Antimicrobial therapy

Antibiotics provide the basis of therapy for septic foals. Initially, a broad-spectrum bactericidal approach must be used based on previous experiences and costs. Antimicrobial therapy should begin immediately in any foal in which sepsis is suspected and should not be delayed pending blood culture results, because sensitivity data typically require 3 to 4 days; therapy can be altered if necessary when these data become available. A minimum therapeutic course of 2 weeks is recommended for bacteremic foals without localizing clinical signs. If localizing signs such as pneumonia or septic arthritis are present, a minimum course of 4 weeks is preferred [26]. The recommended dosages for commonly used antimicrobials are listed in Table 2.

Few published veterinary reports discuss antimicrobial sensitivity of organisms isolated from bacteremic neonatal foals. A common theme is that a lower percentage of gram-negative isolates are sensitive to gentamicin relative to amikacin [2,8,33,36,39]. Paradis [2] has reported that 95% and 91% of gram-negative isolates were sensitive to amikacin and cefotaxime, respectively, whereas sensitivity to gentamicin and trimethoprim-sulfa was much lower. The same study found that the three antimicrobials to which staphylococcal organisms were most sensitive were cephalothin, tetracycline, and chloramphenicol, whereas streptococcal organisms were most sensitive to chloramphenicol, ampicillin, and penicillin. Wilson and colleagues [39] have reported a cumulative sensitivity of all isolates from 33 foals to be greater than 90% for imepenim, ciprofloxacin, ceftriaxone, and ceftazidime; 80% to 89% for amikacin and ceftizoxime; and only 70% to 79% for gentamicin and ceftiofur. Organisms such as *Enterobacter* spp, *Acinetobacter* spp, *Enterococcus* spp, and coagulase-positive *Staphylococcus* spp have demonstrated substantial resistance [8]. *Enterobacter* spp also

Table 2
Recommended antimicrobial dosages

Agent	Preparation	Route	Frequency (h)	Dosage (/kg)	References
Amikacin	Sulfate	IV, IM	24	21–25 mg	[75,76]
Gentamicin	Sulfate	IV, IM	24	6.6 mg	
Ampicillin	Sodium	IV, IM	6	25 mg	
Ampicillin	Trihydrate	IM	12	25 mg	
Penicillin G	Potassium	IV	6	22,000–40,000 IU	
Penicillin G	Procaine	IM	12–24	22,000 IU	
Cefotaxime			6	40 mg	[40,77]
Ceftiofur	Sodium	IV, IM	12	2.2–4.4 mg	[78]

Abbreviations: IM, intramuscular; IV, intravenous.

demonstrated increasing resistance to amikacin, gentamicin, and trimethoprim-sulfa in another study [36]. Interestingly, a recent study [33] from the University of Georgia has revealed considerable gram-positive and -negative resistance to cefotaxime but no amikacin resistance to *Enterococcus* spp. The same study revealed an efficacy of at least 70% against all organisms for chloramphenicol or ceftiofur.

Thus, based on available data, a recommended initial therapeutic approach involves combining amikacin or a third-generation cephalosporin with penicillin or ampicillin. The use of amikacin should be tempered in light of the foal's cardiovascular and renal status. If a foal is severely hypovolemic and azotemic, cephalosporin would be a safer initial choice. If amikacin is used, therapeutic drug monitoring is recommended to ensure appropriate dosing for each individual. An additional recommendation is to serially monitor creatinine levels every 2 to 3 days or perform serial urinalyses that include sediment examination to monitor for potential renal side effects. Cefotaxime is a good choice for foals with gram-negative meningitis [40] or those with unresponsive pneumonia.

Unfortunately, the range of oral antibiotics is limited in horses. Because of significant resistance, trimethoprim-sulfa combinations should not be used in septic foals without documented sensitivity and then only as a long-term option after initial parenteral therapy. Several aminobenzyl penicillins (amoxicillin and ampicillin) and first-generation cephalosporins (cefadroxyl and cephradine) have good bioavailability in young foals (in contrast to older foals and adult horses) but have a limited gram-positive spectrum of activity [41–44]. Cefpodoxime proxetil, a third-generation cephalosporin available for oral administration, was recently shown to be effective against 90% of *Klebsiella* spp, *Pasteurella* spp, and β-hemolytic streptococci [45]. An increase in the frequency of administration would likely increase the effectiveness of this drug against *E coli*. Fluoroquinolones, such as enrofloxacin, have an excellent spectrum of activity against gram-negative and some gram-positive organisms but have been associated with arthropathy in foals [46,47]. Thus, the use of this agent should be reserved for those cases with documented resistance to other antimicrobial agents and informed owner consent.

Antiendotoxin therapy

Not surprisingly, many septic foals have detectable plasma endotoxin concentrations [27]. Recent in vitro work also has shown that β-lactam antimicrobials appear more likely than aminoglycosides (alone or in combination with ampicillin) to induce endotoxemia and tumor necrosis factor-α activity during the treatment of *E coli* sepsis [7]. Agents commonly used for the treatment of endotoxemia include flunixin meglumine, pentoxifylline, and polymyxin B sulfate [48,49]. None of these agents has been scientifically evaluated for the treatment of endotoxemia in foals; thus recommendations are extrapolated from work in vitro and in adult horses. Flunixin and polymyxin B are potentially nephrotoxic and thus should be used with caution. Flunixin also has the potential for gastric ulceration. Pentoxifylline also has been shown to reduce mortality without adverse effects in septic neonates [50] but not adults [51].

Antifungal therapy

Attempted medical treatment options for systemic candidiasis include fluconazole, itraconazole, miconazole, and amphotericin B [38,52]. Fungal sensitivity profiles may help direct therapy if they are available. The pharmacokinetic actions of these drugs have not been established in foals. Amphotericin B has been administered intravenously (IV) at a range of 0.1 to 0.5 mg/kg once a day, starting therapy at the lower dose and increasing by 0.1-mg/kg increments per day [38]. Because this drug can cause potentially life-threatening nephrotoxicity, serum creatinine levels, urine production, and urinalysis should be monitored closely. Fluconazole has previously been administered orally at 4 to 10 mg/kg SID. This agent is less expensive, easier to administer, and has fewer side effects. Miconazole also has been used at a dosage of 1 mg/kg IV Q8 hr [38]. Voriconazole also has been used anecdotally.

Cardiovascular support

Fluid therapy is critical in foals with hypovolemia, acid–base disorders, septic shock, or hypotension. In-depth discussions of fluid therapy [53] and the use of inotropes and vasopressors [54] in the neonatal foal have been presented recently. These are two of the most important concepts in the initial treatment of sepsis, and the reader is directed to the above-mentioned references for additional information. When a foal presents in septic shock, fluid resuscitation is critical. Initial choices commonly include a combination of crystalloid (such as lactated Ringer's solution) and colloid (such as hydroxyethyl starch) preparations. Arterial or venous lactate concentration, systemic blood pressure, cardiac output, and central venous pressure can provide additional information regarding volume status and estimation of tissue perfusion [55]. Once normovolemia has been restored, neonates typically require approximately 100 mL/kg/day (5 L/d for a 50-kg foal) to maintain adequate hydration. Clinicopathologic variables to continuously monitor in septic foals include arterial or venous blood gas (depending on pulmonary status), electrolytes (especially sodium and potassium), and glucose. Physical parameters of importance include careful examination for the development of edema (conjunctiva, distal limbs, and other signs), urine output, vital signs, and temperature of the distal limbs. Derangements in any of the monitored parameters should be addressed as they arise to maintain optimal tissue perfusion.

Antiacid therapy

Although they are uncommon, sick foals can develop gastric ulcers, especially in the glandular region of the stomach. The use of prophylactic antiacid therapy is controversial and depends on the preference of the clinician. The gastric pH level in critically ill foals can differ greatly from that seen in healthy foals. Severely ill, predominantly recumbent patients frequently have predominantly alkaline pH patterns [56]. In addition, sick foals capable of acid production respond more variably to IV ranitidine administration than the normal cohorts. Thus, glandular ulcer disease in sick neonates is likely not strictly an acid-related problem, and factors such as alterations in mucosal blood flow may contribute. In addition, gastric alkalinization can contribute to bacterial translocation [57]. Primary options for acid suppression in the neonatal foal include omeprazole and ranitidine [56,58,59]. Sucralfate remains a possible alternative for ulcer prophylaxis, especially in foals receiving nonsteroidal anti-inflammatory drugs. For a more complete discussion of this topic, the reader is directed to the article on nondiarrheal gastrointestinal disorders elsewhere in this issue.

Experimental therapy

Although experimental agents have shown promise, few have resulted in reduced mortality in large-scale human clinical trials. Recombinant activated protein C has shown a consistent decrease in mortality, especially in the most severely affected patients [60]. This agent, however, has been associated with significant side effects and is currently not a viable option in foals. Although high-dose corticosteroid administration has demonstrated increased mortality, hydrocortisone administered at physiologic doses has been shown to decrease mortality attributable to septic shock in human patients [61].

Focal infection and potential sequelae

Signs consistent with a secondary focus of infection, such as pneumonia, septic arthritis, osteomyelitis, omphalitis, and meningitis, also may occur. In-depth discussions of the various complications are provided elsewhere.

Respiratory involvement

The lungs are a very common location of focal infection in the septic foal, with a reported incidence of pneumonia ranging from 28% [12] to 50% [62]. Respiratory rate and effort, thoracic auscultation, and rectal temperature often can alert the clinician to the possibility of pneumonia in a given animal. Respiratory function is best assessed in septic foals through arterial blood gas analysis [2,55]. Thoracic radiographs can provide an estimation of disease severity and distribution. In addition to hematogenously acquired pneumonia, septic foals can be at risk for aspiration of either meconium or milk, depending on their presentation. Directed antimicrobial therapy and the maintenance of an acceptable arterial oxygen tension with intranasal oxygen insufflation are the most commonly administered forms of therapy. In those foals with severe hypercapnia in addition to hypoxemia, mechanical ventilation may be necessary.

Gastrointestinal involvement

Diarrhea or enteritis also is very common in septic foals, with reported incidence of between 16% and 38% [12,26,62,63]. In the Ohio State University study [12], foals with *Actinobacillus* sp-induced bacteremia were six times more likely to have diarrhea than those with other isolates. With or without enteritis, septic foals also can display signs of ileus or colic. Most of these problems resolve with symptomatic treatment and systemic improvement. One must carefully monitor fluid, electrolyte, and acid–base status in foals with diarrhea and account for ongoing losses. Options for analgesic therapy in colicky foals are somewhat limited, and flunixin meglumine should be used cautiously because of the potential for gastric ulceration. Opiates such as butorphanol provide a reasonable short-term option in such cases.

Umbilical involvement

Omphalitis refers to infection of umbilical structures. Umbilical remnant infections are considered to be a common source of continued bacterial shedding and have been reported to occur in 13% of septic foals [63]. Ultrasonographic evaluation of these structures is critical because external signs (pain, heat, and swelling) are frequently absent. Treatment options include long-term antibiotic therapy or surgical resection. Many septic foals will develop a patent urachus without involvement of other structures. The reported incidence in septic foals is 21% [63]. This problem will often resolve with continued antibiotic therapy, with or without topical therapy.

In one study [64], uroperitoneum was diagnosed in 2.5% of hospitalized neonates, and foals with uroperitoneum were less likely to survive if they had a positive versus negative sepsis score. An interesting note from that study was that, presumably, septic foals receiving fluid therapy were typically older and less likely to have the classic electrolyte abnormalities associated with uroperitoneum. This suggests that the septic foals were diagnosed earlier, but the condition occurred later in life. Thus ischemia and subsequent necrosis of the bladder or urachus may account for uroperitoneum in the septic population. Because of these risks, routine ultrasonographic assessment of the umbilical structures is recommended in all hospitalized neonates in whom sepsis is either confirmed or suspected. The frequency of repeat ultrasound exams is dependent upon the individual foal's clinical progression.

Septic arthritis and osteomyelitis

Orthopedic infections are common in septic foals and represent one of the most important life-threatening and performance-limiting complications. The reported incidence of septic arthritis ranges from 26% to 33% [12,63,65] and that of osteomyelitis ranges from 11% to 12% [63,65]. Clinical signs include lameness and joint effusion, thus daily palpation of every joint in all hospitalized neonates is imperative. Any sign of lameness or joint effusion in a neonate should be considered septic until proven otherwise.

Bone infections normally occur at the epiphysis of long bones, the metaphyseal side of growth plates, costochondral junctions, and the articular facets of vertebral bodies. At the University of Florida, osteomyelitis or infectious synovitis occurred in 80% of foals, from which *Salmonella* spp were isolated from blood cultures (Sanchez and Lester, unpublished observations, 2003). This was, by far, the most striking association between a particular isolate and a focus of infection. A detailed discussion of the diagnosis, treatment, and prognosis associated with orthopedic infections is provided elsewhere in this issue.

Meningitis

Meningitis is a rare but extremely serious complication. Major clinical signs include seizures and severe depression, although this condition is somewhat difficult to assess in a severely compromised foal. Other signs include head tilt, strabismus, nystagmus, and extensor rigidity, depending on the areas of involvement. Analysis of cerebrospinal fluid normally provides a definitive diagnosis, with a pleocytosis (normally neutrophilic) being the typical abnormality. Prognosis is poor to grave, but if therapy is attempted, third-generation cephalosporins (such as cefotaxime) have been recommended [40]. The major differential diagnosis for neurologic signs in a septic neonate is hypoxic-ischemic encephalomyelopathy (HIE). Typically, foals with HIE present within 24 to 48 hours after birth, whereas the age of foals with meningitis is more variable. A recent report [12] has noted that foals with gram-negative bacteremia were less likely to have seizures than those with other isolates.

Ocular involvement

The most common ocular complication in the septic foal is corneal ulceration. Ulceration can occur because of entropion in a dehydrated foal or, more commonly, because of trauma. Because foals do not always show clinical signs of corneal ulceration, a daily ophthalmic examination, including fluorescein staining, should be performed in all hospitalized foals. Another ophthalmic complication is uveitis. When uveitis occurs, it is typically an ocular extension of the systemic disease process.

Coagulopathy

Disorders of coagulation can occur in septic foals, manifested clinically by either hemorrhage or thrombosis. The most common abnormality probably is jugular venous thrombosis at the site of an indwelling venous catheter. Other areas of thrombosis include the brachial artery, digital artery, metatarsal and metacarpal arteries, diffuse vascular thromboses throughout the distal limb, the aortic termination, the lungs, and the colon [27,66–69].

Prognosis and outcomes

Survival rates have increased from the rate of 25% reported in the early 1980s [28]. More recent retrospective studies have reported short-term survival rates ranging from 45% to 55% [12,33,63,70]. Other investigators have reported survival rates as low as 32% [27] and as high as 70% to 72% [35,62,71]. Approximately 50% to 60% of all bacteremic foals admitted to the University of Florida neonatal unit survive to discharge (Sanchez and Lester, unpublished observations, 2003).

Several factors have been associated with survival in retrospective studies. Barton and coworkers [27] have found that foals infected with gram-negative organisms are more likely to die than those with gram-positive infections. In a Texas study [63], the duration of illness before admission was inversely related to survival, whereas the ability of a foal to stand on admission was positively correlated with survival. A recent study [33] of septic foals at the University of Georgia found that foals were more likely to survive if they had a sepsis score less than 11, a negative blood culture at admission, a serum glucose level of greater than 60 mg/dL, a body temperature greater than 100°F, a total CO_2 greater than 15 mmol/L, or a low or normal level of fibrinogen. In the Florida study [12], the prognosis worsened if multiple organisms were isolated from the blood or if multiple foci of infection were involved (Sanchez and Lester, unpublished observations, 2003). In the Ohio State study, foals with multiple blood isolates had longer periods of hospitalization, but not decreased survival. Corley and coworkers [29] have found that a normal arterial lactate concentration either at admission or 18 to 36 hours after admission was a good predictor of survival, whereas elevated lactate was not a good predictor of nonsurvival.

Few studies have addressed the long-term survival and performance of neonatal (N)ICU survivors, much less those specifically of septic foals. In a summary of septic thoroughbred foals admitted to the University of Florida, approximately 75% of short-term survivors are registered, and approximately 50% start at least one race (Sanchez and Lester, unpublished observations, 2003). This observation is similar to that reported for overall NICU survivors, in which the percentage of starters was lower than the control population, but performance over a 2-year period was not different in those animals able to make at least two starts [71]. Similar findings have been reported for foals with neurologic disease and those with pneumonia caused by *Rhodococcus equi* [72,73].

Preventive strategies

Clearly, given the wide range of potentially devastating problems associated with sepsis, prevention will always outweigh treatment, but no single program will eliminate totally the risk of sepsis. Not surprisingly, methods of prevention coincide with the documented risk factors and routes of infection discussed previously. The following suggestions comprise a basic guide one can offer to clients. Although many of the options presented make sense, none of them has been proven to reduce the incidence of sepsis. Thus, the decision to implement some or all of these practices will depend on the individual farm scenario.

Maintain a clean environment

Although this is one of the most basic concepts in all of medicine, its importance cannot be overemphasized. With specific reference to the foaling situation, foaling stalls should be thoroughly cleaned and disinfected between mares. For each inhabitant, the stall should be cleaned at least daily, if not twice daily, and plentiful clean, dry, fresh bedding should be provided for the mare and foal.

Reduce the potential bacterial load introduced during udder seeking

As Madigan [19] suggests, ideally, the mare's hindquarters, perineum, and udder should be thoroughly cleaned with soap and water after foaling but before the foal's introduction. The key feature to this step, which often is overlooked, is that the mare also must be dried. Drying should be performed just outside the stall, rather than in the stall, to prevent contamination of the foal's new environment, which is the point of the exercise. This step requires a great deal of commitment on the part of the farm because it is labor intensive.

Ensure rapid gastrointestinal intake

The volume, quality, and timing of colostrum administration are all likely important factors, rather than just the quality. The ideal scenario involves feeding 6 to 8 ounces of good quality colostrum as soon as the foal develops a good, strong suckle reflex. One of the main concerns with this recommendation is the risk of milk aspiration when untrained individuals are trying to bottle feed newborn, potentially weak foals. Thus, colostrums should be administered through nasogastric intubation in those foals with a suboptimal or absent suckle reflex.

Ensure adequate passive transfer of IgG

Traditionally, passive transfer of maternal IgG to the foal has been considered to be the most important factor in disease prevention. Although other factors clearly play a role, adequate IgG transfer should still be assessed and treated, if necessary. A complete discussion of treatment of FPT is included in the article on immunity in this issue.

Ensure appropriate umbilical care

This recommendation is followed by most horse owners, from the backyard stable client to the large breeding operation. No published studies in foals have critically evaluated the different preparations used for routine umbilical care. In human neonates, surprisingly few randomized, double-blinded clinical trials have broached this issue. In a recent review of published studies [74], 4% chlorhexidine was a popular choice and was shown to consistently reduce the risk of umbilical and periumbilical infections. This concentration of chlorhexidine also is used commonly for foals and thus appears to be a better alternative to the povidone-iodine solutions that were used previously.

Summary

Neonatal infection remains a leading cause of morbidity and mortality in the equine industry, despite advances in prevention and treatment. Many factors can influence a foal's risk for the development of sepsis in the peripartum period. This article discusses those factors as well as causative organisms and therapeutic options. In addition, factors influencing prognosis as well as potential preventative strategies are addressed.

References

[1] Carter GK, Martens RJ. Septicemia in the neonatal foal. Compendium on Continuing Education for the Practicing Veterinarian 1986;8:S256–70.
[2] Paradis MR. Update on neonatal septicemia. Vet Clin North Am Equine Pract 1994;10: 109–35.
[3] Bone RC, Balk RA, Cerra FB, et al for the American College of Chest Physicians/Society of Critical Care Medicine. Definitions for sepsis and organ failure and guidelines for the use of innovative therapies in sepsis: the ACCP/SCCM Consensus Conference Committee. Chest 1992;101:1644–55.
[4] Roy MF. Sepsis in adults and foals. Vet Clin North Am Equine Pract 2004;20:41–61.
[5] Bone RC. Sir Isaac Newton, sepsis, SIRS, and CARS. Crit Care Med 1996;24:1125–8.
[6] Moore JN, Morris DD. Endotoxemia and septicemia in horses: experimental and clinical correlates. J Am Vet Med Assoc 1992;200:1903–14.
[7] Bentley AP, Barton MH, Lee MD, et al. Antimicrobial-induced endotoxin and cytokine activity in an in vitro model of septicemia in foals. Am J Vet Res 2002;63:660–8.
[8] Marsh PS, Palmer JE. Bacterial isolates from blood and their susceptibility patterns in critically ill foals: 543 cases (1991–1998). J Am Vet Med Assoc 2001;218:1608–10.
[9] Bone RC, Grodzin CJ, Balk RA. Sepsis: a new hypothesis for pathogenesis of the disease process. Chest 1997;112:235–43.
[10] McKenzie HC, Furr MO. Equine neonatal sepsis: the pathophysiology of severe inflammation and infection. Compendium on Continuing Education for the Practicing Veterinarian 2001;23:661–70.
[11] MacKay RJ. Inflammation in horses. Vet Clin North Am Equine Pract 2000;16:15–27.
[12] Stewart AJ, Hinchcliff KW, Saville WJA, et al. Actinobacillus sp bacteremia in foals: clinical signs and prognosis. J Vet Intern Med 2002;16:464–71.
[13] LeBlanc MM, Macpherson M, Sheerin P. Ascending placentitis: what we know about pathophysiology, diagnosis, and treatment. In: Proceedings of the 50th Annual Convention of the American Association of Equine Practitioners, Denver, CO. 2004; p. 127–43.
[14] Raidal SL. The incidence and consequences of failure of passive transfer of immunity on a thoroughbred breeding farm. Aust Vet J 1996;73:201–6.
[15] Tyler-McGowan CM, Hodgson JL, Hodgson DR. Failure of passive transfer in foals: incidence and outcome on four studs in New South Wales. Aust Vet J 1997;75:56–9.
[16] Robinson JA, Allen GK, Green EM, et al. A prospective study of septicaemia in colostrum-deprived foals. Equine Vet J 1993;25:214–9.
[17] Clabough DL, Levine JF, Grant GL, et al. Factors associated with failure of passive transfer of colostral antibodies in Standard bred foals. J Vet Intern Med 1991;5:335–40.
[18] Baldwin JL, Cooper WL, Vanderwall DK, et al. Prevalence (treatment days) and severity of illness in hypogammaglobulinemic and normogammaglobulinemic foals. J Am Vet Med Assoc 1991;198:423–8.
[19] Madigan JE. Method for preventing neonatal septicemia, the leading cause of death in the neonatal foal. In: Proceedings of the 43th Annual Convention of the American Association of Equine Practitioners, Denver, CO. 1997; p. 17–9.
[20] Staley TE, Jones EW, Corley LD. Attachment and penetration of Escherichia coli into intestinal epithelium of the ileum in newborn pigs. Am J Pathol 1969;56:371–92.
[21] Vellenga L, Mouwen JM, van Dijk JE, et al. Biological and pathological aspects of the mammalian small intestinal permeability to macromolecules. Vet Q 1985;7:322–32.
[22] Rundell JO, Lecce JG. Independence of intestinal epithelial cell turnover from cessation of absorption of macromolecules (closure) in the neonatal mouse, rabbit, hamster and guinea pig. Biol Neonate 1972;20:51–7.

[23] Jeffcott LB. Studies on passive immunity in the foal. II. the absorption of 125I-labeled PVP (polyvinyl pyrrolidone) by the neonatal intestine. J Comp Pathol 1974;84:279–89.
[24] Jeffcott LB. Passive immunity and its transfer with special reference to the horse. Biol Rev Camb Philos Soc 1972;47:439–64.
[25] Raidal SL, McTaggart C, Yovich JV, et al. Effect of withholding macromolecules on the duration of intestinal permeability to colostral IgG in foals. In: Proceedings of the 46th Annual Convention of the American Association of Equine Practitioners, Denver, CO. 2000; p. 260–3.
[26] Brewer BD. Neonatal infection. In: Koterba AM, Drummond WH, Kosch PC, editors. Equine Clinical Neoatology, 1st edition. Philadelphia: Lea & Febiger; 1990. p. 295–316.
[27] Barton MH, Morris DD, Norton N, et al. Hemostatic and fibrinolytic indices in neonatal foals with presumed septicemia. J Vet Intern Med 1998;12:26–35.
[28] Koterba AM, Brewer BD, Tarplee FA. Clinical and clinicopathological characteristics of the septicaemic neonatal foal: review of 38 cases. Equine Vet J 1984;16:376–82.
[29] Corley KT, Donaldson LL, Furr MO. Arterial lactate concentration, hospital survival, sepsis and SIRS in critically ill neonatal foals. Equine Vet J 2005;37:53–9.
[30] Wilson WD, Madigan JE. Comparison of bacteriologic culture of blood and necropsy specimens for determining the cause of foal septicemia: 47 cases (1978–1987). J Am Vet Med Assoc 1989;195:1759–63.
[31] Brewer BD, Koterba AM. Development of a scoring system for the early diagnosis of equine neonatal sepsis. Equine Vet J 1988;20:18–22.
[32] Brewer BD, Koterba AM, Carter RL, et al. Comparison of empirically developed sepsis score with a computer generated and weighted scoring system for the identification of sepsis in the equine neonate. Equine Vet J 1988;20:23–4.
[33] Henson S, Barton MH. Bacterial isolates and antibiotic sensitivity patterns from septicemic neonatal foals: a 15 year retrospective study (1986–2000). In: Proceedings of the Dorothy Havemeyer Foundation Neonatal Septicemia Workshop 3, Talliores, France. 2001. p. 350–52.
[34] Corley KTT, Furr MO. Evaluation of a score designed to predict sepsis in foals. Journal of Veterinary Emergency and Critical Care 2003;13:149–55.
[35] Raisis AL, Hodgson JL, Hodgson DR. Equine neonatal septicaemia: 24 cases. Aust Vet J 1996;73:137–40.
[36] Sanchez LC, Lester GD. Equine neonatal sepsis: microbial isolates, antimicrobial resistance, and short and long term outcomes. In: Proceedings of the 18th Annual American College of Veterinary Internal Medicine Forum, Seattle, WA. 2000. p. 223–4.
[37] McClure JJ, Addison JD, Miller RI. Immunodeficiency manifested by oral candidiasis and bacterial septicemia in foals. J Am Vet Med Assoc 1985;186:1195–7.
[38] Reilly LK, Palmer JE. Systemic candidiasis in four foals. J Am Vet Med Assoc 1994;205: 464–6.
[39] Wilson WD, Durando MM, Mihalyi JE. The bacteriology of septicaemia as a basis for antibiotic selection in neonatal foals. In: Proceedings of the 2nd International Society of Veterinary Perinatology Conference, Cambridge, England. 1990.
[40] Morris DD, Rutkowski J, Lloyd KC. Therapy in two cases of neonatal foal septicaemia and meningitis with cefotaxime sodium. Equine Vet J 1987;19:151–4.
[41] Henry MM, Morris DD, Lakritz J, et al. Pharmacokinetics of cephradine in neonatal foals after single oral dosing. Equine Vet J 1992;24:242–3.
[42] Duffee NE, Stang BE, Schaeffer DJ. The pharmacokinetics of cefadroxil over a range of oral doses and animal ages in the foal. J Vet Pharmacol Ther 1997;20:427–33.
[43] Duffee NE, Christensen JM, Craig AM. The pharmacokinetics of cefadroxil in the foal. J Vet Pharmacol Ther 1989;12:322–6.
[44] Brown MP, Gronwall R, Kroll WR, et al. Ampicillin trihydrate in foals: serum concentrations and clearance after a single oral dose. Equine Vet J 1984;16:371–3.

[45] Carrillo NA, Giguere S, Gronwall RR, et al. Disposition of orally administered cefpodoxime proxetil in foals and adult horses and minimum inhibitory concentration of the drug against common bacterial pathogens of horses. Am J Vet Res 2005;66:30–5.

[46] Davenport CL, Boston RC, Richardson DW. Effects of enrofloxacin and magnesium deficiency on matrix metabolism in equine articular cartilage. Am J Vet Res 2001;62:160–6.

[47] Vivrette SL, Bostian A, Bermingham E, et al. Quinolone-induced arthropathy in neonatal foals. In: Proceedings of the 47th Annual Convention of the American Association of Equine Practitioners, Denver, CO. 2001. p. 376–7.

[48] Baskett A, Barton MH, Norton N, et al. Effect of pentoxifylline, flunixin meglumine, and their combination on a model of endotoxemia in horses. Am J Vet Res 1997;58: 1291–9.

[49] Durando MM, MacKay RJ, Linda S, et al. Effects of polymyxin B and Salmonella typhimurium antiserum on horses given endotoxin intravenously. Am J Vet Res 1994;55: 921–7.

[50] Haque K, Mohan P. Pentoxifylline for neonatal sepsis. Cochrane Database Syst Rev 2003;4: CD004205.

[51] Staubach KH, Schroder J, Stuber F, et al. Effect of pentoxifylline in severe sepsis: results of a randomized, double-blind, placebo-controlled study. Arch Surg 1998;133:94–100.

[52] Hendrix DVH, Ward DA, Guglick MA. Disseminated candidiasis in a neonatal foal with keratomycosis as the initial sign. Vet Ophthalmol 1997;7:10–3.

[53] Palmer JE. Fluid therapy in the neonate: not your mother's fluid space. Vet Clin North Am Equine Pract 2004;20:63–75.

[54] Corley KT. Inotropes and vasopressors in adults and foals. Vet Clin North Am Equine Pract 2004;20:77–106.

[55] Magdesian KG. Monitoring the critically ill equine patient. Vet Clin North Am Equine Pract 2004;20:11–39.

[56] Sanchez LC, Lester GD, Merritt AM. Intragastric pH in critically ill neonatal foals and the effect of ranitidine. J Am Vet Med Assoc 2001;218:907–11.

[57] Dinsmore JE, Jackson RJ, Smith SD. The protective role of gastric acidity in neonatal bacterial translocation. J Pediatr Surg 1997;32:1014–6.

[58] Sanchez LC, Lester GD, Merritt AM. Effect of ranitidine on intragastric pH in clinically normal neonatal foals. J Am Vet Med Assoc 1998;212:1407–12.

[59] Sanchez LC, Murray MJ, Merritt AM. Effect of omeprazole paste on intragastric pH in clinically normal neonatal foals. Am J Vet Res 2004;65:1039–41.

[60] Rice TW, Bernard GR. Therapeutic intervention and targets for sepsis. Annu Rev Med 2005; 56:225–48.

[61] Minneci PC, Deans KJ, Banks SM, et al. Meta-analysis: the effect of steroids on survival and shock during sepsis depends on the dose. Ann Intern Med 2004;141:47–56.

[62] Freeman L, Paradis MR. Evaluating the effectiveness of equine neonatal care. Veterinary Medicine 1992;87:921–6.

[63] Gayle JM, Cohen ND, Chaffin MK. Factors associated with survival in septicemic foals: 65 cases (1988–1995). J Vet Intern Med 1998;12:140–6.

[64] Kablack KA, Embertson RM, Bernard WV, et al. Uroperitoneum in the hospitalised equine neonate: retrospective study of 31 cases, 1988–1997. Equine Vet J 2000;32:505–8.

[65] Paradis MR. Septic arthritis in the equine neonate: a retrospective study. In: Proceedings of the 9th Annual American College of Veterinary Internal Medicine Forum, New Orleans, LA. 1991. p. 458–9.

[66] Triplett EA, O'Brien RT, Wilson DG, et al. Thrombosis of the brachial artery in a foal. J Vet Intern Med 1996;10:330–2.

[67] Forrest LJ, Cooley AJ, Darien BJ. Digital arterial thrombosis in a septicemic foal. J Vet Intern Med 1999;13:382–5.

[68] Brianceau P, Divers TJ. Acute thrombosis of limb arteries in horses with sepsis: five cases (1988–1998). Equine Vet J 2001;33:105–9.

[69] Moore LA, Johnson PJ, Bailey KL. Aorto-iliac thrombosis in a foal. Vet Rec 1998;142: 459–62.

[70] Brewer BD, Koterba AM. Bacterial isolates and susceptibility patterns in foals in a neonatal intensive-care unit. Compendium on Continuing Education for the Practicing Veterinarian 1990;12:1773–81.

[71] Axon J, Palmer J, Wilkins P. Short- and long-term athletic outcome of neonatal intensive care unit survivors. In: Proceedings of the 45th Annual Convention of the American Association of Equine Practitioners, Denver, CO. 1999. p. 224–5.

[72] Bryant JE, Bernard W, Wilson WD, et al. Race earnings as an indicator of future performance in neonatal foals treated for neurological disorders. In: Proceedings of the 40th Annual Convention of the American Association of Equine Practitioners, Denver, CO. 1994. p. 198.

[73] Ainsworth DM, Eicker SW, Yeagar AE, et al. Associations between physical examination, laboratory, and radiographic findings and outcome and subsequent racing performance of foals with *Rhodococcus equi* infection: 115 cases (1984–1992). J Am Vet Med Assoc 1998;213: 510–5.

[74] Mullany LC, Darmstadt GL, Tielsch JM. Role of antimicrobial applications to the umbilical cord in neonates to prevent bacterial colonization and infection: a review of the evidence. Pediatr Infect Dis J 2003;22:996–1002.

[75] Bucki EP, Giguere S, Macpherson M, et al. Pharmacokinetics of once-daily amikacin in healthy foals and therapeutic drug monitoring in hospitalized equine neonates. J Vet Intern Med 2004;18:728–33.

[76] Magdesian KG, Wilson WD, Mihalyi J. Pharmacokinetics of a high dose of amikacin administered at extended intervals to neonatal foals. Am J Vet Res 2004;65:473–9.

[77] Gardner SY, Sweeney RW, Divers TJ. Pharmacokinetics of cefotaxime in neonatal pony foals. Am J Vet Res 1993;54:576–9.

[78] Meyer JC, Brown MP, Gronwall RR, et al. Pharmacokinetics of ceftiofur sodium in neonatal foals after intramuscular injection. Equine Vet J 1992;24:485–6.

VETERINARY
CLINICS
Equine Practice

Vet Clin Equine 21 (2005) 295–312

ELSEVIER
SAUNDERS

Neonatal Foal Diarrhea

K. Gary Magdesian, DVM

Department of Medicine and Epidemiology, University of California
School of Veterinary Medicine, 1 Garrod Drive, Davis, CA 95616, USA

Diarrhea is a significant cause of morbidity and mortality in the neonatal foal [1]. Altered fecal consistency in the foal may be a manifestation of simple diarrhea or enteritis, in which the latter is associated with a systemic inflammatory response syndrome. Foals with enteritis or enterocolitis develop varying degrees of endotoxemia and suffer a number of metabolic complications, including acidosis, hypovolemic shock, hypotension, and bacteremia. Numerous noninfectious and infectious agents are responsible for enterocolitis and enteritis in the newborn foal. This article provides an overview of the differential diagnoses for neonatal diarrhea and general and specific guidelines for therapy.

Noninfectious diarrhea

Foal heat diarrhea

Mild diarrhea is common in foals aged 5 to 15 days and is termed "foal heat" diarrhea. This form of diarrhea occurs without signs of systemic disease or inflammation and is usually not severe. Foals remain bright and alert, maintain normal hematology and laboratory results, and continue to nurse. The term foal heat is a misnomer. Because of a temporal association, this early onset diarrhea was initially believed to be caused by alterations in the composition of milk during the mare's first estrous period after parturition, hence the term foal heat. However, orphan foals raised on milk replacement formulas also develop diarrhea during this period. An analysis of mares' milk composition during the postpartum period and first estrous cycle has demonstrated that milk is not a factor in foal heat diarrhea [2]. Results of one study [3] have suggested that the developmental or maturational changes of the gastrointestinal (GI) tract that are associated with the initiation of feed ingestion and inoculation of microflora are responsible for the changes in fecal composition during this period. Fecal

E-mail address: kgmagdesian@ucdavis.edu

composition during foal heat diarrhea is suggestive of a secretory-type diarrhea, with higher electrolyte concentrations than is normal [3]. In addition, the fecal pH level was found to be alkaline, and fecal osmolality and volatile fatty acid concentrations decreased with the onset of diarrhea. The authors concluded that their data suggests a hypersecretion in the small intestinal mucosa, which was not compensated for by the immature colon [3]. These findings, along with a temporal association with coprophagy, suggest that the diarrhea occurs in response to the establishment of normal GI flora. Such foals do not require therapy, although they should be monitored closely because early forms of enteritis can mimic foal heat diarrhea. Any signs of systemic disease, including depression or reduced appetite should warrant close investigation of such a neonate.

Asphyxia-associated gastroenteropathies

One of the most common causes of diarrhea is asphyxial gut injury secondary to hypoxic or ischemic insult that is believed to occur as part of a peripartum asphyxia syndrome, also referred to as hypoxic-ischemic encephalopathy. At-risk foals include those born as a result of dystocia or cesarean section, those with umbilical cord problems during delivery, and those with abnormal oxygenation in the immediate postpartum period. Gastroenteropathies may result from hypoperfusion, hypoxic-ischemic and reperfusion injury, and inflammatory mediators. The resulting clinical effects of ischemic enterocolitis include gastroduodenal reflux, ileus, intolerance to enteral feeding, colic, abdominal distention, and diarrhea. Because the organ injury is not limited to the gut, these foals require intensive care. Concurrent organ dysfunction includes neurologic dysfunction, nephropathies, and cardiac or endocrine disorders. As far as the gastrointestinal tract is concerned, foals with asphyxia-associated diarrhea should be checked for nasogastric reflux, may require prokinetic drugs, and should be fed very conservatively through the enteral route. Severely affected foals benefit from parenteral nutrition, with only small volumes of enteral milk to provide local nutrients to enterocytes. Because affected foals are at high risk of developing sepsis, they should be treated with broad-spectrum systemic antimicrobials. Ultrasonography is a useful means of monitoring the progress of GI dysfunction in these foals.

Necrotizing enterocolitis

Necrotizing enterocolitis (NEC) is the most serious gastrointestinal emergency of human infants under intensive care [4]. NEC consists of necrotic injury to the mucosal and submucosal layers of the GI tract. Although the entire GI tract, from the stomach to the rectum, is susceptible, the distal small intestine and proximal colon are most frequently involved. Symptoms of NEC in human neonates include abdominal distention, ileus, hematochezia, and emesis, along with signs of sepsis. Suspected cases often present with nonspecific signs, including food intolerance, gastric residuals, GI bleeding, and sepsis. Foals may develop a similar syndrome. Despite decades of research and clinical investigation, a complete understanding of the pathogenesis of NEC remains unclear. The syndrome involves a complex interaction of immaturity, previous gastrointestinal mucosal injury, enteral milk feeding, and bacterial invasion [4]. The majority (70%–90%) of infants with NEC are born preterm, highlighting the importance of GI maturation to the syndrome [4]. The incidence of NEC varies inversely with gestational age and birth weight. Premature infants may experience vasoconstriction, hypotension, and thrombosis leading to decreased GI perfusion [4]. Additional contributors to reduced mucosal perfusion in preterm infants include umbilical artery catheters and patent ductus arteriosus, with the use of indomethacin possibly contributing to NEC risk [4]. There are some notable differences in NEC that affect preterm and term neonates. NEC in very low-birth weight infants occurs later than in older and larger infants. The onset of NEC is often insidious in preterm infants, with sudden signs occurring more often in older neonates. Risk factors differ as well; those for full-term infants include congenital heart disease, polycythemia, coexisting conditions such as hypothyroidism, Down syndrome or gastroschisis, aggressive enteral feedings, and conditions compromising GI oxygenation such as supraventricular tachycardia.

Mucosal injury is the second factor in the development of NEC. Mucosal compromise is associated with impaired circulation dynamics, for example, hypoxic-ischemic insults. Other forms of injury are inflammatory, with release of interleukins (IL) such as IL-6. Histologic findings include ulceration, edema, hemorrhage, congestion, and in severe cases, transmural coagulation necrosis with perforation. The initial mucosal injury produced by ischemia in an immature infant was believed to predispose the infant to bacterial invasion. Milk was thought to serve as a substrate for bacterial proliferation and subsequent infection, the final factors known to contribute to development of NEC. Abnormal intestinal gas produced by the bacteria then appears as pneumatosis intestinalis or portal venous gas on abdominal radiography or ultrasonography. These risk factors have been questioned recently because of cases of NEC in full term infants and those that were never fed enterally. However, prematurity remains the primary risk factor, because most cases are seen among immature infants.

Necrotizing enterocolitis has been reported in equine neonates [5]. This report describes two foals with a gastrointestinal syndrome characterized by ileus, gastric reflux, intolerance to enteral feeding, and pneumatosis intestinalis on radiography. Both foals developed perforations of the ventral colon. One of the foals was preterm, and the other was full term but had experienced a prolonged delivery and suspected hypoxia. Foals with suspected NEC should be withheld from enteral feeding and instead be placed on parenteral nutritional support. Antimicrobials that target anaerobic overgrowth are likely indicated, as are broad-spectrum anti-microbials to guard against sepsis.

Prevention in at-risk foals should include monitoring for gastric residuals. A nasogastric (NG) tube placed too high (in the esophagus or upper stomach segments) may fail to accurately measure residuals. Both the syringe diameter and the size of the NG tube may affect the volume of aspirate. Residuals should be measured before each feeding, and the meal should be withheld if significant amounts of milk or fluid are aspirated. The ideal feeding volume and maximal allowable residuals have not been calculated in foals. Certainly, a gradual or slow advancement of feedings and small frequent meals or continuous feeding should be applied to pre-mature foals or those with suspected mucosal injury [6]. Foals with ileus, as reflected by hypomotility on ultrasonographic examination, persistent reflux or residuals, abdominal distention, gaseous distention of the GI tract on abdominal radiography, and the absence of stool passage should not be fed enterally. In addition to the amount of feed, the type of enteral nutrition also is important in the prevention of NEC. In humans, a number of studies [4] have demonstrated that breast milk is more protective than formula. Extrapolating this to foals, mare's milk should be used whenever possible, particularly for preterm foals and those with GI injury. The dams of compromised neonates can be milked by hand or with syringes every 1 to 2 hours to provide enteral nutrition for their foals.

Gastroduodenal ulceration and diarrhea

Common signs of gastric ulcers include bruxism, ptyalism, dorsal recumbency, colic, poor thrift, and lethargy. One of the less consistent clinical signs of gastric ulcer syndrome includes diarrhea. In addition, foals with enteritis are at an increased risk for developing ulcers, particularly in the glandular region of the stomach. This occurs secondary to physiologic stress, including hemodynamic derangements, anorexia, inflammatory mediators, and endocrine perturbations [7]. Severe diarrhea therefore warrants consideration of the prophylactic use of antiulcer medications.

Mechanical enterocolitis

Pica, an inappropriate appetite, can result in diarrhea. The ingestion of abnormal material can result in the accumulation of these foreign substances within the GI tract. Most commonly, sand and dirt are implicated in causing diarrhea, because they can result in mechanical irritation to the GI tract and subsequent diarrhea [8]. Diagnosis is easily made with gentle manual (digital) palpation of the rectum, with an evaluation of the feces. Abdominal radiography is definitive for radio-dense material such as sand [8]. Recently, serial monitoring of the evacuation of sand through ultrasonography has been described [9]. Bedding and other materials, such as rice or almond hulls, also can cause diarrhea and enteritis when inappropriately ingested. Colic and abdominal distention are commonly present with these forms of diarrhea.

The treatment of foals with sand accumulation includes good supportive care consisting of intravenous fluid therapy and enteral laxatives, including mineral oil. Although controversy exists regarding the efficacy of psyllium hydrophilic mucilloid in eliminating sand impactions, the present author does recommend its use. It was temporally effective in alleviating sand accumulation as the primary therapy in one filly with sand-induced diarrhea [9]. Caution should be used in the amount of psyllium administered. Occasionally, foals with pica and sand impactions require surgical evacuation. The response to analgesics, medical therapy, and degrees of abdominal distention and pain are important considerations when contemplating surgery.

Nutritional or dietary causes of diarrhea

Dietary intolerances can cause diarrhea in orphan or hospitalized foals receiving enteral nutrition other than mare's milk. Foals fed with milk replacers develop loose feces more often than those on mare's or goat's milk do, particularly if the replacer is prepared using a solution that is too concentrated or too diluted [10]. The energy content of milk replacers should be evaluated in comparison with mare's milk because some may be more energy dense, which necessitates lower volumes of feeding. Bovine milk also may result in diarrhea, most likely from the higher fat content compared with mare's milk.

Diarrhea caused by infectious agents may be compounded by secondary lactase deficiency [11]. Any condition leading to the loss of the small intestinal mucosal brush border may cause lactose intolerance, but rotavirus and *Clostridium difficile* are particularly noted to cause lactase deficiency in foals [10,11]. Supplementation with a lactase enzyme (6000 Food Chemical Codex units/50-kg foal, orally [PO], every 3–8 h) is indicated in foals with suspected lactase deficiency. Lactose intolerance can be confirmed with a lactose tolerance test, but this is usually not necessary because supplementation is very inexpensive and practical [10,11].

Infectious diarrhea

Clostridial enteritis caused by Clostridium difficile and Clostridium perfringens

Clostridial organisms are common causes of enterocolitis in the neonate, and *Clostridium perfringens* and *C difficile* are the most common clostridial agents involved. Although both species cause diarrhea in the adult horse secondary to antimicrobial or other stressor-induced colonic flora disruption and colitis, they can act as primary pathogens in foals without any preceding risk factors. Host, agent, and environmental factors play a role in determining whether these two agents cause diarrhea because both can be found in clinically healthy foals [12].

   C perfringens causes diarrhea both sporadically and in outbreak situations. Some strains of the microorganism, particularly type A isolates, are part of the normal gastrointestinal microflora of horses and foals and can be cultured readily from feces. However, other strains are pathogenic; the number of colony-forming units (CFU) per gram of feces is another determinant of whether colonization is associated with clinical disease. Concentrations less than 10^2 CFU/mL are consistent with benign colonization, whereas most foals with clinical disease show concentrations greater than 10^3 CFU/mL [13]. C perfringens isolates are typed as A, B, C, D, and E, based on the production of one or more large protein exotoxins (α, β, β-2, ε, and enterotoxin). Types A and C are most commonly associated with diarrhea in foals less than 10 days of age. Type A produces α toxin, whereas type C produces both α and β toxins. Enterotoxin is variably produced by all types of C perfringens but most commonly by type A isolates. Typing of isolates is performed using polymerase chain reaction analysis for toxin gene sequences after isolates are cultured [13]. Commercial immunoassays for toxin detection in feces are available only for enterotoxin, which is present only in a minority of cases. Type C causes hemorrhagic and often severe diarrhea, with a higher mortality than type A [13]. Other clinical signs associated with C perfringens infection include colic, dehydration, tachypnea, and obtunded mentation. In the study by East and colleagues [14], foals born on dirt, sand, or gravel and those kept stalled or in dry-lot conditions during the first 3 days of life were found more likely to develop C perfringens-associated disease. Most foals in one study were less than 6 days of age on presentation, and 88% manifested acute onset disease ($\leq$24 h) [13]. Common hematologic findings include an increased number of band neutrophils, leukopenia with neutropenia, toxic cytologic changes, and hyperfibrinogenemia [13]. Hypoproteinemia also is common, although this can be masked on presentation caused by hemoconcentration. Interestingly, most foals (96% in one study [13]) demonstrate adequate passive transfer of colostral antibodies [13]. This has led some authors to speculate that trypsin inhibitors in colostrum may protect against gastric degradation of toxins, thereby potentiating toxigenicity [13]. The serum biochemistry profile of affected foals is variable, but severely affected foals may have hyper-bilirubinemia, azotemia, and increased hepatic enzymes if they exhibit severe sepsis or systemic inflammatory response syndrome (SIRS) [13]. Abdominocentesis can reflect an exudate in foals with severe enteritis. Abdominal ultrasonography and radiography may show gas- and fluid-distended small and large intestines. In the study by East and colleagues [13], the overall mortality rate of foals with C perfringens infections was 54%; those with type A had a 28% mortality (including both death and euthanasia), whereas those with type C had a mortality rate of 83%. In that study, treatment did not appear to alter the mortality rate for most foals that had a positive culture for type C [13], highlighting the importance of early and aggressive intervention. A predominance of large, gram-positive rods or spores found on a fecal smear or Gram stain may suggest the presence of clostridial overgrowth and allows for an early clinical suspicion of infection [13].

C difficile also can produce enteritis, with severe, watery to hemorrhagic diarrhea. Like *C perfringens,* it also can affect foals sporadically or in outbreak situations. Toxins A (enterotoxin) and B (cytotoxin) and binary (ADP ribosyltransferase) toxins play an important role in the pathogenesis of enterocolitis caused by *C difficile.* They alter epithelial cytoskeletal integrity, increase mucosal permeability, and incite inflammation. Interestingly, foals may be asymptomatic carriers of *C difficile* as well, and it has been hypothesized that they may serve as potential reservoirs of infection for their dams [12,15]. Up to 29% of healthy foals less than 14 days of age, in one study, were found to be culture-positive for *C difficile* [12]. This same phenomenon occurs in group-housed human infants. It is unknown why human infants and some foals can become asymptomatically colonized with toxigenic *C difficile,* whereas others develop severe disease. Diarrheal disease also can be experimentally reproduced in foals [16]. *C difficile* can act as a primary pathogen in neonates, without requiring antimicrobial administration as a risk factor, as in most adult horses [16–18]. Specific tests include fecal culture and toxin assays. These tests should be coupled because nontoxigenic isolates cannot be differentiated from toxigenic isolates based on culture alone. Commercial immunoassays for toxins A or B and fecal cell culture cytotoxin assays (for toxin B) allow for the differentiation between toxigenic and nontoxigenic infections. Either toxin A or B alone can provide enough virulence to cause disease, and both are not required as believed previously. As for *C perfringens,* a fecal smear showing large numbers of gram-positive rods or spores suggests clostridial overgrowth, although this is not specific for either organism.

The therapy of foals with clostridial enterocolitis includes intensive and supportive care in addition to specific therapies. Supportive measures include correction of fluid, acid–base, and electrolyte derangements. Hemodynamic support in the form of inotrope and vasopressor therapy may be needed if the volume replacement is not enough to normalize blood pressure. The correction of low oncotic pressure from hypoproteinemia or hypoalbuminemia is performed by administering plasma or synthetic colloids. Affected foals should be monitored for the development of coagulopathy, for which plasma or low-molecular weight heparin may be necessary. Specific therapy includes the early use of metronidazole (10–15 mg/kg intravenous [IV] or PO, every 8–12 h). Bacitracin is not recommended in horses (unlike human patients with *C difficile* infections) because of a high prevalence of resistance among equine *C difficile* isolates

[12,19]. Some *C difficile* isolates from foals have been reported to be resistant to metronidazole, and vancomycin has been used in those circumstances [19,20]. This finding is of concern and is somewhat unusual relative to human isolates. Fortunately, resistance appears to be geographic, because other authors have not found equine isolates in their hospitals to be metronidazole-resistant [12]. Nasogastric administration of di-tri-octahedral smectite (Biosponge, Platinum Performance, Buellton, CA) may be indicated as evidenced by the in vitro neutralization of *C difficile* toxins A and B and *C perfringens* enterotoxins [21]. Plasma products are controversial, but anecdotal or empirical use of *C perfringens* type C and D antitoxin has been reported in foals [13]. Slow administration and pretreatment with diphenydramine are warranted. Foals with *C difficile* enteritis can develop lactase deficiency secondary to the loss of small intestinal mucosal brush border. The supplementation of foals with lactase enzyme (Lactaid tablets, 6000 U/50-kg foal PO, every 3–8 h) may be helpful.

Preventing clostridial enteritis depends on good hygiene, particularly in the foaling area. Strict isolation protocols should be maintained. Vaccination of mares with *C perfringens* type C and D toxoid has been tried on farms with a history of affected foals, but the documentation of the safety and efficacy of such measures are not available. Spores are virtually impossible to eliminate totally, but their numbers can be reduced with good manure control and the use of scrubbing with subsequent disinfection with bleach.

Other bacterial causes

Salmonellosis can cause enterocolitis in horses of any age [22]. Affected foals usually demonstrate signs ranging from sepsis to sepsis syndrome, including fever, diarrhea, depression, and hypotensive shock. Colic and hemorrhagic diarrhea are variable findings. Foals with salmonellosis should be monitored closely for signs of localized infection, including uveitis, synovitis, osteomyelitis, and physitis. The greatest risk for bacteremia and sepsis are posed by enteroinvasive serotypes of salmonellae, including those belonging to group B, such as *Salmonella typhimurium*. All neonatal foals with enteric salmonellosis should therefore be treated with systemic antimicrobials that are effective against salmonellae, including aminoglycosides or third-generation cephalosporins.

Even though *Escherichia coli* is one of the most common causes of sepsis in foals, it has only rarely been associated with diarrhea. *E coli* isolates, particularly enterotoxigenic strains with attaching, effacing, and Shiga-like toxin genes, have been suspected to be associated with sporadic cases of diarrhea in foals [23]. *E coli* is commonly cultured from the feces of horses and foal; therefore, if *E coli* is suspected as a cause of diarrhea, the culture isolate should be further investigated using polymerase chain reaction analysis for toxin genes. The exact role of *E coli* in neonatal diarrhea thus remains to be elucidated.

Other bacteria have been suspected to be associated with diarrhea in foals, but their roles remain undefined. Browning and colleagues [24] found a prevalence of 9% of *Aeromonas hydrophila* among diarrheic foals, but its exact role in diarrhea is currently unknown [24]. *Streptococcus durans* has been isolated from one foal with profuse, watery diarrhea [25] and was subsequently associated with severe diarrhea when inoculated into seven healthy experimental foals.

Anaerobes other than *C difficile* and *C perfringens* have been speculated to play a role in neonatal foal diarrhea. Both *C sordelli* and *Bacteroides fragilis* have been reported as rare or sporadic potential pathogens [26,27]. The diagnosis of diarrhea caused by *Bacteroides* spp is difficult because the microorganism can be isolated from normal, healthy foals, and not all isolates are enterotoxigenic. Enterotoxigenic *B fragilis* often is present with other potential pathogens, including salmonellae and rotavirus [26]. Treatment should include administration of metronidazole, as for clostridiosis.

Septic foals may develop diarrhea from hemodynamic perturbations leading to GI mucosal hypoperfusion, inflammatory mediators associated with SIRS, and dysmotility. Foals with bacteremia caused by *Actinobacillus* sp were found to be six times more likely to have diarrhea compared with foals with bacteremia caused by other bacterial agents, in one study [28].

Viral enteritis

Rotavirus is the most common viral cause of neonatal diarrhea. Equine rotaviruses belong to group A rotaviruses, with a number of different serotypes identified, including G3, G5, G10, G13, G14, P7, P12, and P18 [29,30]. Rotavirus infections often occur as outbreaks on farms. Experimentally, the incubation period appears to be as short as 2 days [31]. Most affected foals are between 5 and 35 days old but the majority are at the younger end of this range [31]. It appears that older foals (up to 60 days old) can be infected, although diarrhea tends to be milder in this age group, but they can serve as reservoirs for neonates and should be isolated when identified. Transmission occurs directly by animal-to-animal and indirectly through personnel or fomites. Clinical signs of rotaviral diarrhea are similar to those of other infectious diarrheas, with a wide range from mild diarrhea to severe, watery diarrhea with dehydration. Some clinicians have suggested an association between gastroduodenal ulcer syndrome and rotaviral infections, although this requires study [10]. The virus affects the small intestine, causing blunting of the microvillus. Maldigestion and malabsorption result. With villous atrophy and compensatory crypt cell proliferation, a net decrease in fluid absorption and an increase in secretion occur. With maldigestion, lactose may enter the colon, with subsequent fermentation and osmotic contribution to diarrhea.

Rotaviral infections are diagnosed through the demonstration of virus particles in feces using commercial immunoassays or electron microscopy.

The virus is highly contagious and warrants strict isolation protocols of affected foals. Morbidity can approach 100% of neonates in outbreak situations. Disinfection should include the use of substituted phenolic compounds or quaternary ammonium disinfectants. The virus can persist for several months in the environment. The mortality rate of rotavirus is lower than with clostridiosis and, in general, is considered low, particularly with good supportive care. The treatment of rotaviral diarrhea is largely supportive.

Prevention of rotavirus outbreaks includes the use of rotavirus vaccines in mares during gestation. Studies [29,30] have demonstrated a variable reduction in morbidity, length of diarrhea, and degree of shedding of viral particles in foals resulting from vaccinated dams. One study [30] has revealed no apparent adverse reactions with the vaccine. Antibody titers were significantly increased at the time of foaling in vaccinated mares and for 90 days after birth in their foals compared with the nonvaccinated group. The incidence of rotaviral diarrhea was lower in foals born to vaccinated mares compared with foals born to controls; however, the difference was not statistically significant [30]. The administration of bovine colostral immunoglobulins has been used in an effort to reduce the prevalence of diarrhea on endemic farms. In one study [32], the morbidity of diarrhea was lower during the year after initiating a protocol of administering bovine colostral immunoglobulin powder orally to all foals compared with a preceding year when it was not administered. However, this was not a randomized or controlled study, and therefore, conclusions are difficult to make. Further study is required.

Coronavirus is another cause of viral enteritis in foals, but it has been reported in only a few studies [33,34]. Foals appear to be most susceptible to coronavirus during the neonatal period. Equine coronavirus is molecularly similar to bovine and human coronaviruses and is a member of mammalian group 2 coronaviruses. One case report [33] describes a 5-day-old foal with severe diarrhea, dehydration, hypoalbuminemia, anemia, and thrombocytopenia. The foal was euthanized when the hoof wall detached from the sensitive laminar structures. Ischemic necrosis of the distal extremities, with reddening of the coronary band and loss of hoof integrity, was found [33]. An antemortem diagnosis of coronaviral enteritis can be made using fecal-capture ELISA, electron microscopy, and serology using bovine assays [33,34]. Immunohistochemistry can be used at postmortem examination. The highest viral load appears to be shed in the feces during the acute stages, highlighting the importance of an early diagnosis and isolation.

The exact role of adenovirus in neonatal equine diarrhea is unknown. It has been identified in the intestinal epithelium of a 9-month-old foal with chronic diarrhea [35]. In addition to that report, intestinal lesions in Arabian foals with severe, combined immunodeficiency syndrome (SCID) with diarrhea have been reported as exfoliated duodenal epithelial cells containing inclusion bodies consistent with adenovirus [36].

Parasitic and protozoal agents of diarrhea

The role of *Strongyloides westeri* in diarrhea of the neonatal foal is unclear. It is unlikely to cause diarrhea except when present in very large numbers because even foals passing high egg counts can be asymptomatic. In one study [37], *Str westeri* was associated with diarrhea only when more than 2000 eggs/g of feces were detected. Although patent infestations are rare in horses older than 6 months of age, foals can establish patent infestations, with embryonated eggs passed in the feces at approximately 10 to 14 days postpartum. The major source of infection to the foal is the mare's milk, caused by arrested larvae in the mammary tissues that become activated during lactation [38]. Ivermectin, administered to the mare shortly after delivery, is effective as a dewormer to reduce the passage of larvae through the milk.

Cryptosporidium parvum was initially regarded as a pathogen of immunocompromised foals, such as those with SCID. However, more recently it has been associated with both sporadic and outbreak cases of diarrhea in even immunocompetent foals [39,40]. Most foals are 4 to 21 days of age when they show clinical signs. Supportive care and the use of bovine colostrum have been the primary focus of therapy in foals. The diagnosis is made by fecal sample evaluation for oocysts by means of acid-fast staining, immunofluorescence assay, electron microscopy, or flow cytometry [39]. Exposure to cattle is a controversial risk factor [40]. Treatment is largely supportive, but specific drug therapy with the aminoglycoside paromomycin could be attempted, although data in foals are lacking [10]. Because *Cryptosporidium parvum* is both contagious and zoonotic, affected foals should be isolated and handled with caution. Other protozoa, including *Giardia* sp and *Eimeria leukarti* oocysts can be found in both healthy and diarrheic foals, but their causal role in diarrhea has not been established.

Principles of management of the foal with diarrhea

Specific therapy

Specific therapies are available for some of the causes of diarrhea, as discussed above. For example, metronidazole is indicated in treating clostridiosis.

Fluid balance

The neonate with enteritis can have significant fluid derangements. Severe sepsis, septic shock, and hypovolemic shock are often present. A combination of crystalloids and colloids are preferred by the present author for volume resuscitation of such foals. The use of crystalloids alone may compound hypoproteinemia and hypo-oncotic states because most foals with enteritis have at least some degree of protein-losing enteropathy. The types, volumes, and rates of fluid administration are highly variable, and the ideal selections are best tailored to the individual foal. However, as general guidelines, good replacement crystalloid choices for the foal with enteritis include lactate Ringer's solution, Normosol R, and Plasma-Lyte 148. Physiologic saline (0.9%) is another choice but is considered less ideal by this author because of its high chloride (154 mEq/L) relative to normal foal plasma. This makes saline mildly acidifying by decreasing the strong ion difference. Saline may be indicated, however, in the hyperkalemic foal because the other commercial replacement fluids contain potassium. Hyperkalemia may be present in the foal with concurrent acute renal disease or hyperkalemic periodic paralysis. Saline also is indicated in the concurrently hyponatremic and hypochloremic foal, in which both are decreased to the same relative extent. Isotonic bicarbonate is another replacement fluid that can be used in the foal with severe metabolic acidemia that is inorganic in origin. Hypertonic saline (7%) also is available as a rapid and temporary expander of intravascular volume. However, serum sodium concentrations should be monitored closely to avoid marked swings. Doses for hypertonic saline include 2 to 4 mL/kg.

Recommendations for volume are based on estimates of hypovolemia and dehydration. As general guidelines, rates of 10 to 20 mL/kg given as slow boluses (over 20–30 min) can be used until signs of hypovolemia improve or plateau, urine is produced, and central venous pressures (CVP) approach maximum (10 cm H_2O). Central venous pressures are measured easily in the neonatal foal through the use of 20-cm jugular catheters.

Colloid options include plasma and synthetic colloids, particularly hetastarch. If these fluids are used then volumes should be used that are lower than those for crystalloids are. In contrast to replacement crystalloids, which distribute to the entire extracellular fluid space (ECF), colloids are largely limited to the intravascular space, assuming relatively normal capillary integrity. Therefore, boluses of 3 to 5 mL/kg colloids should be used. Plasma should be administered slowly to avoid or minimize the risks for anaphylactoid reactions. It can be administered at a rate of 10 mL/kg/h for a total volume of 1 to 2 L, or alternatively it can be used as a constant rate infusion (CRI) of 1 to 2 mL/kg/h as needed for colloid and albumin replacement. Plasma is a cost-effective colloid in foals and has the additional benefit of providing antibodies, clotting factors, antithrombin, and other proteins. Hetastarch can be used in small boluses; however, a total volume of 10 mL/kg/day should not be exceeded, to avoid coagulopathy. Hetastarch causes a decrease in von Willebrand's factor and clotting factor VIII concentrations when administered at volumes at or above 15 mL/kg. Hetastarch should not be used in the hypocoagulable or thrombocytopenic foal.

Once hypovolemia has been corrected, fluid therapy should consist of a maintenance rate combined with estimates of ongoing losses. Relatively hypotonic maintenance fluids should be used for the maintenance portion of fluid therapy if the foal is fed by routes other than orally. These include Plasma-Lyte 56, Normosol M, or 0.45% saline/2.5% dextrose. The ongoing GI losses, however, should be replaced with a replacement fluid because they represent losses from the ECF.

Acid–base balance

The foal with severe diarrhea often has metabolic acidemia. If the acidosis is caused by hypoperfusion (hyperlactatemia), the primary treatment consists of reversing the circulatory perturbations. Treatment consists of volume replacement until no further correction in blood pressure occurs, blood lactate concentrations improve (≤ 2 mmol/L), or alternatively, until CVP approaches 10 cm H_2O. Once these occur, inotropes and vasopressors should be used if perfusion is still inadequate. Dobutamine (2–10 µg/kg/min, CRI) is an excellent inotrope. If pressures and perfusion are still inadequate, vasopressors such as norepinephrine or vasopressin can be tried. Norepinephrine should be diluted in 5% dextrose and is administered at a rate of 0.01 to 0.1 µk/kg/min. Vasopressin has been used more recently in foals, and a suggested dose range is 0.25 to 0.5 mU/kg/min. During vasopressor therapy, the foal should be monitored for excessive vasoconstriction and worsening of hypoperfusion, despite showing increases in blood pressure by monitoring serial blood lactate concentrations, urine output, and clinical parameters of perfusion. A word of caution should be added about lactate: Many foals with SIRS or sepsis remain hyperlactatemic despite volume replacement because of inflammatory mediator-induced decreases in pyruvate dehydrogenase (through activation of pyruvate dehydrogenase kinase) or increases in the production of lactate caused by catecholamine stimulation of the sodium–potassium ATP pump activity. Therefore, urine production and clinical signs of perfusion parameters are very important monitoring tools in addition to blood pressure.

If the acidemia is a result of hyponatremia or relative hyperchloremia, the treatment consists of sodium bicarbonate. The amount of bicarbonate needed is calculated as 0.3 × body weight (kg) × base deficit. Sodium bicarbonate should be administered slowly and carefully because of the potential drawbacks to rapid administration, including hypernatremia, hyperosmolarity, hypokalemia, ionized hypocalcemia, a left shift in the oxygen dissociation curve, and paradoxical intracellular acidosis.

Electrolytes

Foals with enteritis develop a number of electrolyte derangements. Sodium derangements are common, particularly hyponatremia. Neurologic signs may be present in foals with diarrhea and sodium concentrations below a range of 110 to 115 mEq/L [41]. Sodium concentrations can be corrected fairly rapidly up to 115 to 120 mEq/L in order to correct neurologic deficits, but beyond this amount, concentrations should be corrected slowly, at approximately 0.5 mEq/h to avoid central pontine myelinolysis. Serum sodium concentrations should be monitored frequently to avoid overcorrection. Occasionally, hypernatremia may be encountered, particularly if foals have been oversupplemented with oral sodium-containing fluids before presentation. Hypernatremia should also be corrected slowly to avoid increases in intracranial pressure (0.5 mEq/h).

Potassium disorders also may be present in foals with diarrhea. Hyperkalemia is common with concurrent renal disease or with significant inorganic acidemia. Hypokalemia may be present if the foal has been anorexic for prolonged periods, with potassium loss in the diarrheic fluids.

Gastrointestinal protectants

Enteral protective modalities include kaolin/pectin compounds and bismuth subsalicylate. Bismuth is believed to coat the mucosa, whereas the salicylate portion has antiprostaglandin activity. Kaolin/pectin combinations act primarily as mucosal coating agents. Care should be taken to stagger these medications with other oral drugs to avoid nonspecific binding and a reduction in bioavailability of the concurrently administered drugs. These agents are administered at 0.5 to 4 mL/kg, once to four times daily [42].

Activated charcoal and di-tri-octahedral smectite are adsorbents that can bind endotoxin and reduce its absorption. Smectite also has been shown to neutralize toxins of *C difficile* and *C perfringens* in vitro [21].

The modulation of enteric flora with the use of probiotics is a controversial area in equine medicine. Documentation of efficacy is lacking. There is currently on going investigation in this area, including the use of the yeast *Saccharomyces boulardii* for use in enteric clostridiosis. Probiotics must be used with caution in the neonatal foal, particularly the foal less than 24 h of age, because of a potential for bacterial or fungal translocation. Information on gastrointestinal protectants and probiotics is described elsewhere [42].

Gastric ulcer medications

The prophylactic use of antiulcer medications is controversial. However, because foals with enteritis are at risk for developing ulcers, particularly glandular ulcers, this author currently recommends the use of ulcer medications in these foals [7]. Medications may consist of histamine type-2 receptor antagonists, sucralfate, or proton pump inhibitors. Histamine type-2 antagonists include ranitidine (1.5 mg IV, every 8–12 h or 6.6 mg/kg PO, every 8 h) and famotidine (2.8 mg/kg PO, every 12 h or 0.3 mg/kg IV, every 12h). Omeprazole, the most commonly used proton pump inhibitor, has been studied recently in the healthy neonatal foal. A dose of 4 mg/kg PO, every 24 h, increases the gastric pH level within 2 h of administration and for 22 hours [43]. Sucralfate has a number of advantages, including binding glandular ulcers and increasing local prostaglandin E production, thereby increasing mucosal blood flow and mucus and bicarbonate secretion. The recommended dosage of sucralfate is 10 to 20 mg/kg PO, every 6 to 8 h.

Antiendotoxin measures

Most of the antiendotoxin modalities used in adult horses have not been studied in foals. The present author prefers not to use flunixin meglumine in the neonatal foal because of the potential for reducing gastrointestinal perfusion. Polymyxin B has been studied experimentally in older foals [44].

Nutrition

Nutritional support is a very important aspect of managing the neonatal foal with diarrhea. Foals with abdominal distention, gastric residuals, ileus, or colic should be withheld from milk temporarily. Foals with profuse diarrhea, particularly those types of diarrhea suspected to be associated with lactose intolerance or an osmotic diarrhea, should be restricted at least partially in terms of milk intake. In these cases, parenteral nutrition should be provided. Dextrose supplementation (4–8 mg/kg/min with frequent monitoring of blood glucose concentrations) of crystalloids can be used in the short term (first 12–24 h). If enteral nutrition is not tolerated by this time, parenteral nutrition should be instituted. This author uses the following formula as a starting point for making a total parenteral nutrition solution: 1000 mL 50% dextrose + 1500 mL 8.5% amino acid solution + 500 mL 20% intralipid to make a total volume of 3000 mL.

This solution has a caloric content of 1.07 kcal/mL digestible energy, 0.0425 g/mL amino acids, and 0.033 g/mL lipid. The energy requirements of the neonatal foal with diarrhea are unknown. General guidelines for the energy requirements of the neonatal foal include a range of 45 to 50 kcal/kg/day for basal energy requirement and 100 to 170 kcal/kg/day for normal, healthy foals. This author usually targets a value between these amounts, approximately 70 to 75 kcal/kg/day, with gradual advancement as parenteral nutrition is tolerated. Vitamins and minerals must be added to this solution or alternatively to the crystalloids being administered. Serum glucose, serum triglycerides, electrolytes, and acid–base status should be monitored closely in foals receiving parenteral nutrition. Foals intolerant of glucose may benefit from insulin (regular insulin, 0.005–0.01 IU/kg/h, titrated to glucose concentrations). The lipid fraction is decreased if triglyceride concentrations exceed 200 mg/dL. Information on foal nutrition and parenteral nutrition has been described elsewhere [45,46].

Parenteral nutrition should only be viewed as a bridge to enteral nutrition. For foals tolerant of minimal enteral nutrition, even small volumes frequently are beneficial for providing local nutrition to enterocytes.

The neonate should be fed conservatively at first, and volumes should be advanced gradually as enteral feedings are tolerated. A reasonable starting point is 10% of body weight per day divided into hourly or 2-hour feeding intervals through a nasogastric tube. Foals that are bright and strong enough to nurse should be allowed to do so.

Systemic antimicrobials

Broad-spectrum antimicrobials should be administered to the neonatal foal with enteritis because of the risks of bacterial translocation across the compromised GI barrier. Choices include a combination of aminoglycoside (such as amikacin or gentamicin) and β-lactam, or alternatively a third-generation cephalosporin. Foals receiving aminoglycoside therapy should undergo therapeutic drug monitoring to ensure adequate peak and trough plasma concentrations of drug, as well as monitoring of renal function.

References

[1] Cohen ND. Causes of and farm management factors associated with disease and death in foals. J Am Vet Med Assoc 1994,204.1644–51.

[2] Johnston RH, Kamstra LD, Kohler PH. Mares' milk composition as related to "foal heat" scours. J Anim Sci 1970;31:549–53.

[3] Masri MD, Merritt AM, Gronwall R, et al. Faecal composition in foal heat diarrhea. Equine Vet J 1986;18:301–6.

[4] Noerr B. Part 1. current controversies in the understanding of necrotizing enterocolitis. Adv Neonatal Care 2003;3:107–20.

[5] Cudd T, Pauly TH. Necrotizing enterocolitis in two equine neonates. Compendium on Continuing Education for the Practicing Veterinarian 1987;9:88–96.

[6] Paradis MR. Nutritional support: enteral and parenteral. Clin Tech Eq Pract 2003;2:87–96.

[7] Furr MO, Murray MJ, Ferguson DC. The effects of stress on gastric ulceration, T3, T4, reverse T3 and cortisol in neonatal foals. Equine Vet J 1992;37–40.

[8] Ramey DW, Reinertson EL. Sand-induced diarrhea in a foal. J Am Vet Med Assoc 1984;185: 537–8.

[9] Korolainen R, Kaikkonen R, Ruohoniemi M. Ultrasonography in monitoring the resolution of intestinal sand accumulations in the horse. Equine Veterinary Education 2003;5:423–32.

[10] Lester GD. Foal diarrhea. In: Robinson NE, editor. Current therapy in equine medicine. 5th edition. Philadelphia: WB Saunders; 2003. p. 677–80.

[11] Weese JS, Parsons DA, Staempfli HR. Association of *Clostridium difficile* with enterocolitis and lactose intolerance in a foal. J Am Vet Med Assoc 1999;214:229–32.

[12] Baverud V, Gustafsson A, Franklin A, et al. Clostridium difficile: prevalence in horses and environment, and antimicrobial susceptibility. Equine Vet J 2003;35:465–71.

[13] East LM, Savage CJ, Traub-Dargatz JL, et al. Enterocolitis associated with *Clostridium perfringens* infection in neonatal foals: 54 cases (1988–1997). J Am Vet Med Assoc 1998;212: 1751–6.

[14] East LM, Dargatz DA, Traub-Dargatz JL, et al. Foaling-management practices associated with the occurrence of enterocolitis attributed to *Clostridium perfringens* infection in the equine neonate. Prev Vet Med 2000;46:61–74.

[15] Baverud V, Franklin A, Gunnarsson A, et al. Clostridium difficile associated with acute colitis in mares when their foals are treated with erythromycin and rifampicin for *Rhodococcus equi* pneumonia. Equine Vet J 1998;30:482–8.

[16] Arroyo LG, Weese JS, Staempfli HR. Experimental *Clostridium difficile* enterocolitis in foals. J Vet Int Med 2004;18:734–8.

[17] Jones RL, Shideler RK, Cockerell GL. Association of *Clostridium difficile* with foal diarrhea. In: Proceedings of the 5th International Conference of Equine Infectious Diseases 1988; 236–40.

[18] Jones RL, Adney WS, Shideler RK. Isolation of *Clostridium difficile* and detection of cytotoxin in the feces of diarrheic foals in the absence of antimicrobial treatment. J Clin Microbiol 1987;25:1225–7.

[19] Jang SS, Hansen LM, Breher JE, et al. Antimicrobial susceptibilities of equine isolates of *Clostridium difficile* and molecular characterization of metronidazole-resistant strains. Clin Infect Dis 1997;25(Suppl 2):S266–7.

[20] Magdesian KG, Hirsh DC, Jang SS, et al. Characterization of *Clostridium difficile* isolates from foals with diarrhea: 28 cases (1993–1997). J Am Vet Med Assoc 2002;220:67–73.

[21] Weese JS, Cote NM, deGannes RVG. Evaluation of in vitro properties of di-tri-octahedral smectite on clostridial toxins and growth. Equine Vet J 2003;35:638–41.

[22] Walker RL, Madigan JE, Hird DW, et al. An outbreak of equine neonatal salmonellosis. J Vet Diagn Invest 1991;3:223–7.

[23] Holland RE, Sriranganathan N, DuPont L. Isolation of enterotoxigenic *Escherichia coli* from a foal with diarrhea. J Am Vet Med Assoc 1989;194:389–91.

[24] Browning GF, Chalmers RM, Snodgrass DR, et al. The prevalence of enteric pathogens in diarrhoeic Thoroughbred foals in Britain and Ireland. Equine Vet J 1991;23:405–9.

[25] Tzipori S, Hayes J, Sims L, et al. *Streptococcus durans:* an unexpected enteropathogen of foals. J Infect Dis 1984;150:589–93.

[26] Myers LL, Shoop DS, Byars TD. Diarrhea associated with enterotoxigenic *Bacteroides fragilis* in foals. Am J Vet Res 1987;48:1565–7.

[27] Hibbs CM, Johnson DR, Reynolds K, et al. *Clostridium sordelli* isolated from foals. Equine Practice 1977;72:256–8.

[28] Stewart AJ, Hinchcliff KW, Saville WJA, et al. *Actinobacillus* sp. Bacteremia in foals: clinical signs and prognosis. J Vet Int Med 2002;16:464–71.

[29] Barrandeguy M, Parreno V, Lagos Marmol M, et al. Prevention of rotavirus diarrhoea in foals by parenteral vaccination of the mares: field trail. Dev Biol Stand 1998;92:253–7.

[30] Powell DG, Dwyer RM, Traub-Dargatz JL, et al. Field study of the safety, immunogenicity, and efficacy of an inactivated equine rotavirus vaccine. J Am Vet Med Assoc 1997;211:193–8.

[31] Conner ME, Darlington RW. Rotavirus infection in foals. Am J Vet Res 1980;41: 1699–703.

[32] Watanabe T, Ohta C, Shirahata T, et al. Preventive administration of bovine colostral immunoglobulins for foal diarrhea with rotavirus. J Vet Med Sci 1993;55:1039–40.

[33] Davis E, Rush BR, Cox J, et al. Neonatal enterocolitis associated with coronavirus infection in a foal: a case report. J Vet Diagn Invest 2000;12:153–6.

[34] Guy JS, Breslin JJ, Breuhaus B, et al. Characterization of a coronavirus isolated from a diarrheic foal. J Clin Microbiol 2000;38:4523–6.

[35] Corrier DE, Montgomery D, Scutchfield WL. Adenovirus in the intestinal epithelium of a foal with prolonged diarrhea. Vet Pathol 1982;19:564–7.

[36] McChesney AE, England JJ, Rich LJ. Adenoviral infection in foals. J Am Vet Med Assoc 1973;162:545–9.

[37] Netherwood T, Wood JLN, Townsend HGG, et al. Foal diarrhoea between 1991 and 1994 in the United Kingdom associated with *Clostridium perfringens*, rotavirus, *Strongyloides westeri*, and *Cryptosporidium sp.* Epidemiol Infect 1996;117:375–83.

[38] Ludwig KG, Craig TM, Bowen JM, et al. Efficacy of ivermectin in controlling *Strongyloides westeri* infections in foals. Am J Vet Res 1983;44:314–6.

[39] Cole DJ, Cohen ND, Snowden K, et al. Prevalence of and risk factors for fecal shedding of *Cryptosporidium parvum* oocysts in horses. J Am Vet Med Assoc 1998;213:1296–302.

[40] Grinberg A, Oliver L, Learmonth JJ, et al. Identification of *Cryptosporidium parvum* 'cattle' genotype from a severe outbreak of neonatal foal diarrhoea. Vet Rec 2003;153:628–31.

[41] Lakritz J, Madigan J, Carlson GP. Hypovolemic hyponatremia and signs of neurologic disease associated with diarrhea in a foal. J Am Vet Med Assoc 1992;200:1114–6.

[42] Tillotson K, Traub-Dargatz JL. Gastrointestinal protectants and cathartics. Vet Clin North Am Equine Pract 2003;599–615.

[43] Sanchez LC, Murray MJ, Merritt AM. Effect of omeprazole paste on intragastric pH in clinically normal neonatal foals. Am J Vet Res 2004;65:1039–41.

[44] Durando MM, MacKay RJ, Linda S, et al. Effects of polymyxin B and *Salmonella typhimurium* antiserum on horses given endotoxin intravenously. Am J Vet Res 1994;55:921–7.

[45] Magdesian KG. Nutrition for critical gastrointestinal illness: feeding horse with diarrhea or colic. Vet Clin North Am Equine Pract 2003;19:617–45.

[46] Dunkel BM, Wilkins PA. Nutrition and the critically ill horse. Vet Clin North Am Equine Pract 2004;20:107–27.

VETERINARY
CLINICS
Equine Practice

Vet Clin Equine 21 (2005) 313–332

Nondiarrheal Disorders of the Gastrointestinal Tract in Neonatal Foals

Clare A. Ryan, DVM, L. Chris Sanchez, DVM, PhD*

*Department of Large Animal Clinical Sciences,
College of Veterinary Medicine, University of Florida, 2015 SW 16th Avenue,
Box 100136, Gainesville, Florida 32610-0136, USA*

With the exception of diarrhea, which is covered elsewhere in this issue, primary disorders of the gastrointestinal tract are relatively uncommon in neonatal foals. This body system is predisposed to a variety of secondary complications, however, which can drastically alter an individual foal's clinical course. An understanding of the perceived pathophysiology of these issues and implementation of preventative measures can improve short- and long-term outcome for many neonatal patients. Other primary events are discussed according to anatomic location.

Physical examination and routine monitoring

The gastrointestinal tract should always be considered during examination of the equine neonate, whether for routine examination of a perceived healthy foal or for examination of a neonate with systemic illness. The initial examination should include observation of the foal's interaction with the mare, including its ability and desire to find the udder, demonstration of an appropriate suckle reflex, ability to suckle effectively from the udder, ability to swallow ingested milk, and ability to drain the udder appropriately. If any aspect of the foal's nursing behavior raises concern, one can auscult the foal's trachea during suckling to detect subtle aspiration. Thorough examination of the head should include manual palpation of the hard palate and soft palate extending to the caudal border of the soft palate. Small defects in the palate may require endoscopy for detection, but large defects should be evident with careful examination.

---

* Corresponding author.
E-mail address: sanchezl@mail.vetmed.ufl.edu (L.C. Sanchez).

0749-0739/05/$ - see front matter
doi:10.1016/j.cveq.2005.04.005

Objective monitoring of abdominal size is indicated in any neonate considered at risk for gastrointestinal disease. Such individuals include any critically ill foal, especially those that are predominantly recumbent, or any foal that has displayed signs of colic. Abdominal circumference can be measured easily with a measuring tape. One should take care to make marks with clippers or a permanent marker on the lateral aspect of each of the foal's sides to ensure locational consistency between measurements. A trend of increasing circumference often precedes outward signs of colic and should prompt re-evaluation of the patient.

Other diagnostic procedures that are not specific to the gastrointestinal tract but can provide additional information for individual patients include basic blood work (complete blood cell count [CBC], biochemical profile, and arterial or venous blood gas), abdominal ultrasound, nasogastric intubation, endoscopy of the upper airway or proximal gastrointestinal tract, plain or contrast radiography, and, occasionally, exploratory celiotomy. Indications for each of these procedures are detailed in the following sections.

Oral cavity

Cleft palate

Routine physical examination of the neonatal foal should include oral examination for congenital deformities, including, most commonly, cleft palate. A range of locations and sizes of cleft palate (palatoschisis) has been reported in foals [1,2]. Primary cleft palate involves the lip and external nares and has not been reported in foals. Secondary cleft palate involving the hard or soft palate may require additional tests, such as upper airway endoscopy or skull radiographs, for definitive diagnosis. The rate of cleft palate in foals has been reported as 24 (0.268%) per 8954 necropsies of horses less than 1 year of age [1], 2 (0.31%) in 640 necropsies of fetuses or foals [3], and 1 (0.1%) per 1000 hospital admissions [4].

Most foals with cleft palate display clinical signs of dysphagia while nursing, including coughing or milk at the nares after nursing, but the severity of clinical signs is extremely variable. Signs are usually noted shortly after birth but may go unnoticed for some time if the defect is small. Compromised ability to suckle may predispose the foal to partial or complete failure of passive transfer. Most foals develop some degree of aspiration pneumonia, and pneumonia may even be the presenting complaint. Therefore, appropriate diagnosis and treatment of this complication (thoracic radiographs or ultrasound, CBC, and broad-spectrum antimicrobial therapy) should be implemented if surgical correction of the defect is pursued.

The prognosis is generally poor but depends on the location and size of the defect. Various approaches to surgical correction have been discussed in the literature [5–11]. Difficulty in exposure of the site during surgery and a high rate of dehiscence make repair difficult. For these reasons, survival rates have historically been low. If surgical correction is pursued, ethical ramifications should be discussed with the owner, especially regarding use of the affected individual for future breeding purposes because of the possibility that these disorders could be inherited.

Dysphagia

Causes of dysphagia in neonatal foals are more limited than those reported in adult horses, but the initial diagnostic approach begins in a similar fashion. This approach should include a thorough oral examination, neurologic examination (with specific attention to the cranial nerves), observation of the foal during suckling, and external palpation of the larynx and proximal esophagus followed by upper airway endoscopy. Clinical signs include coughing while suckling, regurgitation of milk through the mouth or nares, and, occasionally, ptyalism. Specific causes of dysphagia in neonates can be broken down into morphologic and functional abnormalities.

Morphologic abnormalities resulting in dysphagia in the foal include cleft palate, as discussed previously, physical obstruction of the larynx from a focal mass, and generalized inflammation of the pharynx or larynx. Less common morphologic abnormalities of the upper airway include subepiglottic cysts [12], congenital dorsal displacement of the soft palate [13], and persistent frenulum of the epiglottis [14]. Pharyngitis or arytenoid chondritis can occur as an iatrogenic complication after nasogastric intubation or as a result of external trauma. Upper airway endoscopy, alone or in combination with radiography, can often confirm a diagnosis.

Common functional abnormalities include generalized weakness and a variety of neurologic deficits. Normal suckling in foals requires a complex interaction of cortical (necessary for affinity to the mare and recognition of the udder) and cranial nerve function. Normal function of cranial nerves V, VII, and XII is required for suckling as well as normal input from the pons, hindbrain, and cerebrum. Cranial nerves IX and X and the hindbrain are necessary for swallowing. Many primary diseases in foals, such as sepsis and prematurity, can cause generalized weakness resulting in functional dysphagia. For this reason, it is imperative to monitor foals with these problems before allowing suckling from the mare and to use extreme caution if attempting bottle feeding. Dysphagia resulting from generalized weakness usually resolves as the foal recovers from the primary disease, and specific therapy is not indicated [15]. An alternate means of nutrition should be provided, however, comprising enteral feeding via a nasogastric tube alone or in conjunction with parenteral nutrition.

One of the more common neurologic causes of dysphagia is hypoxic ischemic encephalomyelopathy. This problem is covered in depth in the article in this issue on neurologic disorders, but the ability to suckle appropriately (along with affinity for the mare) is often one of the first normal behaviors lost and one of the last to return. Other neuromuscular causes of dysphagia include botulism and white muscle disease. Botulism occurs with the highest frequency in Kentucky and the Middle Atlantic region, causes progressive neuromuscular weakness, and can result in dysphagia and respiratory difficulty or failure [16]. Because of the progressive nature of the disease, botulism does not typically cause dysphagia alone without other associated lesions. White muscle disease, also known as nutritional myodegeneration, can cause dysphagia, often in addition to generalized muscle weakness [17]. White muscle disease is typically associated with selenium-deficient soils and has been reported in North America, Europe, Australia, and New Zealand.

Regardless of the cause, dysphagia can result in aspiration pneumonia. Thus, if a dysphagic foal has been allowed to suckle, additional diagnostic procedures should include thoracic radiographs or ultrasound to investigate this potential complication.

Thrush (oral candidiasis)

Severely ill or immunocompromised foals may develop oral fungal plaques, commonly called "thrush." Oral lesions may appear as focal white plaques or diffuse thick pseudomembranous coatings of the oral cavity. These are mainly associated with opportunistic organisms ubiquitous in the local environment. *Candida* spp, especially *Candida albicans*, a dimorphic fungus, are commonly identified causative agents. In the yeast phase, *Candida* normally inhabits the upper respiratory, alimentary, and genital mucosa of mammals. *Candida* does not normally cause a reaction, and fungal plaques on the tongue are unlikely to be of consequence primarily. Nevertheless, their presence should prompt an investigation of the foal's overall immune status and raise the possibility of systemic fungal infection, which has previously been described in the foal [18,19]. One report describes the colonization of hyperkeratotic mucosa surrounding ulcers in the esophagus and stomach of foals with colic that was nonresponsive to medical treatment [20]. In another report, ulcerative keratitis was the initial indication of systemic candidiasis [21]. Predisposing factors may include immunodeficiency, antimicrobial therapy, corticosteroid administration, and administration of parenteral nutrition.

Culture of the organism is easy to perform because it grows readily on a blood agar plate. If oral thrush is noted, one should evaluate for the presence of fungal organisms in blood or other sources deemed clinically significant, such as intravenous catheter tips, indwelling urinary catheters, endotracheal tubes, or specific foci of suspected infection (eg, synovial fluid, umbilical remnants). If an indwelling venous catheter is affected, it must be removed and, if possible, not replaced. Infections of the synovium or bone should be treated similar to bacterial septic arthritis with joint lavage and, possibly, intravenous regional limb or interosseous perfusion [22].

Attempted medical treatment options include fluconazole, itraconazole, voriconazole, and amphotericin B [19,21]. Fungal sensitivity profiles may help to direct therapy if an organism has been definitively identified, but pharmacokinetics of these drugs have not been established in foals. Amphotericin B has been administered intravenously at a range of 0.1 to 0.5 mg/kg/d, starting therapy at the lower dose and increasing by 0.1-mg/kg increments each day [19]. Because this drug can have potentially life-threatening toxic effects on the kidney, creatinine, urine production, and urinalysis should be monitored closely throughout therapy. Fluconazole has previously been administered orally at a rate of 4 to 10 mg/kg/d. If culture of the organism indicates sensitivity, treatment with fluconazole may be more appropriate than amphotericin B because it is less expensive, easier to administer, and has far fewer side effects. Miconazole has also been used at a dose of 1 mg/kg administered intravenously every 8 hours. [19].

Esophagus

Disorders of the esophagus in foals are uncommonly reported but may be categorized as a physical obstruction (intra- or extraluminal) or a disorder of motility. Reported diseases include congenital esophageal stenosis, tubular duplication of the esophagus, vascular ring anomalies, esophageal ectasia, megaesophagus, choke, trauma, stenosis, and stricture [23–28]. Although differing in cause, each of these disorders may present with common clinical signs of milk, feed, or saliva at the nares (bilateral and often noted when the head is lowered); ptyalism; a palpable "mass" or distention in the cervical region of the esophagus; or cough. Other clinical signs are related to secondary aspiration pneumonia (fever, lethargy, anorexia, tachycardia, tachypnea, or abnormal lung sounds).

Careful palpation of the cervical region may reveal a firm mass in the case of choke, firm painful swelling in the case of traumatic injury, or soft fluctuant mass in the case of megaesophagus and fluid accumulation orad to the lesion. In the case of obstruction, attempts at passing a nasogastric tube are unsuccessful if the tube is larger than the diameter of the esophagus at the affected region. Care should be taken not to apply too much pressure during intubation so as to avoid iatrogenic esophageal rupture. The esophagus should be fully examined by endoscopy when possible. The endoscope should be advanced to the stomach (or to the level of the obstruction if complete passage is not possible) and backed out slowly. The examiner should look for mucosal or submucosal defects, narrowing of the esophageal lumen, or abnormal dilations with lack of motility. If possible, sedation should be avoided when assessing motility because it may affect esophageal motility and cause transient dilation. Lateral radiographs of the cervical and thoracic portions of the esophagus can be taken. One may occasionally identify a lesion with plain radiographs; however, contrast is commonly required to identify strictures or megaesophagus [29]. Foals with these disorders may be at increased risk of aspiration, and appropriate contrast medium should be selected. Fluoroscopy or serial radiographs may be helpful in identifying abnormalities of esophageal motility. Vascular ring anomalies may require intravenous contrast with fluoroscopy or CT to identify the aberrant vessel.

With cases of mucosal erosion, foals may be temporarily managed by feeding via a nasogastric tube, thus allowing for a period of esophageal rest. Disruptions in the mucosa may benefit from treatment with sucralfate. In the case of abnormal motility, medical therapy has been attempted with varying degrees of success. Permanent feeding practice changes may be required, including feeding gruels or finely chopped hay. Elevation of the horse's front feet may allow for gravity-assisted transit down the esophagus. The presence of aspiration pneumonia should be assessed and managed with appropriate antibiotic therapy if necessary. Long-term survival depends on the ability to resolve the primary defect or to manage the foal's diet adequately. In many cases, repeated episodes of choke lead to eventual euthanasia.

Stomach

Gastric ulceration

Gastric ulceration is a well-recognized and frequently treated phenomenon in foals. The reported prevalence of gastric ulceration in foals has ranged from 25% to 57% [30,31]. In one large study involving 75 Thoroughbred foals from 2 to 85 days of age without clinical signs of ulceration, the prevalence of gastric ulceration was 51% [32]. Ulceration was most often noted in the squamous mucosa adjacent to the margo plicatus along the greater curvature of the stomach, with involvement of the squamous fundus, glandular fundus, and squamous mucosa along the lesser curvature noted less frequently [32]. In another study, squamous ulceration was noted more commonly in older asymptomatic foals, whereas glandular ulceration, especially in the cardiac region, occurred more commonly in neonates with another primary clinical disorder [31]. Duodenal ulceration can occur in neonatal foals, but the syndrome of gastroduodenal ulceration (GDUD) typically occurs in foals between 2 and 6 months of age, and is thus beyond the scope of this discussion.

Gastric ulceration is of particular concern in neonatal foals because clinical signs are often not evident until ulceration is severe and, in some cases, are not evident until gastric rupture has occurred. Neonates with gastric ulceration occasionally become inappetent or show signs of colic, but they do not frequently display clinical signs associated with gastric ulceration in older foals, such as bruxism or ptyalism [33]. A definitive diagnosis of gastric ulceration is made via gastric endoscopy. Even in an average 45- to 50-kg newborn foal, a 1-m endoscope does not allow for complete evaluation of the entire stomach, although such a unit is likely to allow viewing of the squamous and glandular mucosa along the greater curvature. Because of their liquid diet, neonatal foals do not require an extended period of fasting before examination, preferably with an endoscope with a working length of at least a 2 m and a maximum external diameter of 9 mm. It is recommended to examine the entire stomach, including the gastric antrum and pylorus, and the proximal duodenum if at all possible, because some foals may have antral lesions without ulceration elsewhere in the stomach. When examining the stomach of young foals, one must consider that the squamous mucosa is thin at birth, with more of a light pink appearance relative to that of adult horses, but becomes hyperplastic and parakeratotic within days [34]. Because the size of the neonate's stomach is much smaller than that of the adult horse, one must always take care when inflating the stomach during examination and also ensure that insufflated air is removed with suction before removal of the endoscope into the esophagus.

The pathophysiology of ulcer disease in foals is likely complex and multifactorial but is not completely understood. In most forms of the equine gastric ulcer syndrome (EGUS), hydrochloric acid has been described as a major intrinsic contributing factor [35,36]. Horses secrete gastric acid continuously, and foals are able to maintain an acidic stomach environment by 2 days of age [37]. Pony foals were reported to have an increased pH during the first day of life [38], but some critically ill foals have demonstrated periods of acidity on the first day of life [39]. The ontogeny of gastric acid production in foals has not been established, but premature human infants are capable of acid secretion by 28 weeks of gestation [40]. Suckling has an immediate profound effect on intragastric pH in neonatal foals, raising pH from approximately 1.5 to 2.5 to 5 to 6 within 30 seconds of suckling after a period of recumbency [37]. Other intrinsic factors that may contribute to ulcer formation include pepsin and bile salts [41]. Extrinsic factors reportedly contributing to ulcer formation include administration of nonsteroidal anti-inflammatory drugs (NSAIDs), "stress," factors related to diet or management, other gastrointestinal disorders (especially those resulting in delayed gastric emptying), and, in humans, *Helicobacter pylori* [42,43]. To date, although PCR fragments unique to gastric-dwelling *Helicobacter* species have been identified in horses, an association between *H pylori* and ulceration has not been established in adult horses or foals [44,45]. In human neonates, stress associated with a primary clinical disorder has been strongly associated with the development of gastric ulceration [46]. Primary intrinsic gastric protective factors include adequate mucosal blood flow, mucus and bicarbonate secretion, mucosal epidermal growth factor and prostaglandin E_2 production, and gastric and duodenal motility [42].

An imbalance between protective mechanisms and ulcerogenic factors can lead to ulcer formation. Because many of the mucosal protective factors are concentrated within the glandular epithelium, their deficiency would theoretically lead to glandular ulceration. Alternatively, because much of the squamous mucosa is not normally exposed to acidic gastric contents, factors leading to such exposure may contribute to ulceration of this region. Hypovolemia and hypotension commonly accompany many of the primary conditions for which neonatal foals require intensive care. Thus, perfusion to the gastrointestinal tract and other vital organs can become compromised. Recent work has shown that the 24-hour intragastric pH profile in severely ill recumbent foals remains primarily alkaline, whereas the profile of foals able to ambulate more closely mimics that seen in healthy foals [39] Also, a retrospective study revealed no correlation between the incidence of gastric ulcer disease and administration of pharmacologic prophylaxis [47]. When considered together, these factors suggest that alterations in gastric perfusion play a more significant role than hydrochloric acid in the development of gastric ulcers in the severely compromised neonatal foal. This would also support the authors' clinical impression that the incidence of perforated gastric ulcers in hospitalized foals has decreased in conjunction with overall improvements in neonatal supportive care. Nevertheless, one must also consider that the prophylactic administration of acid-suppressive drugs is commonplace at many institutions.

When considering treatment of gastric ulcers in young foals, one must consider two different scenarios: the need for prophylactic therapy in foals treated for other primary disorders and therapeutic administration to those foals in which gastric ulcers have been documented or are suspected. Prophylactic therapy in neonatal foals remains controversial for several reasons. Prolonged periods of gastric alkalinity potentially could allow for alteration of bacterial flora within the gastrointestinal tract, thus increasing the propensity for bacterial translocation across a compromised gastrointestinal mucosal barrier [48]. This is primarily a theoretic concern in the foal, because such a risk has not yet been definitively identified.

The foal's age, condition, and primary disorder should be considered before commencement of therapy. In the severely compromised recumbent neonate, supportive care likely provides more protection against ulcer formation than would any medication directed at the suppression of hydrochloric acid. In this group, hydration, blood pressure, and perfusion should be monitored as closely as possible, with therapeutic alterations made as deemed appropriate. Monitoring of central venous pressure and cardiac output can supplement the more frequently used parameters, such as palpation of peripheral pulses, temperature of the extremities, vital signs, indirect blood pressure, and arterial and venous blood gas analysis, with particular attention to lactate. In the future, methods of monitoring gastric perfusion, such as measurement of intragastric partial pressure of carbon dioxide (pCO_2), may provide more information regarding organ perfusion.

For less severely affected hospitalized foals, documented gastric acidity is contrasted with the reduced frequency of reported ulceration. Thus, prophylactic treatment of this group remains debatable. In ambulatory foals receiving repeated administration of NSAIDs (eg, for musculoskeletal abnormalities) or those with diarrheal disorders, additional ulcerogenic risk factors may warrant prophylactic treatment.

Options for therapy in the foal are similar to those reported in older horses. Histamine type 2 antagonists, such as ranitidine, cimetidine, and famotidine, inhibit gastric acid secretion by competing with histamine type 2 (H_2) receptor sites on the parietal cell [49]. Ranitidine has been shown to increase intragastric pH effectively in normal foals after intravenous (2 mg/kg) or oral (6.6 mg/kg) administration for 4 and 8 hours, respectively [37]. Intravenous administration of ranitidine at the same dose to critically ill foals did not result in a similar consistent response, however [39]. Altered dosing requirements of H_2 receptor antagonists in critically ill human neonates have also been reported [50].

Proton pump inhibitors, such as omeprazole, block hydrogen secretion by irreversibly binding to the hydrogen-potassium-ATPase pump in the gastric glands of functional parietal cells. Omeprazole is the only proton pump inhibitor currently approved by the US Food and Drug Administration (FDA) for use in horses, and oral administration at 4 mg/kg has been shown to increase intragastric pH in normal foals significantly for up to 23 hours [51]. Pantoprazole, another proton pump inhibitor, is available in intravenous and oral preparations. Pantoprazole has recently been evaluated in healthy foals, increasing intragastric pH for at least 24 hours after intravenous or intragastric administration [52]. Because a commercially available intravenous preparation of omeprazole is not currently available, pantoprazole could provide a therapeutic alternative in foals with suspected ulceration in which oral therapy is not possible, such as those with concurrent ileus.

Sucralfate provides an alternative means of therapy. Its postulated mechanism of action involves adherence to ulcerated mucosa, stimulation of mucus secretion, and enhancement of prostaglandin E and epidermal growth factor synthesis [53]. Because these mechanisms primarily relate to glandular mucosa, sucralfate may provide a means of ulcer prophylaxis in severely ill foals without increasing the risk of pathogenic gastric colonization [54], although this risk has not been demonstrated in foals. The recommended dose of sucralfate in foals is 10 to 20 mg/kg administered orally every 6 to 8 hours. Concerns regarding the efficacy of sucralfate in an alkaline gastric environment are controversial but currently seem to be unwarranted [55–57].

Because intravenously administered ranitidine is the only product that has been evaluated in an abnormal population of foals, the application of dosing regimens of all other products to abnormal foals is currently speculative.

Small intestine

Ileus

There are many causes of ileus in neonatal foals. Strangulating obstructive diseases are inherently surgical and are covered in detail in the article in this issue on abdominal surgery. Ileus is a common secondary complication in critically ill human patients and is also common in foals suffering from prematurity, sepsis, or hypoxic-ischemic syndrome (HIS) [58]. Recent investigations into the distribution of interstitial cells of Cajal (ICC) in the equine fetus and neonate have demonstrated that the small intestinal ICC network is relatively advanced in the late-term fetus and neonate at the time of birth [59]. Thus, ICC immaturity is not likely to contribute to ileus in the mild to moderately premature foal.

The cause of damage to the intestinal tract in foals with HIS is likely related to tissue hypoxia, with or without subsequent reperfusion injury. When ischemia and/or reperfusion injury to the gastrointestinal tract is severe, ileus may be mediated in part by upregulation of inducible nitric oxide synthase 2 [60]. Acute hemorrhagic shock can result in an intercellular adhesion molecule-1 (ICAM-1)–mediated intestinal inflammatory response and subsequent ileus in other species [61]. In human beings, the neonatal intestine has low vascular resistance, thus making the newborn gut particularly sensitive to systemic hypotension and hypoxemia [62]. The intestinal tract of foals with sepsis may suffer from an insult directly related to inflammation caused by exposure to bacteria or from the effects of the systemic inflammatory response syndrome.

The pathophysiology of sepsis-induced ileus is currently under intense investigation. Many products of inflammation can result in an alteration of motility [63–66]. Exogenous lipopolysaccharide (LPS) administration results in activation of macrophages within the intestinal muscularis, elaboration of various inflammatory substances, and subsequent recruitment of leukocytes [64,66]. Mediators like prostaglandins and nitric oxide can alter the kinetic properties of intestinal smooth muscle cells [67,68], and inflammatory cytokines can alter enteric neurotransmission [69–71]. In dogs, endotoxin administration abolishes interdigestive migrating motility complexes (MMCs) and decreases interdigestive and digestive duodenal and jejunal action potentials [72]. The pathophysiologic mechanisms of motility alteration differ in models of polymicrobial sepsis-induced ileus from those seen in LPS-induced ileus, however [65]. In these models, neutrophilic infiltration in the jejunal muscularis predominates [65]. Poor organ perfusion, hypoxemia, and resultant interruption of metabolic processes within the body may contribute to further tissue damage, and early hypoperfusion of the gut and resultant ileus can contribute to subsequent multiple organ failure [73].

Clinical signs associated with the development of ileus include gastric reflux or abdominal distention. Often, overt signs of colic are not seen in severely ill foals despite significant reflux or intestinal distention attributable to the obtunded or depressed mentation of the patient. It is therefore crucial to monitor the foal for reflux frequently, especially before each enteral feeding, and to routinely monitor abdominal circumference as described previously.

In critically ill foals, especially when recumbent, enteral feeding is often not well tolerated, especially at the volumes required to provide adequate nutrition. An initial starting point for enteral nutrition in severely ill foals depends somewhat on the individual animal and the clinician's preference. In recumbent foals, the authors prefer to initiate feedings at no more than 5% of the foal's body weight per day, spaced at 1- to 2-hour intervals. This may be gradually increased if the foal is tolerating enteral feedings, especially if the foal is making other clinical improvements. This small amount of milk or milk replacer is insufficient for complete nutrient requirements, however, and should be supplemented with dextrose-containing fluids or partial or total parenteral nutrition. The increased metabolic demands of sepsis should be taken into account when calculating caloric requirements of a septic neonate.

If the foal develops reflux (characterized by a volume of > 50–100 mL of fluid before a feeding), feedings should be discontinued until reflux is no longer obtained and some evidence of motility is noted (increased intestinal borborygmi, passage of feces, or ultrasonographic assessment of motility). Abdominal circumference can be used to determine if distention is becoming significant. Careful evaluation of the abdomen should be performed by ultrasound if possible. With ileus, the small intestine may seem to be filled with fluid and may be hypo- or amotile. Usually, bowel wall thickness is normal with a simple ileus. A thickened intestinal wall may indicate an obstructive disease affecting vasculature or an impending enteritis, and further diagnostics may be necessary. The stomach may be assessed for distention and may indicate the need for further removal of fluid via a nasogastric tube. The presence of increased free abdominal fluid also warrants further investigation.

One should attempt to continue some degree of enteral feeding, even in small volumes, if at all possible. Although the foal can successfully be maintained with parenteral nutrition alone, trophic feeding of enterocytes has been proven to be beneficial to the health and development of the intestinal tract [74,75]. Supportive care, including maintenance of adequate tissue perfusion, normovolemia, normothermia, and nutritional support, is also critical in these foals.

Colon, rectum, and anus

Meconium impaction

Meconium impaction is the most common cause of colic in neonatal foals. Meconium is formed during fetal development and is present in the large colon of the foal at birth. It is made up of sloughed cells, swallowed amniotic fluid, and mucus from the intestinal tract. It is normally passed by the foal beginning within the first few hours of birth and should be passed completely within 48 hours of birth. Recently, the colonic network of ICC has been shown to be immature in the full-term neonate; thus, an immature pacemaker-generating region in the large colon may contribute to meconium retention [59]. Signs of colic in impacted foals may begin several hours to approximately 2 days after birth, but they typically begin from 12 to 24 hours of age. A breed predilection has not been identified, but colts may be overrepresented [76]. Affected foals may display a wide variety of colic signs ranging from decreased suckling and depression to severe signs of pain, such as rolling and marked abdominal distention. Many foals frequently posture and attempt to defecate. A frequently raised tail, tail-flagging even while recumbent, and restlessness may all be signs of colic from meconium impaction. If attempts to defecate are frequent or cannot be distinguished from attempts to urinate, a ruptured bladder should also be considered. The two diseases may occur simultaneously, possibly with a ruptured bladder occurring secondary to an affected foal repeatedly straining to defecate. In sick recumbent neonates with profound depression or abnormal mentation, signs of colic may be more subtle. The foal may have repeated abdominal efforts but an inability to pass feces. Alternately, the only signs may be the foal turning the head to rest on its side or dorsum or attempting to position itself in dorsal recumbency.

Many farms have engaged in the practice of administering prophylactic enemas, often commercially available products, such as Fleet (C.B. Fleet Company, Inc., Lynchburg, Virginia). If meconium impaction is suspected, caretakers should be questioned about the administration of the product, because repeated use of over-the-counter phosphate-containing enema solutions may cause electrolyte disturbances, including, most notably, hyperphosphatemia [77,78].

A diagnosis of meconium impaction may be made based on history, signs of colic, and age of the foal. Per rectum palpation with a gloved well-lubricated finger may reveal the presence of firm meconium at the pelvic inlet. If the foal is relaxed and/or sedated enough to allow for external abdominal palpation, the presence of firm meconium in the large colon or rectum may be felt. If the clinician is still unsure of the location or extent of the impaction, contrast radiography can be used to help identify the impaction [79]. This procedure may also help to distinguish impaction from other diseases, such as colonic atresia or aganglionosis.

Most meconium impactions can be medically managed. First, adequate supportive care should be provided. If the foal is dehydrated, intravenous fluid therapy should be initiated to restore circulating volume. If the foal does not respond to initial therapy and requires continued withdrawal of milk, supplemental nutritional support should be provided in the form of intravenous fluids with dextrose for shorter periods or total parenteral nutrition (TPN) if required. Pain control should be considered for foals that do not respond to an initial enema. Appropriate analgesia may significantly reduce the amount of straining and may allow the bowel to relax. Commonly used analgesics include NSAIDs, such as flunixin meglumine (1 mg/kg administered intravenously up to every 12 hours), and opiates, most commonly butorphanol (2–4 mg administered intravenously or intramuscularly for a typical 50-kg foal). When flunixin is administered, one should always consider the potential for gastric ulceration and nephrotoxicity. Normal hydration status should be maintained, especially if there is concomitant administration of other possible nephrotoxic drugs, such as aminoglycosides. Butorphanol can produce profound sedation, and foals that are still allowed to suckle should be monitored for aspiration if sedative effects are observed and withheld from suckling if aspiration is noted. If the impaction has been long standing or the severity of pain is enough to cause ileus, some foals develop gastric reflux. Thus, in foals with overt abdominal distention or those with repeated discomfort, a nasogastric tube should be placed and the reflux removed intermittently to relieve pain and prevent gastric rupture. If reflux is not present, foals may be administered mineral oil via a nasogastric tube to serve as a laxative. Repeated measurement of abdominal circumference can be used to assess abdominal distention objectively. If bowel distention is severe, the foal should be monitored for tachypnea and dyspnea, because pressure on the diaphragm may affect the foal's ability to properly ventilate.

Enemas are the treatment of choice for meconium retention. Initially, a warm soapy water enema may be administered using a gentle nonirritating soap, such as Ivory (The Proctor & Gamble Company, Cincinatti, Ohio). The enema may be administered with the foal standing or in lateral recumbency. Soft flexible tubing, such as a Foley or stallion catheter, is generously lubricated and gently inserted into the rectum until resistance is met. This can often be a distance of 6 to 10 inches into the rectum, and care should be taken to not use excessive force, thus avoiding rectal tears. A volume of 500 to 1000 mL for a 50-kg foal may be administered by gravity flow only. During administration, the foal may push some fluid out around the sides of the tubing; this should be allowed. After administration, the foal may benefit from standing or walking. If the initial enema is unsuccessful in resolving the impaction, this procedure may be repeated several times. It should be noted that repeated enemas may cause rectal irritation and should be administered only if clinically warranted.

If routine enemas are unsuccessful in resolving the impaction, a retention enema with acetylcysteine may be administered. For this procedure, the foal is sedated and placed in lateral recumbency. A lubricated Foley catheter is inserted into the rectum, and the cuff is inflated to prevent backflow. A mixture of warm water (160 mL) mixed with commercial 20% acetylcysteine (40 mL) is commonly recommended for infusion, with a final concentration of 4% acetylcysteine. If possible, sodium bicarbonate (20 g) should be added to the mixture to adjust pH to an optimum of 7 to 9 [76,80]. The Foley catheter should remain in place for 30 to 45 minutes; the cuff should then be deflated and the catheter removed. Retention enemas have been widely used since their introduction to equine medicine [80]. In a recent retrospective study, 41 of 44 foals responded to medical therapy that included one to three retention enemas [76]. The 3 remaining foals had surgery performed at the request of the owner without acetylcysteine enema therapy. Interestingly, 3 foals (treated medically) from that study developed bladder rupture, which was treated successfully with surgery [76]. This was an improved rate of successful medical therapy relative to previous work in which 8 of 24 foals required surgery [81]. The use of acetylcysteine was initially applied from its use orally and rectally in management of meconium impaction in human infants [82–84]. Acetylcysteine works by cleaving disulfide bonds and decreasing the viscosity of meconium [84]. The mucolytic effect increases along with pH, however, and the maximum effect requires at least 30 minutes of contact.

In occasional severe cases, the impaction may not resolve with medical therapy and may require surgical intervention. Specific discussion of surgical treatment is discussed elsewhere in this issue in the article on abdominal surgery.

Intestinal atresia

Various locations of intestinal atresia have been documented in the foal [85–87]. Atresia of the colon has been reported as an uncommon congenital defect of the foal. The Purdue University Veterinary Medical database (1964–1993) reported occurrence in only 12 of 10,000 horses examined. Other sources indicate an incidence of 3.1% of 1130 horses with congenital abnormalities [1]. The most widely accepted theory of the pathogenesis of intestinal atresia implicates an ischemic vascular event affecting a segment of the bowel during gestation [88,89]. It is theorized that the ischemic event halts growth, causing atrophy and resorption of the affected segment of the bowel. Possible causes for these ischemic events could be volvulus and intussusception. Per rectum palpation of the amniotic vesicle for a pregnancy examination between day 36 and day 42 of gestation has been associated with intestinal atresia in calves [90], but this association has not been found in horses.

Typically foals present within the first 2 to 48 hours of life with progressive signs of colic and abdominal distention. Foals do not pass meconium but may have mucus in the rectum. Attempts to relieve a meconium impaction with an enema are unproductive, and there is a lack of fecal staining in the enema fluid. Foals may also display signs of tenesmus, tachycardia and tachypnea, dehydration, weakness, and anorexia. Contrast radiography may be helpful in positively identifying an atretic colon or in differentiation from other causes of colic. Atresia of the proximal colon, however, may not be identifiable by this method.

Five categories of atresia have been identified in horses. Type I is membrane atresia, in which a membranous diaphragm occludes the lumen of the intestine. Type II is cord atresia, characterized by a fibrous or muscular cord-like remnant of intestine connecting the blind ends of the proximal and distal segments. Type IIIa is blind-end atresia, in which a segment of intestine is absent, the blind ends are disconnected, and the mesentery has a defect that corresponds to the missing intestinal segment. Type IIIb is similar to type IIIa, except that the intestinal segment distal to the mesenteric defect is coiled. In type IV, there are multiple sites of atresia (which can consist of any of the other types) [91]. Surgery is required to determine the extent and exact location of the atresia. Survival is not possible without surgical correction, and the prognosis is guarded even with surgical intervention [87].

Aganglionosis

Intestinal aganglionosis is most commonly seen in foals with the lethal white syndrome (often referred to as the overo lethal white syndrome or lethal white foal syndrome [LWFS]). This defect has recently been described as an autosomal recessive missense mutation in the endothelin B receptor gene [92–94]. Affected foals lack submucosal and myenteric ganglia from the distal small intestine to the large colon [92]. The problem is most commonly seen in American Paint horses born to overo-overo cross-matings but has also been reported in a foal born to a registered Quarter Horse mare [95]. One Clydesdale foal has also been reported with colonic hypoganglionosis, but this does not seem to be the same defect as that seen in foals with LWFS [96]. Foals with LWFS are predominantly white in color and present with signs of colic within 12 to 24 hours of life. Because of the extent of the aganglionosis, effective therapy is not available and euthanasia is recommended. Genetic testing is available and recommended for at-risk horses. An important fact for consideration is that all white foals are not necessarily afflicted with LWFS; thus, one should perform a thorough clinical evaluation or genetic testing before humane destruction of such a foal.

Peritoneal disorders

Chyloabdomen

Few cases of chyloabdomen have been reported in the literature [97,98]. It is an uncommon cause of colic in neonatal foals. Diagnosis is made based on the detection of chylous abdominal fluid. Suspected causes include trauma and congenital defects within the gastrointestinal lymphatic structures. Treatment depends on the causative factors and is not recommended in cases involving congenital defects. For those with suspected trauma, treatment is predominantly supportive.

Septic peritonitis

Septic peritonitis is an infrequent event in the neonatal foal. When present, it can be associated with gastric rupture secondary to gastric ulceration and contamination of the peritoneal cavity secondary to septic omphalitis or omphalophlebitis, especially after surgery to remove affected structures [99–101]. Less common causes are numerous but include trauma and severe enterocolitis resulting in bacterial translocation. Clinical signs include colic, fever, depression, and other clinical signs associated with sepsis or endotoxemia. Diagnosis is based on ultrasonographic findings and results of abdominocentesis. Treatment is not indicated in cases of gastrointestinal rupture, and the prognosis is poor regardless of the inciting cause.

Summary

Neonates can have a variety of gastrointestinal disorders, primary and secondary in nature. Important primary disorders include congenital abnormalities and meconium retention. One of the most important secondary lesions is generalized ileus. Gastric ulceration can occur as a primary or secondary event. This article addresses the pathophysiology, diagnosis, and treatment of gastrointestinal problems commonly observed in neonatal foals.

References

[1] Crowe MW, Swerczek TW. Equine congenital defects. Am J Vet Res 1985;46:353–8.
[2] Gaughan EM, DeBowes RM. Congenital diseases of the equine head. Vet Clin North Am Equine Pract 1993;9:93–110.
[3] Platt H. Etiological aspects of perinatal mortality in the Thoroughbred. Equine Vet J 1973; 5:116–20.
[4] Batstone JH. Cleft palate in the horse. Br J Plast Surg 1966;19:327–31.
[5] Bowman KF, Tate LP Jr, Evans LH, et al. Complications of cleft palate repair in large animals. J Am Vet Med Assoc 1982;180:652–7.
[6] Cook WR. Surgical repair of cleft soft palate in the horse. Vet Rec 1977;100:326.
[7] De Geus JJ, Jones RS, Lovius BB, et al. Surgical repair of cleft soft palate in the horse. Vet Rec 1977;100:145.
[8] Jones RS. Surgical repair of cleft palate in the horse. Equine Vet J 1975;7:86–90.
[9] Kirkham LE, Vasey JR. Surgical cleft soft palate repair in a foal. Aust Vet J 2002;80:143–6.
[10] Mason TA, Speirs VC, Maclean AA, et al. Surgical repair of cleft soft palate in the horse. Vet Rec 1977;100:6–8.
[11] Stickle RL, Goble DO, Braden TD. Surgical repair of cleft soft palate in a foal. Vet Med Small Anim Clin 1973;68:159–62.
[12] Stick JA, Boles C. Subepiglottic cyst in three foals. J Am Vet Med Assoc 1980;177:62–4.
[13] Shappell KK, Caron JP, Stick JA, et al. Staphylectomy for treatment of dorsal displacement of the soft palate in two foals. J Am Vet Med Assoc 1989;195:1395–8.
[14] Yarbrough TB, Voss E, Herrgesell EJ, et al. Persistent frenulum of the epiglottis in four foals. Vet Surg 1999;28:287–91.
[15] Barton MH. Nasal regurgitation of milk in foals. Compend Contin Educ Pract Vet 1993;15: 81–91.
[16] Wilkins PA, Palmer JE. Botulism in foals less than 6 months of age: 30 cases (1989–2002). J Vet Intern Med 2003;17:702–7.

[17] Lofstedt J. White muscle disease of foals. Vet Clin North Am Equine Pract 1997;13:169–85.

[18] McClure JJ, Addison JD, Miller RI. Immunodeficiency manifested by oral candidiasis and bacterial septicemia in foals. J Am Vet Med Assoc 1985;186:1195–7.

[19] Reilly LK, Palmer JE. Systemic candidiasis in four foals. J Am Vet Med Assoc 1994;205: 464–6.

[20] Gross TL, Mayhew IG. Gastroesophageal ulceration and candidiasis in foals. J Am Vet Med Assoc 1983;182:1370–3.

[21] Hendrix DVH, Ward DA, Guglick MA. Disseminated candidiasis in a neonatal foal with keratomycosis as the initial sign. Vet Comp Ophthalmol 1997;7:10–3.

[22] Madison JB, Reid BV, Raskin RE. Amphotericin-B treatment of Candida-arthritis in 2 horses. J Am Vet Med Assoc 1995;206:338–41.

[23] Gaughan EM, Gift LJ, Frank RK. Tubular duplication of the cervical portion of the esophagus in a foal. J Am Vet Med Assoc 1992;201:748–50.

[24] Rohrbach BW. Congenital esophageal ectasia in a thoroughbred foal. J Am Vet Med Assoc 1980;177:65–7.

[25] Clabough DL, Roberts MC, Robertson I. Probable congenital esophageal stenosis in a thoroughbred foal. J Am Vet Med Assoc 1991;199:483–5.

[26] Smith TR. Unusual vascular ring anomaly in a foal. Can Vet J 2004;45:1016–8.

[27] Bowman KF, Vaughan JT, Quick CB, et al. Megaesophagus in a colt. J Am Vet Med Assoc 1978;172:334–7.

[28] Murray MJ, Ball MM, Parker GA. Megaesophagus and aspiration pneumonia secondary to gastric ulceration in a foal. J Am Vet Med Assoc 1988;192:381–3.

[29] King JN, Davies JV, Gerring EL. Contrast radiography of the equine oesophagus: effect of spasmolytic agents and passage of a nasogastric tube. Equine Vet J 1990;22:133–5.

[30] Murray MJ, Murray CM, Sweeney HJ, et al. Prevalence of gastric lesions in foals without signs of gastric disease: an endoscopic survey. Equine Vet J 1990;22:6–8.

[31] Murray MJ. Endoscopic appearance of gastric lesions in foals: 94 cases (1987–1988). J Am Vet Med Assoc 1989;195:1135–41.

[32] Murray MJ, Grodinsky C, Cowles RR, et al. Endoscopic evaluation of changes in gastric lesions of Thoroughbred foals. J Am Vet Med Assoc 1990;196:1623–7.

[33] Cudd TA. Gastrointestinal system dysfunction. In: Koterba AM, Drummond WH, Kosch PC, editor. Equine clinical neonatology. 1st edition. Philadelphia: Lea & Febiger; 1990. p. 367–442.

[34] Murray MJ, Mahaffey EA. Age-related characteristics of gastric squamous epithelial mucosa in foals. Equine Vet J 1993;25:514–7.

[35] Murray MJ. Aetiopathogenesis and treatment of peptic ulcer in the horse: a comparative review. Equine Vet J Suppl 1992;13:63–74.

[36] Andrews FM, Bernard WV, Byars TD, et al. Recommendations for the diagnosis and treatment of equine gastric ulcer syndrome (EGUS). Equine Vet Educ 1999;1:122–34.

[37] Sanchez LC, Lester GD, Merritt AM. Effect of ranitidine on intragastric pH in clinically normal neonatal foals. J Am Vet Med Assoc 1998;212:1407–12.

[38] Baker SJ, Gerring EL. Gastric pH monitoring in healthy, suckling pony foals. Am J Vet Res 1993;54:959–64.

[39] Sanchez LC, Lester GD, Merritt AM. Intragastric pH in critically ill neonatal foals and the effect of ranitidine. J Am Vet Med Assoc 2001;218:907–11.

[40] Kuusela AL. Long-term gastric pH monitoring for determining optimal dose of ranitidine for critically ill preterm and term neonates. Arch Dis Child Fetal Neonatal Ed 1998; 78(Suppl):F151–3.

[41] Argenzio RA. Comparative pathophysiology of nonglandular ulcer disease: a review of experimental studies. Equine Vet J Suppl 1999;(29):19–23.

[42] Mertz HR, Walsh JH. Peptic ulcer pathophysiology. Med Clin North Am 1991;75:799–814.

[43] Murray MJ. Pathophysiology of peptic disorders in foals and horses: a review. Equine Vet J Suppl 1999;(29):14–8.

[44] Green EM, Sprouse RF, Jones BD. Is *Helicobacter (Campylobacter) pylori* associated with gastritis/ulcer disease in asymptomatic foals [abstract]? Proc Equine Colic Res Symp 1991; 4:27.

[45] Scott DR, Marcus EA, Shirazi-Beechey SSP, et al. Evidence of Helicobacter infection in the horse. In: Proceedings of the American Society of Microbiology 2001. p. D-56.

[46] Nord KS. Peptic ulcer disease in the pediatric population. Pediatr Clin North Am 1988;35: 117–40.

[47] Barr BS, Wilkins PA, Del Piero F, et al. Is prophylaxis for gastric ulcers necessary in critically ill equine neonates?: a retrospective study of necropsy cases 1989–1999 [abstract]. J Vet Intern Med 2000;14(3):328.

[48] Cothran DS, Borowitz SM, Sutphen JL, et al. Alteration of normal gastric flora in neonates receiving ranitidine. J Perinatol 1997;17:383–8.

[49] Feldman M, Burton ME. Histamine 2-receptor antagonists. Standard therapy for acid-peptic diseases. 1. N Engl J Med 1990;323:1672–80.

[50] Harrison AM, Lugo RA, Vernon DD. Gastric pH control in critically ill children receiving intravenous ranitidine. Crit Care Med 1998;26:1433–6.

[51] Sanchez LC, Murray MJ, Merritt AM. Effect of omeprazole paste on intragastric pH in clinically normal neonatal foals. Am J Vet Res 2004;65:1039–41.

[52] Ryan CA, Sanchez LC, Giguere S, et al. Pharmacokinetics and pharmacodynamics of pantoprazole in clinically normal neonatal foals. Equine Vet J 2005;37(4), in press.

[53] Ogihara Y, Okabe S. Effect and mechanism of sucralfate on healing of acetic acid-induced gastric ulcers in rats. J Physiol Pharmacol 1993;44:109–18.

[54] Ephgrave KS, Kleiman-Wexler R, Pfaller M, et al. Effects of sucralfate vs antacids on gastric pathogens: results of a double-blind clinical trial. Arch Surg 1998;133:251–7.

[55] Danesh BJ, Duncan A, Russell RI. Is an acid pH medium required for the protective effect of sucralfate against mucosal injury? Am J Med 1987,83:11–3.

[56] Danesh JZ, Duncan A, Russell RI, et al. Effect of intragastric pH on mucosal protective action of sucralfate. Gut 1988;29:1379–85.

[57] Konturek SJ, Brzozowski T, Mach T, et al. Importance of an acid milieu in the sucralfate-induced gastroprotection against ethanol damage. Scand J Gastroenterol 1989;24:807–12.

[58] Bauer AJ, Schwarz NT, Moore BA, et al. Ileus in critical illness: mechanisms and management. Curr Opin Crit Care 2002;8:152–7.

[59] Fintl C, Pearson GT, Ricketts SW, et al. The development and distribution of the interstitial cells of Cajal in the intestine of the equine fetus and neonate. J Anat 2004;205:35–44.

[60] Hassoun HT, Weisbrodt NW, Mercer DW, et al. Inducible nitric oxide synthase mediates gut ischemia/reperfusion-induced ileus only after severe insults. J Surg Res 2001;97:150–4.

[61] Kalff JC, Hierholzer C, Tsukada K, et al. Hemorrhagic shock results in intestinal muscularis intercellular adhesion molecule (ICAM-1) expression, neutrophil infiltration, and smooth muscle dysfunction. Arch Orthop Trauma Surg 1999;119:89–93.

[62] Reber KM, Nankervis CA, Nowicki PT. Newborn intestinal circulation. Physiology and pathophysiology. Clin Perinatol 2002;29:23–39.

[63] Eskandari MK, Kalff JC, Billiar TR, et al. LPS-induced muscularis macrophage nitric oxide suppresses rat jejunal circular muscle activity. Am J Physiol 1999;277:G478–86.

[64] Eskandari MK, Kalff JC, Billiar TR, et al. Lipopolysaccharide activates the muscularis macrophage network and suppresses circular smooth muscle activity. Am J Physiol 1997; 273:G727–34.

[65] Overhaus M, Togel S, Pezzone MA, et al. Mechanisms of polymicrobial sepsis-induced ileus. Am J Physiol Gastrointest Liver Physiol 2004;287:G685–94.

[66] Schwarz NT, Engel B, Eskandari MK, et al. Lipopolysaccharide preconditioning and cross-tolerance: the induction of protective mechanisms for rat intestinal ileus. Gastroenterology 2002;123:586–98.

[67] Nathan CF. Secretory products of macrophages. J Clin Invest 1987;79:319–26.

[68] Sweet MJ, Hume DA. Endotoxin signal transduction in macrophages. J Leukoc Biol 1996; 60:8–26.

[69] Hurst S, Collins SM. Interleukin-1 beta modulation of norepinephrine release from rat myenteric nerves. Am J Physiol Gastrointest Liver Physiol 1993;264:G30–5.

[70] Galeazzi F, Haapala EM, van Rooijen N, et al. Inflammation-induced impairment of enteric nerve function in nematode-infected mice is macrophage dependent. Am J Physiol Gastrointest Liver Physiol 2000;278:G259–65.

[71] Lodato RF, Khan AR, Zembowicz MJ, et al. Roles of IL-1 and TNF in the decreased ileal muscle contractility induced by lipopolysaccharide. Am J Physiol 1999;276:G1356–62.

[72] Cullen JJ, Ephgrave KS, Caropreso DK. Gastrointestinal myoelectric activity during endotoxemia. Am J Surg 1996;171:596–9.

[73] Hassoun HT, Kone BC, Mercer DW, et al. Post-injury multiple organ failure: the role of the gut. Shock 2001;15:1–10.

[74] Buchman AL, Moukarzel AA, Bhuta S, et al. Parenteral nutrition is associated with intestinal morphologic and functional changes in humans. Journal of Parenteral and Enteral Nutrition 1995;19:453–60.

[75] Wildhaber BE, Yang H, Spencer AU, et al. Lack of enteral nutrition—effects on the intestinal immune system. J Surg Res 2005;123:8–16.

[76] Pusterla N, Magdesian KG, Maleski K, et al. Retrospective evaluation of the use of acetylcysteine enemas in the treatment of meconium retention in foals: 44 cases (1987–2002). Equine Vet Educ 2004;16:133–6.

[77] Marraffa JM, Hui A, Stork CM. Severe hyperphosphatemia and hypocalcemia following the rectal administration of a phosphate-containing Fleet pediatric enema. Pediatr Emerg Care 2004;20:453–6.

[78] Hickman SA, Gill MS, Marks SL, et al. Phosphate enema toxicosis in a pygmy goat wether. Can Vet J 2004;45:849–51.

[79] Fischer AT, Yarbrough TY. Retrograde contrast radiography of the distal portions of the intestinal tract in foals. J Am Vet Med Assoc 1995;207:734–7.

[80] Madigan JE, Goetzman BW. Use of acetylcysteine solution enema for meconium retention in the neonatal foal. Proc Am Assoc Equine Pract 1990;36:117–9.

[81] Hughes FE, Moll HD, Slone DE. Outcome of surgical correction of meconium impactions in 8 foals. J Equine Vet Sci 1996;16:172–5.

[82] Burke MS, Ragi JM, Karamanoukian HL, et al. New strategies in nonoperative management of meconium ileus. J Pediatr Surg 2002;37:760–4.

[83] Lillibridge CB, Docter JM, Eidelman S. Oral administration of N-acetyl cysteine in the prophylaxis of "meconium ileus equivalent." J Pediatr 1967;71:887–9.

[84] Shaw A. Safety of N-acetylcysteine in treatment of meconium obstruction of the newborn. J Pediatr Surg 1969;4:119–25.

[85] Anderson WI, King JM, Rothwell JT. Segmental atresia of the transverse colon in a foal with concurrent equine herpes virus-1 infection. Cornell Vet 1987;77:119–21.

[86] van der Gaag I, Tibboel D. Intestinal atresia and stenosis in animals: a report of 34 cases. Vet Pathol 1980;17:565–74.

[87] Young RL, Linford RL, Olander HJ. Atresia coli in the foal: a review of six cases. Equine Vet J 1992;24:60–2.

[88] Louw JH. Investigations into etiology of congenital atresia of colon. Dis Colon Rectum 1964;7:471–8.

[89] Louw JH, Barnard CN. Congenital intestinal atresia—observations on its origin. Lancet 1955;2:1065–7.

[90] Leipold HW, Saperstein G, Johnson DD, et al. Intestinal atresia in calves. Vet Med Small Anim Clin 1976;71:1037–9.

[91] Benamou AE, Blikslager AT, Sellon DC. Intestinal atresia in foals. Compend Contin Educ Pract Vet 1995;17:1510–7.

[92] Metallinos DL, Bowling AT, Rine J. A missense mutation in the endothelin-B receptor gene is associated with Lethal White Foal Syndrome: an equine version of Hirschsprung disease. Mamm Genome 1998;9:426–31.

[93] Santschi EM, Purdy AK, Valberg SJ, et al. Endothelin receptor B polymorphism associated with lethal white foal syndrome in horses. Mamm Genome 1998;9:306–9.

[94] Yang GC, Croaker D, Zhang AL, et al. A dinucleotide mutation in the endothelin-B receptor gene is associated with lethal white foal syndrome (LWFS); a horse variant of Hirschsprung disease. Hum Mol Genet 1998;7:1047 52.

[95] Lightbody T. Foal with Overo lethal white syndrome born to a registered quarter horse mare. Can Vet J 2002;43:715–7.

[96] Murray MJ, Parker GA, White NA. Megacolon with myenteric hypoganglionosis in a foal. J Am Vet Med Assoc 1988;192:917–9.

[97] Campbell-Beggs CL, Johnson PJ, Wilson DA, et al. Chyloabdomen in a neonatal foal. Vet Rec 1995;137:96–8.

[98] Hanselaer JR, Nyland TG. Chyloabdomen and ultrasonographic detection of an intra-abdominal abscess in a foal. J Am Vet Med Assoc 1983;183:1465–7.

[99] Becht JL, Byars TD. Gastroduodenal ulceration in foals. Equine Vet J 1986;18:307–12.

[100] Murray MJ. Gastric ulceration in horses: 91 cases (1987–1990). J Am Vet Med Assoc 1992; 201:117–20.

[101] Reef VB, Collatos C, Spencer PA, et al. Clinical, ultrasonographic, and surgical findings in foals with umbilical remnant infections. J Am Vet Med Assoc 1989;195:69–72.

VETERINARY
CLINICS
Equine Practice

ELSEVIER
SAUNDERS

Vet Clin Equine 21 (2005) 333–355

Maturity of the Neonatal Foal

Guy D. Lester, BVMS, PhD

*Department of Veterinary Clinical Sciences, School of Veterinary and Biomedical Sciences,
Murdoch University, Murdoch 6150, Western Australia*

The immature foal frequently represents a significant management challenge to even the most experienced clinician. The clinical course typically involves complications to a range of body systems, including the musculoskeletal, respiratory, and gastrointestinal tract systems. Before the commencement of treatment, it is important to provide the owner with an estimation of short-term and long-term survival, expected costs, and possible complications. Formulation of an accurate prognosis can be a difficult task but is aided by knowledge not only of normal maturation but of the factors that affect this process.

Normal gestational period

In contrast to most other domesticated species, the duration of the gestational period in mares is variable. The gestational age is typically calculated from the day of insemination to the day of parturition, a value that may overestimate the true gestational period by as much as 7 days. Although the mean gestational length in the Thoroughbred breed is consistently reported to be from 340 to 342 days [1–5], the range of normal gestational ages is wide. In a study from Newmarket in England, 95% of mares foaled from 327 to 357 days of pregnancy [1]. The mean duration of pregnancy also seems to be relatively consistent across breeds. In a study of Friesian births in the Netherlands, the mean length of gestation was 331.6 days [6], whereas another study from the same country reported a figure of 337.7 days [7]. The mean gestational age for Arabian foals in Egypt was 332 days [8], 336.5 days in Dutch Freiberger mares [9], and 343.3 days in draught breeds [7]. Gestational length was shorter in pony mares in studies from the United Kingdom, with a mean of 333 days and a range of 315 to 350 days in one study [5] and a mean of 325 days in another [10]. Bos and van der May [7]

E-mail address: g.lester@murdoch.edu.au

reported values similar to Thoroughbred mares for Haflinger ponies (341.3 days), Fjord ponies (342.2 days), and Shetland ponies (337.2 days) in the Netherlands.

There are several factors that seem to determine the length of gestation in mares. Numerous studies have reported that colts, on average, have a longer gestation than fillies. The reported difference in gestational age between colts and fillies is approximately 1.5 to 2.5 days [2–4,6]. Colts are also heavier than fillies, have a heavier placenta, and take slightly longer to stand [4]. The time of conception within the breeding season has an impact on the duration of the gestational period. Mares that conceive early in the breeding season experience longer pregnancies than those bred toward the end of season. This difference in gestation may be as great as 10 days [1,2]. The year of breeding may influence the duration of pregnancy, but specific year-to-year factors, such as changes in weather patterns or feed, have not been elucidated [3]. Furthermore, this finding has not been consistent in all studies [2].

An influence of the mare, sire, and dam's sire on gestational length was recently reported in Friesian mares [6]. A significant effect of the sire was again reported in the Freiberger breed [9]. An Australian study of Thoroughbred mares concluded that the dam but not the sire, in addition to foal gender and month of conception, had a significant effect on the duration of pregnancy [2]. The age or parity of the mare does not seem to influence the length of gestation [2,3]. Twinning is also an important cause of shortened gestational periods and in utero growth retardation [11].

Definitions and terminology

The terminology associated with birth maturity in most species is straightforward but is clouded in the mare because of the variability in gestational length. Retrospective studies often report wide variability in gestational age but do not report physical characteristics or survival of foals. For example, Hintz and colleagues [3] reported a range of 305 to 365 days based on data collected from a large Canadian Thoroughbred stud over a period of 18 years. An Australian study, again using Thoroughbred data, reported a range of 315 to 387 days [2], and a study of Japanese mares described a range of 286 to 370 days [12]. The term *premature* in human beings and other domesticated animals refers to the birth of an infant or animal after a gestational period shorter than normal. A premature human infant was once classified based on birth weight (less than 2500 g) but is now defined according to gestational age. The Department of Reproductive Health and Research of the World Health Organization in Geneva defines a preterm human infant as one delivered at least 21 days before the mean pregnancy duration of 266 days.

The use of gestational age to classify equine prematurity has been described in the equine literature despite the reported variability in the duration of the normal gestational period. The most commonly used definition is a foal born before 320 days of gestation [5]. This definition was based on studies that reported significantly lower birth weights and poor outcomes of foals born before 320 days [13]. It could also be argued that foals born outside the lower 95% confidence interval of the normal gestational period would best fit the classification of premature; this would be less than 327 days according to Rossdale and Short [1] or less than 325 days using data extrapolated from Hintz and colleagues [3]. It is clear that any precise classification of prematurity based solely on estimated gestational age would falsely classify a small number of appropriately mature animals.

There are similar difficulties in classifying animals that have experienced a longer than normal gestational period. Again, using the upper confidence interval limits based on data collected from Rossdale and Short [1] and extrapolated from Hintz and colleagues [3], foals born after 357 days or after 356 days, respectively, should be regarded as postterm foals. A distinction should be made between postterm and postmature, however, with the latter describing a condition of increased neonatal morbidity as a consequence of failing placental function.

Dysmaturity is a term commonly used to describe foals that have experienced some degree of intrauterine growth retardation. These foals typically demonstrate some signs of physical immaturity, such as low birth weight, despite having a "normal" gestational age.

Other terms that have been used to classify foals with incomplete maturation include *viable* and *nonviable* [13] and *ready* or *unready for birth* [14]. In a review on terminology, Koterba [13] suggested that the terms *viable* and *nonviable* were inappropriate, because the outcomes of premature foals are heavily influenced by access to facilities and the value of the animal. The concept of "readiness for birth" was used to categorize foal outcomes, based primarily on the degree of maturation of the fetal hypothalamus-pituitary-adrenal (HPA) axis. Although this plays a critical role in determining postpartum survival, other factors, including the degree of physical maturation and the consequences of an adverse intrauterine environment, are also highly relevant in determining the ultimate outcome [13]. Premature maturation of the HPA axis often takes place at an inappropriate developmental stage for some body systems, causing asynchrony of organ maturation and significant postnatal problems [15]. Proceeding on from the concept of readiness for birth, Rossdale [5] introduced the term *twilight foals* to describe those foals with accelerated but incomplete maturation of the HPA axis at the time of birth [16].

Physical characteristics

The physical characteristics associated with prematurity include low birth weight and small body size, a short and shiny hair coat, a prominent rounded head, periarticular laxity, and droopy ears (Fig. 1). Premature foals typically have moderate flexor laxity with elevation of the toe, but some have contracture of the fetlock. Muscle development is usually poor. Most demonstrate generalized weakness and hypotonia and have difficulty in standing. Severely premature foals may have eyelids naturally sutured closed and little hair covering of their body (Fig. 2).

Postmature foals usually have an acceptable birth weight, with a large frame but poor muscle development. This gives the foal a lanky appearance. In contrast to premature animals, fetlock contracture is common, although laxity can also be seen. Consistent with their prolonged gestation, postterm or postmature foals often have erupted incisors and a long hair coat. In term foals, the central incisors typically erupt during the first 5 to 7 days of postnatal life.

Causes

The pregnant uterus is highly responsive to contractile agents, such as oxytocin and prostaglandins, throughout gestation. Consequently, one of

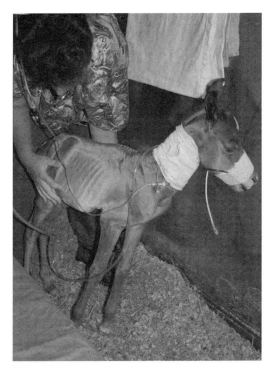

Fig. 1. A Quarter Horse foal demonstrates some of the physical features of immaturity. These include a small body size, domed head, and short and silky hair coat.

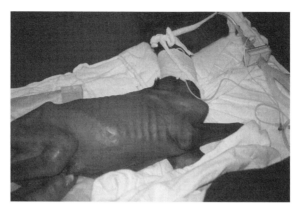

Fig. 2. A premature Thoroughbred foal taken by caesarean section after approximately 275 days of gestation.

the most important causes of premature birth and perinatal morbidity and mortality is the induction of labor with exogenous oxytocin or prostaglandins. Leadon and coworkers [17] highlighted the adverse consequences of premature induction of parturition in a study in which parturition was chemically induced in 49 mares before 300 days of gestation and in 31 mares from 300 to 320 days. The overall survival rate was only 5%, with the youngest surviving animal delivered after 318 days of gestation. Other surviving foals were all delivered after 320 days of gestation. The decision to terminate a pregnancy prematurely may be made deliberately in the normal mare or may be forced on the veterinarian and owner because of catastrophic disease of the mare. The latter frequently involves delivery of a compromised and often premature foal by caesarean section. Chemical induction of parturition has occurred when late pregnancy intestinal disturbances are misinterpreted as ineffective labor.

Premature birth can occur as a sequela to infectious or noninfectious placental problems. These include placental infection, edema, or detachment (premature placental separation). Placental insufficiency attributable to twinning is another cause of intrauterine growth retardation.

The consumption of tall fescue pasture infected with the endophyte *Neotyphodium coenophialum* by pregnant mares leads to range of abnormal signs that include prolongation of gestation, perinatal mortality, and agalactia [18]. The large skeletal frame of the postmature foal predisposes mares to dystocia. The delay in parturition may be attributable to toxin-induced interference with fetal corticotropin-releasing hormone (CRH) and delay in maturation of the HPA axis. Foals born to mares grazing endophyte-infected fescue pasture have normal thyroxine (T4) and reverse tri-iodothyronine (T3) levels but reduced T3 levels compared with control foals [19]. This is also consistent with failure of cortisol-induced maturation of thyroid function. A syndrome of congenital hypothyroidism has been reported in foals in western Canada [20]. Signs include prolonged gestation; dysmaturity; and a range of musculoskeletal abnormalities, including flexural deformities, delayed ossification, and mandibular prognathia. The specific cause has not been determined, although consumption of diets that contain nitrate or are deficient in iodine are suspected [21].

Steroidogenesis during pregnancy

Steroid hormones are synthesized and secreted throughout pregnancy, particularly during the latter half [22]. The fetoplacental unit using precursors secreted by enlarged fetal gonads synthesizes estrogens. Progesterone (P4) and 5α-reduced progestogens are synthesized from maternal precursors (Fig. 3). Progestogens are likely important for maintenance of myometrial quiescence and may inhibit 3β-hydroxysteroid dehydrogenase (HSD), thereby restricting further progestogen synthesis [23].

Interestingly, total progestogen levels can still rise in the face of 3β-HSD blockade, prompting Schtuzer and Holtan [24] to describe an alternative pathway of progestogen metabolism, where pregnenolone (P5) is converted to 3β-hydroxy-5α-pregnan-20-one and then to 5α-pregnane-20-dione by the

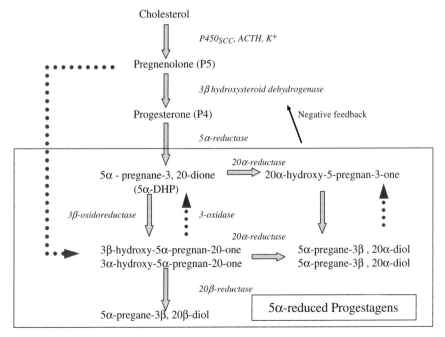

Fig. 3. Pathway of cholesterol metabolism during pregnancy in the mare. (*Adapted from* Ousey JC. Peripartal endocrinology in the mare and foetus. Reprod Domest Anim 2004;39(4):223; with permission.)

enzyme 5α-reductase (see Fig. 3). Near term, additional P5 is secreted by the fetal adrenal glands so that the mare exhibits the unusual phenomenon of foaling while maternal serum progestogen concentrations are increasing and estrogen concentrations are decreasing [25]. The increase in total progestogen concentration during the final weeks of gestation is followed by a rapid decline in the hours to days before birth. The increase in total progestogens coincides with mammary gland development. The decline in concentration before parturition coincides with maturation of the fetal HPA axis and the increase in fetal cortisol.

Maturation of the fetal hypothalamic-pituitary-adrenal axis

The final maturation of several key organ systems seems to be related to changes in the fetal HPA axis that occur in the latter stages of pregnancy [15]. Fetal cortisol is important in terms of organ maturation, but early or excessive levels have been associated intrauterine growth restriction in some species. Consequently, mechanisms are in place to protect the fetus from cortisol during much of gestation. The enzyme 11β-HSD exists in two forms, type 1 and type 2. Type 2 converts excess biologically active cortisol into the inactive 11-oxo derivative cortisone in the placenta, thereby reducing the exposure of the fetus to maternal glucocorticoids during pregnancy. Exposure to prostaglandins before parturition results in upregulation of 11β-HSD type 1, which favors the production of cortisol from cortisone [26]. Reduced placental activity of 11β-HSD type 2 is associated with low birth weight and severe fetal distress in human neonates [27]. The relative proportions of these isoforms have yet to be determined in the equine placenta [22].

The postnatal adrenal gland, under influence of corticotropin (adrenocorticotropic hormone) from the pituitary, can readily synthesize cortisol from cholesterol and P5 (Fig. 4). Several important enzymes are required for this conversion, including 3β-HSD, P450scc, and P450C17. These enzymes are inhibited or deficient during most of pregnancy, again protecting the developing fetus from excessive cortisol exposure during development. Consequently, during most of gestation, the major products of steroidogenesis are P4 and the 5α-reduced progestogens (see Fig. 3) [22].

Foals, like other species studied, undergo enhanced adrenal activity before birth. This is reflected by high plasma cortisol and corticotropin concentrations in term newborn foal plasma in the first hours after birth [28]. There is also a substantial change in the amount and localization within the adrenal gland of 3β-HSD, P450scc, and P450C17 (also referred to as 17α-hydroxylase) around the time of birth [29].

The trigger, or triggers, for the process that results in fetal cortisol production, organ maturation, and birth are not known. Data derived from ovine studies indicate that the process begins with upregulation of CRH mRNA in the fetal hypothalamus and pro-opiomelanocortin (POMC) in the

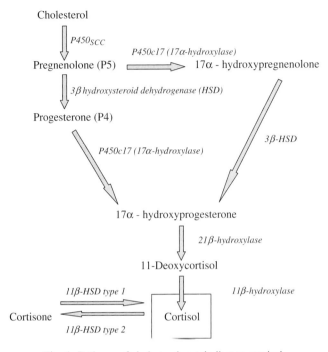

Fig. 4. Pathway of cholesterol metabolism to cortisol.

fetal pituitary gland [15,30]. At the same time, there is upregulation of corticotropin receptors and key steroidogenic enzymes in the fetal adrenal glands. The consequence is a progressive increase in circulating corticotropin and cortisol in the fetus.

According to Challis and his colleagues [15,26,30], the rise in fetal cortisol has a direct effect on the placenta to increase prostaglandin H synthase 2 (PGH_2), leading to secretion of prostaglandins like PGE_2. Prostaglandins further stimulate the fetal HPA axis, stimulate placental 11β-HSD-1 (which favors the production of cortisol from cortisone), and also facilitate the conversion of estrogen from P5. It is arguable whether or not these events also occur in the pregnant mare, but they do seem to be consistent across most species studied. In contrast to other species, the mare foals in the face of a declining concentration of estrogen. Estrogens are clearly important in the birthing process, and several investigators have demonstrated an association with uterine myoelectric activity and the concentration of estradiol-17β [31,32].

An important difference between equids and other species is the timing of these events before parturition [15]. In pregnant ewes, maturation of the HPA axis occurs during the final 20 days of a 150-day gestation. In contrast, the production of significant fetal cortisol seems to occur during the final 48 to 72 hours of pregnancy in mares [33]. There are a number of important maturational events that seem to be tightly associated with the prepartum increase in corticotropin and cortisol [22]. These include changes in red and white blood cell parameters, most notably a large increase in the neutrophil-to-lymphocyte (N/L) ratio [33,34]. Fowden and colleagues [35] reported that hepatic and renal glucose-6-phosphatase, a key enzyme of gluconeogenesis, also increased sharply around the time of birth. This coincided with increases in hepatic and skeletal muscle glycogen stores.

In fetal sheep, the prepartum rise in plasma cortisol induces deiodination of the outer ring of T4 to produce the biologically active T3 [36]. Adequate levels of T3 are required for a number of biologic functions, including postnatal thermogenesis. Normal-term foals have high levels of thyroid hormones, including T3, at the time of birth [37]. These levels decline over the initial weeks or months of postnatal life. A relation between circulating (T3) levels and cortisol was reported in premature, dysmature, and mature foals [16]. The increase in T3 seems to be dependent on maturation of the HPA axis, because adrenalectomy in fetal sheep prevents the prepartum rise [38]. Cortisol and T3 seem to be critical in lung maturation, particularly with respect to the normal postpartum reabsorption of lung liquid [38].

Renal and pulmonary angiotensin-converting enzyme (ACE) levels increase from day 250 to a peak concentration around term before declining during the neonatal period [39]. The increase in pulmonary ACE may be related to the prepartum surge in fetal cortisol, and the authors suggested that premature foals have reduced ACE levels and retardation of the renin-angiotensin system. Fetal blood pressure increases and heart rate falls progressively during late gestation in lambs, and, again, the increase is a direct consequence of maturation of the HPA axis and the production of cortisol [36].

Accelerated maturation of the fetal hypothalamus-pituitary-adrenal axis

There are several factors that can induce premature maturation of the fetal HPA axis. Hypoxemia is a potent stimulator of the axis in sheep, with rises in fetal corticotropin and cortisol [40]. The insult is associated with expression of CRH mRNA in the hypothalamus, POMC mRNA in the pituitary, and upregulation of corticotropin receptors and steroidogenic enzymes in the adrenal cortex [15]. The HPA axis can also be manipulated using exogenous glucocorticoids; betamethasone is commonly administered to women in danger of preterm birth to hasten HPA maturation and therefore improve the chances of postnatal survival. Poor nutrition before and after conception in sheep produces a shortened gestational period and hastened maturation of the fetal HPA axis [30]. Placental or fetal infection also can accelerate maturation of the HPA axis. The cytokines induced by infection increase prostaglandin synthesis and decrease metabolism. Prostaglandins exert a range of actions in addition to promoting cortisol production.

The stimuli associated with precocious HPA axis maturation in foals are not well described. The exception is infection of fetal membranes, where foals are often delivered before term with laboratory findings consistent with axis maturation. Spatial and nutritional deprivation resulting from a Thoroughbred foal placed in a pony uterus using embryo transfer resulted in a premature rise in maternal plasma progestogen concentration consistent with fetal stress and premature maturation of the fetal adrenal, with increased fetal secretion of P5 and subsequent metabolism to reduced progestogens by the placenta [10]. These foals also had increased plasma cortisol consistent with in utero stress [41].

Clinical experience would indicate that many late-gestation maternal problems do not have a significant effect on foal maturity. It is not uncommon for mares to deliver preterm foals after a stressful incident, such as the hypotension and hypoxemia associated general anesthesia. Santschi and coworkers [42] reported that when hypoxemia occurred during colic surgery in mares during the final 60 days of pregnancy, there was a high rate of abortion or preterm delivery of compromised foals that did not survive. It is likely that the insult in these cases was so severe that the interval between surgery and delivery was inadequate for maturation of the axis to occur. Another important consideration in determining outcomes would be the effect of hypoxia or ischemia on other fetal organ systems.

Treatment of the at-risk late pregnant mare

Improvements in human antenatal therapy have reduced the morbidity and mortality associated with preterm birth. The most common approach in human medicine is to administer corticosteroids to the pregnant mother at risk for preterm birth. Administration of corticosteroids to the dam seems to have little effect on maturation of the HPA axis in foals, at least at levels that are considered safe for the mare [5]. Direct injection of corticotropin$_{1-24}$ to the fetus resulted in increases in fetal cortisol, but the effect was dependent on the gestational age of the fetus, with maximal responses occurring at approximately 313 days of gestation. There was no response in cortisol after corticotropin$_{1-24}$ when it was administered before day 295 of gestation [33]. Direct administration of CRH, corticotropin, or betamethasone to the fetus in utero using ultrasound-guided intramuscular injection results in increased maternal progestogen levels consistent with maturation of the fetal adrenal gland [43,44]. The procedure itself was not without risk and resulted in abortion shortly thereafter in a small number of mares. Of interest was the recent work of Ousey and colleagues [45], who investigated the effect of exogenous corticotropin$_{1-24}$ administered to late pregnant pony mares on subsequent gestational length and fetal maturation. The investigators gave Depot corticotropin$_{1-24}$ at a dose of 4 to 5 mg to mares at 300 days, 301 days, and 302 days of gestation and noted shortened gestational length, increased mean corpuscular volume (MCV), and lower body weights consistent with preterm birth. The foals seemed to be hormonally mature. The dose induced mammary gland development and increased maternal cortisol and total progestogens, the latter consistent with accelerated fetal maturation. A significant confounding effect in this study was the time of conception, with the most significant findings observed in mares bred late in the breeding season.

In general terms, it is preferable to maintain the fetus in utero to ensure not only adequate HPA axis maturation but effective ossification and maturation of other body systems. Consequently, the primary focus of therapy for a mare with placental infection is to eliminate infection, reduce inflammation, and maintain the pregnancy. The specific management of placentitis is not the focus of this article, but treatment may involve broad-spectrum antibiotics, nonsteroidal anti-inflammatory drugs, pentoxifylline, β2-adrenoreceptor agonists, and the oral progestogen altrenogest. The use of altrenogest to prolong pregnancy in mares with signs of placentitis has been questioned [22].

The termination of postterm pregnancies is one of the most difficult decisions for equine practitioners, particularly with the angst that is common in many owners. Given the wide variation in gestational range, it is almost always in the best interests of the foal to let the pregnancy continue. If facilities are available, rectal and transabdominal ultrasound assessment of the fetus and chorioallantois should be made, looking carefully for thickening or detachment of the fetal membranes. Ideally, any induction of parturition should be based on appropriate changes in milk electrolytes. Mares grazing endophyte-infected tall fescue can be medicated with dopamine receptor antagonists, such as domperidone [18].

Laboratory assessment

Premature foals that fail to thrive usually demonstrate minimal cortisol secretion in the face of adequate levels of corticotropin. Furthermore, the change in plasma cortisol in response to exogenous corticotropin$_{1-24}$ (0.125 mg administered intramuscularly) is typically inconsistent and usually inadequate [28]. The total white blood cell count, neutrophil and lymphocyte counts, and N/L ratio are important factors to help predict survival. The foal with incomplete adrenal maturation has low total white blood cell and neutrophil counts and an N/L ratio that is often less than 1:1 [34]. It is important to determine if sepsis is present, because neutropenia is also a common hematologic finding of systemic sepsis. Evidence of shifting toward immature cell types and neutrophil toxicity should point the clinician toward primary sepsis or prematurity complicated by sepsis. Premature foals that fail to improve their total white blood cell and neutrophil counts over the initial 24 to 48 hours of treatment usually do not survive (Anne Koterba, DVM, PhD, personal communication, 1989).

Changes in red blood cell indices have also been reported in nonstressed preterm foals [34]. Most notable is an elevated MCV in preterm foals. An elevated plasma fibrinogen concentration is considered to be a good prognostic factor in premature foals because it often reflects prepartum exposure to bacterial infection.

Induced or spontaneously delivered term foals have a significantly higher plasma glucose concentration than premature cohorts [46]. Plasma creatinine levels are often elevated in newly born preterm or dysmature foals because of placental dysfunction. This increase is independent of foal renal function.

Measurement of low cortisol levels coupled with increased progestogens would provide further evidence that effective maturation of the HPA axis has not occurred in the foal before birth [47].

Clinical progression

The clinical progression usually reflects the degree of endocrinologic maturity, additional perinatal stresses (eg, asphyxia, sepsis, meconium aspiration), and extent of physical maturity. Typically, foals born prematurely but chronically exposed to an appropriate in utero stress, such as placental infection, initially seem weak and depressed in the immediate postpartum period. Some require resuscitation. After a longer than normal period of postural adaptation, they usually manage to stand but often require assistance. Suckle reflex and appetite may be reduced or absent, and many need to be fed initially via a nasogastric tube. They frequently have trouble maintaining their body temperature and blood glucose levels. After the initial 24-hour period, many of these foals demonstrate improvement in physical strength and mentation. Their appetite for milk often exceeds that of a healthy "term" foal (Fig. 5).

In contrast, foals with incomplete maturation of the HPA axis frequently require immediate resuscitation. They may mimic the clinical progression of in utero stressed premature foals up until 12 to 18 hours of age, after which a range of progressive abnormalities develop (Fig. 6). These problems are addressed individually elsewhere in this article and include systemic weakness, depression, seizures, respiratory failure, and intolerance to feeding. Cardiovascular collapse may ensue, the first sign of which is a reduc tion in the intensity of peripheral pulses, followed by a reduction or absence of urine flow, subcutaneous edema, and worsening neurologic function. Poor tissue perfusion leads to lactate accumulation and a mixed metabolic and respiratory acidosis. Death occurs without aggressive support, and even with high-level intensive care, mortality rates are high.

Treatment of the premature or dysmature foal

Therapeutic intervention for the premature, dysmature, or postmature foal should be preceded by an investigation of likely causes for the abnormal

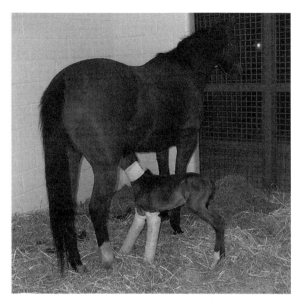

Fig. 5. A premature foal with an excellent appetite for milk.

length of gestation or growth retardation. In most cases, the cause can be elucidated from a careful medical history and gross inspection of the chorioallantois. As discussed previously in this article, the initial clinical course and short-term outcome are determined in large part by evidence of

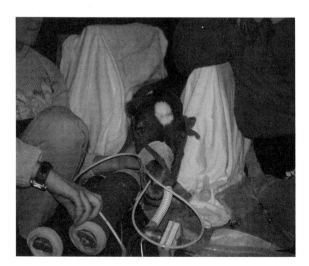

Fig. 6. A premature foal taken by caesarean section that has developed progressive dysfunction of the circulatory, pulmonary, and neurologic systems. Problems attributable to excessive peripartum asphyxia are superimposed on inadequate hormonal maturation in this foal.

HPA axis maturation and the degree of in utero and birth stress. Precocious maturation of fetal HPA function may have little bearing on short-term survival if the foal undergoes prolonged birth asphyxia attributable to premature placental separation or dystocia.

It is also critical to perform a thorough physical examination, because problems of altered maturity can involve many organ systems. Successful outcomes are dependent not only on careful management of identified problems but on predicting the problems that may arise in the hours, days, or weeks to come. For example, a clinician may aggressively and successfully manage pulmonary dysfunction in a dysmature foal only to encounter life-threatening intestinal disease the next day caused by previously overfeeding an immature intestine.

Respiratory system

Most premature and dysmature foals experience some degree of pulmonary insufficiency. There are numerous risk factors that predispose this group to respiratory problems, including incomplete structural and functional maturation, a naive and potentially immature immune system, altered pulmonary vascular reactivity, a highly compliant rib cage, and a propensity for prolonged or persistent recumbency. Maturation of the respiratory system seems to be highly dependent on a functional HPA system.

Dysfunction is confirmed and monitored most commonly by measurement of arterial pH, carbon dioxide, and oxygen concentrations. The low arterial oxygen concentration in newborn foals, relative to adult horses, is further decreased in dysmature or premature foals. Extrapulmonary shunts can account for more than 30% of cardiac output in contrast to less than 10% in normal full-term foals [48]. In addition, ventilation/perfusion mismatching occurs as the result of a poorly reactive pulmonary vasculature and dependent atelectasis. Deficiency of lung surfactant is not likely to play a primary role in respiratory dysfunction in most premature or dysmature foals. Surfactant activity can be detected in the equine fetus by 100 days and is fully developed in most foals by 300 days, although it may be delayed in some foals until after 340 days [49]. Surfactant is produced from type II alveolar epithelial cells and is composed of phospholipids (including dipalmitoyl phosphatidylcholine and phosphatidylglycerol), inert lipids, and protein. It prevents spontaneous collapse of the alveoli by reducing alveolar surface tension.

The most severe form of respiratory failure is known as neonatal respiratory distress syndrome (RDS) or hyaline membrane disease, and it occurs commonly in preterm foals that have not experienced precocious maturation of the HPA axis. Thankfully, RDS occurs relatively rarely in foals older than 300 gestational days, although this author has seen RDS-like signs in foals as advanced as 330 gestational days. The most common clinical scenario for RDS involves foals delivered prematurely by emergency caesarean section because of severe acute maternal illness such as a colonic volvulus. Neonatal RDS is characterized by progressive respiratory difficulty and failure, severe hypoxemia and hypercapnia, coma, and death. A diffuse severe alveolar pattern is a classic radiographic finding of neonatal RDS. Intervention would ideally involve mechanical ventilation, bovine or synthetic surfactant, and glucocorticoids, but outcomes are extremely poor irrespective of the level of care.

Most premature foals demonstrate lung dysfunction characterized by reduced ventilation capacity, tachypnea, hypoxemia, and varying levels of hypercapnia. These foals are more susceptible to the development of dependent lung atelectasis than term foals. The most common radiographic pattern is of the interstitial type. It is important to note that inflammatory lung disease may be difficult, if not impossible, to differentiate from simple atelectasis using imaging techniques. The degree of ventilatory support is obviously dependent on the severity of dysfunction, but most foals benefit from supplemental intranasal oxygen. Initial flow rates of 5 L/min are recommended. Adjustment in flow rate is dictated by positive changes in arterial blood gas analyses or improvement in ventilation rate and depth. It is important to avoid prolonged periods of lateral recumbency to minimize the impact of atelectasis. If the foal is unable to stand, placement in sternal recumbency is recommended. This is made easier by the use of a specially constructed V-pad (Fig. 7). Some foals benefit from mechanical ventilation and airway pressure support with or without nitric oxide, but delivery of this level of care is restricted to a handful of tertiary care hospitals throughout the world.

Many premature and dysmature foals are susceptible to the hypoventilation that commonly occurs after prolonged periods of peripartum asphyxia. These foals typically have erratic or Cheynes-Stokes patterns of breathing, often including long periods of apnea. Arterial blood gas analyses usually reveal moderate to severe hypercapnia with mild hypoxemia. The arterial pH is determined by the degree of metabolic compensation; treatment is indicated with poorly compensated respiratory acidosis and may include intravenous infusion of doxapram hydrochloride or oral caffeine.

Perfusion failure

Failure of the cardiovascular system is common in foals with partial or incomplete maturation of the HPA axis. Management is challenging to say the least, partly because of inconsistent responses to standard vasoreactive therapy. Successful treatment is reliant on early detection of reduced perfusion. This is reflected clinically by cool extremities, the presence of limb and ventral edema, and darkening of the mucous membranes with prolongation of the capillary refill time. As failure ensues, peripheral pulses

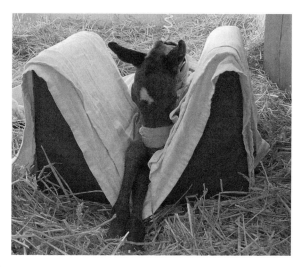

Fig. 7. A dysmature foal positioned in a V-pad to improve ventilation.

become difficult to palpate, blood pH falls, and there are increases in plasma lactate and anion gap. Indirect (or direct) measurement of mean blood pressure along with determination of blood lactate helps to guide therapy. Maintenance of a mean blood pressure greater than 60 mm Hg seems to be important for survival. An initial approach to the treatment of failing perfusion may involve intravenous plasma, followed, if necessary, by dopamine (3–5 µg/kg/min) or dobutamine (5–20 µg/kg/min) infusion.

The volume of fluids given should be carefully monitored, because fluid overload is common in premature foals. This may be related in part to abnormal renal function. Urine output should be appropriate for the volume of fluids administered, and anuria or oliguria should be treated aggressively. This may include "low-dose" dopamine infusion, furosemide boluses or infusion, or mannitol infusion. Establishment of urine flow is critical in terms of survival. The overadministration of replacement solutions, such as lactated Ringer's solution, often results in significant hypernatremia.

Gastrointestinal function

Overt signs of gastrointestinal tract dysfunction are rarely evident on initial assessment of most premature or dysmature foals. The premature or dysmature foal that has incomplete maturation is unable to tolerate aggressive force-feeding. Peripartum asphyxia has an additive effect. These foals commonly develop intestinal stasis with reduced fecal passage, gas accumulation, and gastric distention. The combination of prolonged asphyxia and prematurity is a risk factor for the development of necrotizing enterocolitis in human neonates. This severe intestinal condition is also seen in foals.

Feeding should be restricted to small volumes (eg, 10–20 mL/h) until the foal seems to be systemically stable. Concurrent parenteral nutrition is indicated to prevent loss of body weight. Foals should be monitored closely for signs of gastrointestinal dysfunction irrespective of feeding volume or frequency. This includes assessment of fecal passage, changes in abdomen size (assessed using a measuring tape), testing for gastric reflux if a nasogastric tube is in place, and frequent measurement of intestinal diameter using transabdominal ultrasound.

Regulation of body temperature

Premature and dysmature foals are susceptible to hypothermia. Thermogenic mechanisms develop late in gestation and are related to circulating T3 levels. As discussed previously, thyroid hormone generation is closely tied to maturation of the HPA axis. Consequently, problems with thermogenesis are exacerbated in preterm foals with incomplete adrenal function.

The mature foal is capable of generating body heat through shivering. It is not known if the premature foal shares this capability. Brown adipose tissue is also lacking in premature animals of most species studied, although not quantified in premature foals. Body temperature needs careful management, because rapid warming may result in peripheral vasodilatation and possible cardiovascular collapse. Initially, the foal should be covered by blankets and removed from any drafts. Intravenous and oral fluids should be warmed before use. Once the foal begins to demonstrate vigor, heat lamps and circulating warm-water blankets can be used.

Hypoglycemia

The premature and dysmature foal often has inadequate gluconeogenic enzyme activity and limited glycogen stores at the time of birth. Consequently, most have difficulty in maintaining a normal blood glucose concentration. This is managed acutely by infusion of a 10% dextrose solution over several minutes at a rate of 10 mL/kg, followed by a constant infusion at approximately 6 mg/kg/min (5% dextrose solution at a rate of approximately 200 mL/h to a 30-kg foal). Blood glucose should be monitored regularly to avoid hyperglycemia. Some foals with persistent hyperglycemia benefit from insulin supplementation.

Glucocorticoids

There are numerous problems that can arise during the clinical course of a premature or dysmature foal. The respiratory complications associated with human preterm infants are often managed using exogenous surfactant and glucocorticoid therapy. Dexamethasone has been the preferred drug in human medicine because of its potency, but it is associated with a number of

adverse side effects, including hypertension, hyperglycemia, and catabolism
[50]. Hydrocortisone has a shorter half-life and lower biologic activity and is
as effective for improving lung function in preterm human infants without
the side effects of dexamethasone. A tapering dose of hydrocortisone over
3 weeks beginning at 5 mg/kg/d and ending at 1 mg/kg/d has been
recommended in human preterm neonates. The use of glucocorticoids in
certain premature or dysmature foals is compelling. This is based on our
knowledge of foal in utero maturation as well as borrowing experiences
from our human medicine counterparts. There has also been some interest
in using multiple injections of Depot corticotropin$_{1-24}$ in postpartum
premature foals to accelerate maturation (Anne Koterba, DVM, PhD,
personal communication, 1989).

Musculoskeletal system

Skeletal maturity is most easily assessed by taking radiographs of the
carpus and tarsus for evidence of incomplete ossification (Fig. 8). Precocious
maturation of the HPA axis is critical for development of several key organ
systems. Unfortunately, accelerated ossification does not seem to be a
feature of foals born prematurely after exposure to chronic in utero stress.
Incomplete ossification coupled with periarticular laxity predisposes the
premature or dysmature foal to long-term skeletal problems (Fig. 9).

Management of the foal with incomplete skeletal ossification is
controversial. Restriction of exercise is recommended to minimize collapse
of developing carpal or tarsal bones, but forced recumbency may predispose
the foal to or exacerbate pulmonary disease. Furthermore, normal load
bearing encourages ossification. Periarticular laxity predisposes the premature foal to angular limb deformities that facilitate abnormal load
bearing and increases the risk of cuboidal bone crush injury of the carpus or
hock. Splinting and attention to hoof care are recommended if angular limb
deviation develops.

In most cases, flexural deformities and laxities improve over time. Dorsal
splints are recommended for flexural deformities involving the fetlock, and
heel extensions are helpful in foals with flexural laxity.

Immunity and infection

There are several reasons why colostral transfer of maternal immunoglobulin may not occur in premature foals. Mares may have lactated
prematurely or not at all, the foal may not be able to suck, or the intestinal
tract may not be capable of efficient colostral uptake. Consequently, plasma
transfusion is often indicated even in foals less than 18 to 24 hours of age.

A history of placental infection seems to be a positive factor when
predicting survival in preterm foals. One obvious downside is that many of
these foals are born with aspiration pneumonia or systemic sepsis. This,
coupled with the fact that many foals have an impaired immune system,

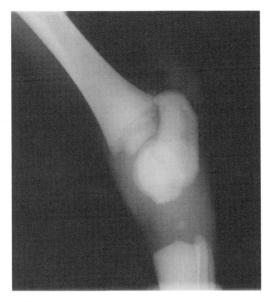

Fig. 8. A lateral radiograph of the hock of a premature foal with incomplete ossification.

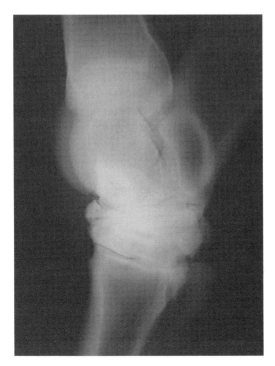

Fig. 9. A young horse with tarsal bone disease that has likely resulted from weight bearing after preterm birth.

warrants the use of broad-spectrum antimicrobial therapy. If aminoglycosides are used, monitoring of peak and trough plasma levels is recommended, because sick premature foals may have poorly predictable pharmacokinetics [51].

Formulating a prognosis

Defining a prognosis for short-term and long-term survival for the premature or dysmature foal can be difficult. With respect to premature foals, it is important to determine the reason for early delivery, estimate what additional stresses may have occurred during the perinatal period (eg, dystocia, premature placental separation), examine essential laboratory data, and determine what resources are available for management.

In a survey of 135 neonates admitted to the University of Florida with a gestational age of 320 days or less, short-term survival was in part predicted by the total white blood cell count, neutrophil count, lymphocyte count, and N/L ratio [52]. The N/L ratio of surviving premature foals (12.5 ± 1.7:1) was well above that reported for normal-term foals (2.5:1) and for nonsurviving premature foals (3.2 ± 1.7:1). Many of the surviving animals were exposed to confirmed or suspected placental infection. Interestingly, the outcome was not affected by gestational age (surviving foals 311 days of gestational age versus nonsurvivors 307 days of gestational age). These data confirm that in utero stress, with probable maturation of the HPA axis, is a good prognostic factor for survival in foals delivered before term. Indeed, in many foals, the greater the neutrophil count, the better is the outlook, at least in terms of survival.

An important area of research is the effect of fetal and perinatal illness on long-term outcomes, specifically athletic and reproductive performance. Most premature or dysmature foals are smaller than their peers for the initial 12 to 18 months of life, but this physical difference becomes less noticeable after that time (Anne Koterba, DVM, PhD, personal communication, 1989). Preliminary data from the University of Florida suggest that surviving premature Thoroughbred foals are less likely to be successful athletes than their siblings, but the numbers are small [52]. There are no data to suggest that surviving female preterm foals are also likely to produce preterm offspring when they become sexually mature.

There are no data on short- or long-term outcomes for postmature foals. It is likely that the outlook would be good once the foal has survived the immediate postpartum period.

Acknowledgment

This article was written by a clinician with a strong interest in perinatal medicine. The significant contributions of Peter Rossdale, Marion Silver (deceased), Abigail Fowden, Jennifer Ousey, and others to our knowledge of fetal maturation are recognized.

References

[1] Rossdale PD, Short RV. The time of foaling of thoroughbred mares. J Reprod Fertil 1967; 13(2):341–3.
[2] Ropiha RT, Matthews RG, Butterfield RM, et al. The duration of pregnancy in Thoroughbred mares. Vet Rec 1969;84:552–5.
[3] Hintz HF, Hintz RL, Lein DH, et al. Length of gestation periods in Thoroughbred mares. J Equine Med Surg 1979;3:289–92.
[4] Campitelli S, Carenzi C, Verga M. Factors which influence parturition in the mare and development of the foal. Applied Animal Ethology 1982;9:7–14.
[5] Rossdale PD. Clinical view of disturbances in equine foetal maturation. Equine Vet J Suppl 1993;14:3–7.
[6] Sevinga M, Barkema HW, Stryhn H, et al. Retained placenta in Friesian mares: incidence, and potential risk factors with special emphasis on gestational length. Theriogenology 2004; 61(5):851–9.
[7] Bos H, van der Mey GJW. Length of gestation periods of horses and ponies belonging to different breeds. Livest Prod Sci 1980;7:181–7.
[8] El-Wishy AB, El-Sayed MAI, Seida AA, et al. Some aspects of reproductive performance in Arabian mares in Egypt. Reprod Domest Anim 1990;25(5):227–34.
[9] Giger R, Meier HP, Kupfer U. Gestation length of Freiberger mares with mule and horse foals. Schweiz Arch Tierheilkd 1997;139(7):303–7.
[10] Allen WR, Wilsher S, Stewart F, et al. The influence of maternal size on placental, fetal and postnatal growth in the horse. II. Endocrinology of pregnancy. J Endocrinol 2002;172(2): 237–46.
[11] Jeffcott LB, Whitwell KE. Twinning as a cause of foetal and neonatal loss in the thoroughbred mare. J Comp Pathol 1973;83(1):91–106.
[12] Sato K, Miyaki M, Sugiyama K, et al. An analytical study of the duration of gestation in horses. Jap J Zoo Tech Sci 1973;44:375–9.
[13] Koterba AM. Definitions of equine perinatal disorders: problems and solutions. Equine Vet Educ 1993;5(5):271–3.
[14] Rossdale PD, Silver M. The concept of readiness for birth. J Reprod Fertil Suppl 1982;32: 507–10.
[15] Challis JR, Sloboda D, Matthews SG, et al. The fetal placental hypothalamic-pituitary-adrenal (HPA) axis, parturition and post natal health. Mol Cell Endocrinol 2001;185(1–2): 135–44.
[16] Silver M, Fowden AL, Knox J, et al. Relationship between circulating tri-iodothyronine and cortisol in the perinatal period in the foal. J Reprod Fertil Suppl 1991;44: 619–26.
[17] Leadon DP, Jeffcott LB, Rossdale PD. Behavior and viability of the premature neonatal foal after induced parturition. Am J Vet Res 1986;47(8):1870–3.
[18] Cross DL, Redmond LM, Strickland JR. Equine fescue toxicosis: signs and solutions. J Anim Sci 1995;73(3):899–908.
[19] Boosinger TR, Brendemuehl JP, Bransby DL, et al. Prolonged gestation, decreased triiodothyronine concentration, and thyroid gland histomorphologic features in newborn foals of mares grazing Acremonion coenophialum-infected fescue. Am J Vet Res 1995;56(1): 66–9.
[20] Allen AL, Doige CE, Fretz PB, et al. Hyperplasia of the thyroid gland and concurrent musculoskeletal deformities in western Canadian foals: reexamination of a previously described syndrome. Can Vet J 1994;35(1):31–8.

[21] Allen AL, Townsend HG, Doige CE, et al. A case-control study of the congenital hypothyroidism and dysmaturity syndrome of foals. Can Vet J 1996;37(6):349–51 354–8.

[22] Ousey JC. Peripartal endocrinology in the mare and foetus. Reprod Domest Anim 2004; 39(4):222–31.

[23] Chavatte P, Holtan D, Ousey JC, et al. Biosynthesis and possible biological roles of progestogens during equine pregnancy and in the newborn foal. Equine Vet J Suppl 1997;24: 89–95.

[24] Schutzer WE, Holtan DW. Steroid transformations in pregnant mares: metabolism of exogenous progestins and unusual metabolic activity in vivo and in vitro. Steroids 1996; 61(2):94–9.

[25] Allen WR. Fetomaternal interactions and influences during equine pregnancy. Reproduction 2001;121(4):513–27.

[26] Alfaidy N, Xiong ZG, Myatt L, et al. Prostaglandin F2alpha potentiates cortisol production by stimulating 11beta-hydroxysteroid dehydrogenase 1: a novel feedback loop that may contribute to human labor. J Clin Endocrinol Metab 2001;86(11):5585–92.

[27] Kajantie E, Dunkel L, Turpeinen U, et al. Placental 11 beta-hydroxysteroid dehydrogenase-2 and fetal cortisol/cortisone shuttle in small preterm infants. J Clin Endocrinol Metab 2003; 88(1):493–500.

[28] Silver M, Ousey JC, Dudan FE, et al. Studies on equine prematurity 2: post natal adrenocortical activity in relation to plasma adrenocorticotrophic hormone and catecholamine levels in term and premature foals. Equine Vet J 1984;16(4):278–86.

[29] Han X, Fowden AL, Silver M, et al. Immunohistochemical localisation of steroidogenic enzymes and phenylethanolamine-N-methyl-transferase (PNMT) in the adrenal gland of the fetal and newborn foal. Equine Vet J 1995;27(2):140–6.

[30] Challis JR, Sloboda DM, Alfaidy N, et al. Prostaglandins and mechanisms of preterm birth. Reproduction 2002;124(1):1–17.

[31] Haluska GJ, Currie WB. Variation in plasma concentrations of oestradiol-17 beta and their relationship to those of progesterone, 13,14-dihydro-15-keto-prostaglandin F-2 alpha and oxytocin across pregnancy and at parturition in pony mares. J Reprod Fertil 1988;84(2): 635–46.

[32] O'Donnell LJ, Sheerin BR, Hendry JM, et al. 24-hour secretion patterns of plasma oestradiol 17beta in pony mares in late gestation. Reprod Domest Anim 2003;38(3):233–5.

[33] Silver M, Fowden AL. Prepartum adrenocortical maturation in the fetal foal: responses to ACTH. J Endocrinol 1994;142(3):417–25.

[34] Jeffcott LB, Rossdale PD, Leadon DP. Haematological changes in the neonatal period of normal and induced premature foals. J Reprod Fertil Suppl 1982;32:537–44.

[35] Fowden AL, Mundy L, Ousey JC, et al. Tissue glycogen and glucose 6-phosphatase levels in fetal and newborn foals. J Reprod Fertil Suppl 1991;44:537–42.

[36] Nathanielsz PW, Berghorn KA, Derks JB, et al. Life before birth: effects of cortisol on future cardiovascular and metabolic function. Acta Paediatr 2003;92(7):766–72.

[37] Irvine CH, Evans MJ. Postnatal changes in total and free thyroxine and triiodothyronine in foal serum. J Reprod Fertil Suppl 1975;23:709–15.

[38] Wallace MJ, Hooper SB, Harding R. Role of the adrenal glands in the maturation of lung liquid secretory mechanisms in fetal sheep. Am J Physiol 1996;270(1 Pt 2):R33–40.

[39] O'Connor SJ, Fowden AL, Holdstock N, et al. Developmental changes in pulmonary and renal angiotensin-converting enzyme concentration in fetal and neonatal horses. Reprod Fertil Dev 2002;14(7–8):413–7.

[40] Matthews SG, Challis JR. Developmental regulation of preproenkephalin mRNA in the ovine paraventricular nucleus: effects of stress and glucocorticoids. Brain Res Dev Brain Res 1995;86(1–2):259–67.

[41] Ousey JC, Rossdale PD, Fowden AL, et al. Effects of manipulating intrauterine growth on post natal adrenocortical development and other parameters of maturity in neonatal foals. Equine Vet J 2004;36(7):616–21.

[42] Santschi EM, Slone DE, Gronwall R, et al. Types of colic and frequency of postcolic abortion in pregnant mares: 105 cases (1984–1988). J Am Vet Med Assoc 1991;199(3):374–7.
[43] Rossdale PD, McGladdery AJ, Ousey JC, et al. Increase in plasma progestogen concentrations in the mare after foetal injection with CRH, ACTH or betamethasone in late gestation. Equine Vet J 1992;24(5):347–50.
[44] Ousey JC, Rossdale PD, Dudan FE, et al. The effects of intrafetal ACTH administration on the outcome of pregnancy in the mare. Reprod Fertil Dev 1998;10(4):359–67.
[45] Ousey JC, Rossdale PD, Palmer L, et al. Effects of maternally administered depot ACTH(1–24) on fetal maturation and the timing of parturition in the mare. Equine Vet J 2000;32(6):489–96.
[46] Fowden AL, Silver M, Ellis L, et al. Studies on equine prematurity 3: insulin secretion in the foal during the perinatal period. Equine Vet J 1984;16(4):286–91.
[47] Houghton E, Holtan D, Grainger L, et al. Plasma progestogen concentrations in the normal and dysmature newborn foal. J Reprod Fertil Suppl 1991;44:609–17.
[48] Rose RJ, Stewart J. Basic concepts of respiratory and cardiovascular function and dysfunction in the full term and premature foal. Proc Am Assoc Equine Pract 1983;29:167–78.
[49] Pattle RE, Rossdale PD, Schock C, et al. The development of the lung and its surfactant in the foal and in other species. J Reprod Fertil Suppl 1975;23:651–7.
[50] van der Heide-Jalving M, Kamphuis PJ, van der Laan MJ, et al. Short- and long-term effects of neonatal glucocorticoid therapy: is hydrocortisone an alternative to dexamethasone. Acta Paediatr 2003;92(7):827–35.
[51] Green SL, Conlon PD. Clinical pharmacokinetics of amikacin in hypoxic premature foals. Equine Vet J 1993;25(4):276–80.
[52] Lester GD. Outcomes in foals with a gestational age less than 320 days. In: Paradis MR, editor. Proceedings of the Neonatal Septicemia Workshop. Dorothy Russell Havemayer Foundation, Inc.; 2001. p. 42–4.

VETERINARY
CLINICS
Equine Practice

Vet Clin Equine 21 (2005) 357–385

Orthopedic Disorders in Neonatal Foals

Troy N. Trumble, DVM, PhD

Department of Large Animal Clinical Sciences, College of Veterinary Medicine,
University of Florida, PO Box 100136, Gainesville, FL 32610-0136, USA

The first month of life is one of the most vulnerable times for any species, and foals are no exception. It is a time where foals must adjust to their environment while still somewhat compromised immunologically, and their musculoskeletal systems are rapidly growing and adjusting to the stresses applied from an increasing amount of exercise. Therefore, if a foal is born with or rapidly acquires an abnormality or disease related to the musculoskeletal system, rapid adjustments must be made to allow the foal to grow and respond so that future athletic performance will be minimally compromised. Problems must be identified early, which requires multiple thorough examinations so that appropriate steps can be taken. When problems are identified, treatment often entails a complex mixture of conservative therapy (eg, exercise adjustment), medical therapy, or surgery.

This article summarizes treatment options for orthopedic disorders that tend to be present or become clinically evident within the first month of life. Those disorders that are likely present but do not manifest clinically until later in life, such as osteochondritis dissecans (OCD), will not be discussed in this chapter.

Congenital anomalies

Congenital anomalies of the equine musculoskeletal system have been described previously [1,2]. These conditions have some type of abnormality in structure or function present at the time of birth. Congenital anomalies of the skeleton are generally sporadic in occurrence, with no known causes [3]. The anomaly may be inherited or result from some environmental insult during gestation. In horses, congenital defects are one of the major reasons for embryonic, fetal, and neonatal mortality and morbidity [1]. Regardless of whether the problem regresses spontaneously or is surgically manipulated, it

E-mail address: TrumbleT@mail.vetmed.ufl.edu

doi:10.1016/j.cveq.2005.04.008

is strongly recommended that these animals be neutered because there may be a genetic component.

One of the most common anomalies of the distal limb is polydactylism, a duplication of all or part of the digit [1,4]. It has been believed that there may be a heritable component to this anomaly because the modern horse likely originated from animals that had multiple phalanges. However, there has not been enough evidence to support a hereditary cause [5]. Often, polydactylism is associated with other congenital deformities such as adactylia (absence of phalanges), arthrogryposis (multiple joint contractures), and jaw anomalies [5,6]. Most of the extra digits are unilateral and originate from either metacarpus II or III [4,7], with 80% on the medial side of the forelimb [7]. However, extra digits can originate from the carpus, including the presence of extra carpal bones. Most of these limbs lack extensor tendons but do have their own superficial and deep digital flexor tendons as well as suspensory ligaments [4]. The limbs usually are not long enough to be weight bearing but can interfere with normal locomotion because of their occupation of space. Surgery can be performed on these horses to improve the appearance of the limb as well as to prevent any lameness that may be associated with the extra limb [8,9].

Any lameness in the foal that is associated with defects in hoof wall growth can be congenital in origin [3,10]. Often, these foals have a noticeable asymmetry in the size of their hoof wall on one limb [10]. Radiographs can be taken to definitively diagnose the deformity. The most common congenital problems identified on radiographs include agenesis or hypoplasia of the middle phalanx, distal phalanx, or the navicular bone, as well as bipartite and tripartite navicular bones [10]. It has been hypothesized that these bones may fail to form correctly because of an alteration in the vascular supply to the digit during embryogenesis [11]. These foals are likely to have permanent lameness.

Congenital anomalies of the head also can occur in horses [1,2,12]. These conditions can occur alone or concurrently with other limb abnormalities [12]. Brachygnathism (parrot mouth) is an overbite in which there is an abnormal shortening of the mandible resulting in malocclusion of the maxillary and mandibular dental arcades [12–14]. This condition is generally referred to as a congenital condition but can actually develop over 3 to 6 months [13,14]. There is little to no effect on the ability of the foal to nurse, so the problem usually goes unnoticed until the foal makes the transition to solid food [12,14]. This condition reportedly will not regress spontaneously, and surgery is required to slow down the premaxillary and maxillary development until the mandibular development can catch up [13,14]. The malocclusion can be reduced by the use of premaxillary tension band wires [13,14]. Correction is best when the surgery is performed within the first 6 months of life, but surgery should not be performed until the foal is 10 weeks of age to allow for the eruption of the second deciduous incisor [13,14].

"Wry nose" is a lateral deviation of the maxilla, nasal, inclusive, and vomer bones on the rostral aspect of the premaxilla, seen in comparison with the mandible [12,15]. It is speculated to be inherited but may be caused by faulty positioning in utero [16]. This deviation usually is important from a cosmetic as well as functional standpoint because many foals will have a respiratory noise present on inspiration and expiration [12,15]. However, these foals tend to suckle normally. Mild deformities of less than 20° reportedly resolve spontaneously with growth and development [16]. For those deformities that are more than 20°, successful surgical correction has been described [15]. Correction can be difficult and tends to require two surgeries, first for the dental malocclusion, followed by the nasal septum.

Congenital malformations of the spine of the horse are rarely observed to occur on their own and usually are combined with limb contracture [17]. The following deformities may occur in the horse: torticollis (rotation of the spine), scoliosis (lateral deviation of the spine), lordosis (ventral curvature of the spine), and "roach back" (dorsal curvature of the spine). The causes of these deformities are unknown, and the severity determines the prognosis because there are no treatments described [17]. Often, because of the nature of these deformities, most of these foals result in a dystocia and need to be delivered through cesarean section or fetotomy. Another congenital malformation related to the spine is occipitoatlantoaxial malformation, which occurs mostly in Arabians and half-Arabians [18,19]. These foals can have a wide range of neurologic deficits, including tetraparesis, ataxia, proprioceptive deficits, cervical scoliosis, and head tilt [18,20]. The prognosis depends on the severity of the clinical signs present.

Congenital syndromes also can occur in the horse when different areas of the skeleton are affected, such as the contracted foal syndrome. Often, these foals have bilateral contracture of multiple joints on the forelimbs, asymmetric formation of the cranium, torticollis, or scoliosis [1]. Contracted foal syndrome has been reported to be one of the most common congenital anomalies diagnosed in the horse [2,21]. However, again, many of these foals require delivery through cesarean section or fetotomy. Another congenital syndrome reported in the horse is congenital hypothyroidism dysmaturity. These foals have mandibular prognathia (under bite), flexural deformities, ruptured extensor tendons, and incompletely ossified carpal or tarsal bones [22,23]. These foals are commonly dysmature, even after a prolonged gestation [24]. For those foals that survive parturition, many will develop other orthopedic problems related to the delayed ossification such as angular limb deformities, juvenile osteoarthritis, tarsal collapse, physitis, and OCD [22].

Septic arthritis and osteomyelitis

Generally, because of its immature immune system, neonatal foals are more likely to be susceptible to infection and subsequently acquire septicemia than adult horses do. A slow rise in endogenous antibodies combined with a rapid decrease in passive antibody levels makes foals more susceptible to infection. In addition, if the foal fails to fully absorb adequate levels of antibodies from colostrum, then sepsis is a common sequela [25]. Septic foci in foals have the tendency to infect other tissues, such as the joints or bones, through hematogenous spread of the bacteria. In retrospective studies [26,27] of foals with septic joints, 50% to 88% were identified with partial (400–800 mg/dL) or complete (≤400 mg/dL) failure of passive transfer. In fact, septic arthritis and osteomyelitis have been reported to be the second most common lesions identified at necropsy in septicemic foals [28]. In two studies [29,30] that have examined foals with confirmed sepsis, 26% and 28% had concurrent septic arthritis or osteomyelitis, respectively. However, it also is important to note that foals also can develop septic joints secondary to trauma. Nonetheless, the bacteria most commonly isolated from septic arthritis or osteomyelitis are the same ones that can cause the initial septicemia [31].

In immature bones and joints, there is a rapid growth phase that requires an increased blood flow through transphyseal vessels to the metaphysis, physis and epiphysis, as well as the joint capsule [32]. This physeal region is more predisposed to developing infection because the blood has a lower oxygen tension as well as a decreased flow, with pooling in sinusoids [33]. Colonization of these vessels can result in thrombosis and ischemic necrosis of the physeal region as well as thrombosis of the vasculature of the synovial membrane. This results in impaired synovial fluid production and exchange because of increased vascular permeability [34]. Prematurity or dysmaturity can actually maintain this vascular pattern for longer than normal, making these foals more prone to joint and bone infections [35]. The normal production and drainage of synovial fluid becomes impaired, which in turn affects cartilage metabolism because cartilage derives its nutrients from synovial fluid. There is an increased influx of serum proteins, white blood cells, and proteolytic enzymes in the synovial fluid that can disrupt the reparative nature of the chondrocytes and cause eventual degradation of articular cartilage. In addition, a decreased synovial fluid pH level can activate the degradative enzymes, contributing to further damage of the cartilage [36].

The identification of septic arthritis or osteomyelitis can be difficult in young foals, especially systemically septic foals, because often, the foal is weak and recumbent. In addition, alterations in the rectal temperature or hemogram are inconsistent and tend to correlate more with the overall systemic condition of the foal; therefore, thorough daily musculoskeletal examinations are very important. Often, the first detectable clinical signs will include one or all of the following: moderate to severe synovial distention or heat, periarticular edema, pain from or restriction to passive movement, and focal pain on palpation of the joint or bone [37]. In fact, lameness takes approximately 8 to 24 hours to develop after sufficient bacteria have colonized the joint [35]. However, lameness caused by sepsis in the synovial cavity has been identified as early as 12 hours after parturition [38,39] and should be considered in any lame foal less than 1 month of age. Any joint or combination of joints can be involved, but usually the larger joints such as the stifle, hock, carpus, and fetlocks are most affected [26,27,40].

When the clinical signs point toward either septic arthritis or osteomyelitis, obtaining radiographs of the joints of interest as soon as possible is important. This is partly because infection of the joint and physeal region are closely related because of the proximity of the vascular network, making it possible to have both problems concurrently [37]. In fact, the relationship between septic arthritis and osteomyelitis has been classified based on clinical, radiographic, and pathologic findings [39]. First, radiographic changes such as concurrent osteomyelitis, physitis, or osteoarthritis also have been reported to be present in 38% to 80% of foals with septic arthritis [26,27,30,41]. Second, if both the bone and joint are infected, the prognosis will be adversely affected. Third, identification of osteomyelitis usually is delayed compared with septic arthritis because it takes 10 to 14 days to observe noticeable radiographic changes [42]. Therefore, if a set of radiographs are taken when the infection is first diagnosed, they can be used as a baseline to determine whether there is any initial bony involvement (at the time of the first examination) and whether further therapy is worth pursuing. If the foal does not respond to therapy or regresses during treatment, more radiographs should be taken and compared with the baseline radiographs. In addition, because radiographs are relatively insensitive to early bone changes, other more advanced diagnostic imaging techniques, such as ultrasonography [42], nuclear scintigraphy (using radionucleotide-labeled leukocytes) [43], or magnetic resonance imaging, could potentially identify osteomyelitis before radiographic changes are seen.

As mentioned earlier, because most of these foals have some sort of multisystemic disease, alterations in the hemogram are relatively unrewarding when trying to diagnose septic joints. In one study [26], the only consistent finding in foals with septic joints was a plasma fibrinogen level greater than 40 g/dL. However, examination of the synovial fluid helps to confirm the diagnosis, monitor the effectiveness of therapy, and potentially identify the causative agent, thereby directing future therapies. Synovial fluid should be collected aseptically to allow for the examination of at least the total white blood cell (WBC) count and total protein but also should preferably have the differential leukocyte count and pH level analyzed as well.

The presence of inflammation within the joint leads to an increase in the permeability of the vasculature of the synovial membrane. This leads to an increase in both total protein and white blood cells within the synovial fluid. The total protein levels increase quickly in response to the inflammation, but the WBC count does not obtain its greatest increase until 12 to 24 hours after the initiation of the infection [44]. Usually, a synovial fluid total protein level greater than 4 g/dL indicates severe inflammation that can be associated with infection [45]. When this is combined with a synovial fluid WBC count of greater than 30,000 μL, infection should be suspected, but a synovial fluid WBC count greater than 100,000 μL is pathognomonic for infection [45]. It is important to note that the presence of fibrin within the joint can produce falsely low WBC counts because the cells can aggregate with the fibrin clots [46]. If a differential analysis of the leukocytes is performed on the synovial fluid, septic arthritis usually contains more than 80% to 90% neutrophils compared with mostly mononuclear cells in normal synovial fluid [44,47]. In addition, septic synovial fluid usually is acidic, with a pH level as low as 6.2 compared with a normal synovial fluid pH level of 7.3 [44].

Synovial fluid also should be collected for bacterial culture to help select the appropriate antibiotic. The sample should be collected even if the foal has been started on antibiotic therapy (as is typical for systemically septic foals), but it is preferable to collect the sample before initiation of antibiotic therapy. To maximize the chance for a positive culture, approximately 5 to 10 mL of synovial fluid should be collected and placed directly into a blood culture medium (thioglycolate broth) [35,37]. This is the same bottle used for systemic blood culture, and it enhances the recovery of many aerobic, microaerophilic, and anaerobic bacteria [37]. The chances of obtaining a positive culture are based partly on the sample handling, the number and virulence of the organisms present, and the defense mechanisms of the organisms [35]. The reported chances of obtaining a positive bacterial culture from synovial fluid range from 64% to 89% [26,27,44,47–49]. This means that 11% to 36% of the time, a negative culture result will be returned, but this does not necessarily mean that there are no bacteria present. Therefore, good general rule is to also collect other synovial samples, such as synovial membrane, fibrin aggregates, or purulent debris, especially if surgery is performed. Although synovial fluid has been shown to yield a greater percentage of positive results compared with synovial membrane cultures [26,48], obtaining as many different samples as possible is best to increase the chances for identification. In fact, the collection of synovial membrane for culture has been shown to increase the chance for isolation of the bacteria by 10% compared with collecting just synovial fluid culture [50]. Commonly, multiple bacterial species are identified in foals with septic arthritis or osteomyelitis [29,37,47]. Presumptive results also can be obtained by analyzing the synovial fluid through Gram staining, which might help guide the initial therapy before the culture results come back [37].

The treatment for septic arthritis in foals, especially neonates, can be difficult because many foals have multisystemic disease. Successful outcomes in these foals often are associated with early diagnosis and aggressive treatment [26,27,40,47]. One form of treatment is not necessarily better than others are, and in reality, combinations of some or all forms of treatment probably lead to the best chance for a successful outcome. Generally, the clinical course and economic situation must be taken into account; in addition, the defense capability of the foal also is important to consider because the treatment choices may need to be altered accordingly.

Systemic antibiotic therapy should be commenced as soon as possible after the diagnosis is confirmed or even presumed. Synovial fluid cultures should be obtained before administration, if at all possible, to isolate the bacteria species and to identify its antibiotic susceptibility. However, culture results generally take approximately 48 hours to obtain. Therefore, the selection of an antibiotic initially will need to be chosen before having knowledge of the infecting organism and should be based on experience of common regional bacterial isolates. Broad-spectrum antibiotics should be chosen because many foals have gram-negative organisms that inoculate the joints [51–53]. Anaerobic infections can occur but tend to be gradual in onset and nonresponsive to appropriate aerobic therapy. When deciding on which broad-spectrum antibiotics to choose, the following points need to be considered [35]. The antibiotic ideally should be bactericidal because the immune system of many of these foals is already compromised. Also, many foals are renally compromised, so the excretion and metabolism of the antibiotics needs to be considered as well. In foals, the most ideal route of administration is either intravenous or oral compared with intramuscular because there is little relative muscle mass. The antibiotic chosen also should have the best opportunity to be delivered to the bone and synovia at adequate therapeutic concentrations.

Cephalosporins, β-lactam, and aminoglycosides have been historically the three most effective classes of broad-spectrum bactericidal drugs used in the treatment of septic joints in foals. The cephalosporins (eg, cefazolin or ceftiofur) and aminoglycosides (eg, gentamicin or amikacin) are efficacious against gram-negative organisms, whereas the β-lactams (penicillins) are better against gram-positive organisms. Most of the time, either a cephalosporin or β-lactam is used in combination with an aminoglycoside, depending on the regional occurrence and availability of the drug. The following are some important considerations when using these antibiotics in septic joints. Little is known about the actual penetration of systemically administered antibiotics into inflamed joints because of the alterations in the blood supply and tissue metabolism in response to the inflammation [54–56]. Penetration becomes an important factor for the aminoglycosides because the bactericidal effect is proportional to the peak drug concentration obtained within the tissues. The acidic environment of the synovial fluid combined with the presence of purulent material also can decrease the efficacy of some antibiotics, aminoglycosides in particular [56,57]. Third-generation cephalosporins (ceftiofur) have been demonstrated to have good penetration into the bone and synovial fluid in normal joints [56], and amikacin has been shown to be the most efficacious aminoglycoside against orthopedic pathogens [58–62]. In addition, bacteria rarely develop resistance to amikacin [62]. However, aminoglycosides such as amikacin need to be used with caution in foals because of their nephrotoxic nature.

Non-steroidal anti-inflammatory drugs (NSAIDs) can be beneficial as well in these cases because of their potent anti-inflammatory properties. In addition, NSAIDs are good for providing musculoskeletal analgesia. The combination of analgesia and decreased inflammation can be valuable in septic joints. This makes it possible to obtain better antibiotic penetration into the synovial fluid by decreasing the degree of vascular thrombosis within the synovial membrane and allowing better clearance of the proinflammatory mediators and degradative enzymes within the synovial fluid through the lymphatic system [63]. In addition, NSAIDs often are antipyretic, presumably because of the mitigation of the effect of endotoxins. The biggest disadvantage of NSAIDs use in systemically compromised foals is their side effects, which include gingival and gastric ulceration, hypoproteinemia, and renal papillary necrosis [64–67]. The ulceration side effects can be decreased by using antiulcer medication in combination with the NSAID. Even if NSAIDs are not used in these foals, one can argue for the administration of antiulcer medication to reduce the pain and stress of constant manipulation. Commonly used antiulcer medications include H2-histamine receptor antagonists (ranitidine and cimetidine), proton pump inhibitors (omeprazole), or ulcer-binding protectants (sucralfate).

Another treatment that can enhance the effectiveness of the systemic antibiotic therapy is joint lavage. Essentially, joint lavage decreases the number of organisms present within the synovial fluid so that the systemic antibiotic potentially is more effective against the decreased numbers. In addition, joint lavage allows for the removal of debris and inflammatory products from the synovial fluid, decreasing the likelihood of osteoarthritis development secondary to enzymatic degradation. Ideally, 1 to 2 L of a balanced, buffered polyionic Ringer's solution or physiologic saline is lavaged through any joint suspected of being infected. This type of lavage can be performed aseptically by placing needles into the joint on heavily sedated or anesthetized foals. Two techniques can be used to perform an adequate joint lavage. The first method is the distention-irrigation technique, in which one large-gauge needle (14–18 gauge) is inserted into the joint. The joint is then alternately infused to distention with the irrigating fluid and then aspirated [27]. The second technique is the through-and-through lavage, in which two or more large-gauge needles (14–18 gauge) are placed as far away from each other as possible in the joint [68]. One needle then functions as ingress and the remaining needle functions as an egress. Generally, the joint lavage will need to be repeated within 48 hours if there is no significant improvement in the amount of effusion or degree of lameness. The number of lavage procedures that need to be performed is based on the individual case. One study [27] has reported that the average required number of lavage procedures was 3.3, with a range of

2 to 11. To have the most beneficial effect, lavage should be performed within the first 24 to 48 hours after the initiation of infection, before accumulation of fibrin [46,69]. Once a significant inflammation is present, the amounts of fibrin and debris become too big or viscous to be removed adequately through the needles [49,70]. At this stage, treatment needs to become more aggressive by combining debridement along with the lavage through an arthrotomy or arthroscopically.

One of the main reasons for treatment failure in septic joints is the inability to eliminate the causative agent [33]. Once fibrin accumulates within the joint, which can occur as quickly as 48 hours, bacteria will congregate around the fibrin aggregates, making it difficult to adequately decrease the number of organisms until the fibrin is removed. If the foal's joint has been lavaged repeatedly with little to no improvement in clinical signs, then debridement must be performed to have a chance at a successful outcome. Arguably, if the septic joint has not been treated for more than 2 days after the initial identification of the infection, then lavage alone will be of limited value. In addition, if the economic value of the foal is high, arthroscopic debridement and lavage can be considered as the first treatment rather than lavage alone. When debridement of the fibrin and debris is required, either arthroscopy or an arthrotomy can be successfully used.

The biggest advantage of arthroscopy is that it allows good debridement of the fibrin, articular cartilage, bone, and synovium because these structures can be directly visualized [27,49,71]. In addition, it allows better access to more remote areas of the joint. The biggest disadvantages of arthroscopy are the cost and the need for the facilities, equipment, and training to be able to adequately perform this surgery. Arthroscopy has been shown to be less effective in eliminating joint infection because it does not provide lavage and continuous drainage as well as an arthrotomy does [68,70,71]. However, the arthroscope also can be used to visualize and debride the appropriate structures and then convert the portals into larger incisions that are left open to drain. If the arthrotomy or arthroscopy incisions are left open to drain, there is a greater risk for an additional ascending bacterial contamination because these foals usually are recumbent for a large amount of time [71]. The biggest advantage to an arthrotomy is that, under aseptic conditions, it can be performed by anyone, at any time, when the need arises. The biggest disadvantage is that greater iatrogenic damage to all components of the joint can occur, and generally the debridement of all aspects of the joint is not as good as arthroscopy. No matter which approach is used, it is important to remember that in those joints that have large distinct dorsal and palmar or plantar pouches (eg, fetlock or tibiotarsal joint), both pouches must be entered and debrided. If only the dorsal pouch is entered, usually significant bacteria remain in the fibrin aggregates in the palmar or plantar pouch and will rapidly re-seed the dorsal pouch.

An additional approach to treating septic joints is to deliver antibiotics in a greater local concentration. Alterations in tissue blood supply, pH level, and metabolism can limit the amount and activity of the systemically administered antibiotic in the actual infected tissue [55,57]. Therefore, the delivery of a high concentration of antibiotics directly to the infected site may be critical for the success of therapy [72]. In addition, because most septic joints are infected through hematogenous spread of bacteria, it is important to treat the surrounding vascular system as aggressively as the septic joint. This local delivery of antibiotics is referred to as regional perfusion. Regional perfusion has proven to be a valuable adjunctive therapy in septic orthopedic conditions [55,73–77]. Regional perfusion can be divided into two basic techniques. The first technique is referred to as distal limb perfusion and is performed by delivering drugs directly into the tissue through the venous system [76,77], whereas the other is referred to as intraosseous perfusion, in which the drugs are administered through the medullary cavity [72,78].

In both techniques, the antibiotic is administered under pressure. With the distal limb perfusion method, a tourniquet is placed proximal to the infected site, and the antibiotic is injected directly into a vein, whereas with the intraosseous technique, a small hole is drilled through one cortex of the bone proximal to the infected joint, and the antibiotic is delivered directly into the medullary cavity. Presumably, by delivering the antibiotic through a pressurized system, a high concentration of antibiotic will diffuse into the ischemic tissues and exudates [79]. In normal tissues, both techniques have provided five to 50 times the recommended peak serum concentration of the antibiotic needed to produce a therapeutic effect in the synovial fluid [78]. The ideal number of regional perfusions that should be performed to clear up septic arthritis or osteomyelitis is unknown [78], but repeat administration often performed within 48 hours, especially if the joint is being lavaged again. For a repeat administration, intraosseous perfusion is easier because access to the veins often is disrupted as a result of edema or localized hemorrhage and thrombophlebitis [78,80].

Because most of the bacterial isolates of septic joints and osteomyelitis will be gram-negative organisms, aminoglycosides such as amikacin and gentamicin are routinely used for regional perfusion. Amikacin generally is used the most because it has demonstrated the greatest efficacy against most equine musculoskeletal disorders, with little development of bacterial resistance [58,59,62]. Generally, 50 mg to 1 g of amikacin or gentamicin in 10, 30, or 60 mL of lactated Ringer's solution (dose and volume generally depend on the size of the horse and the area to be perfused) has been reported to be administered intravenously or intraosseously [72,76–78]. However, there are anecdotal reports of soft tissue sloughing that occur with the administration of more than 1 g of aminoglycosides [76].

Additional therapies that have been reported to be of some benefit in septic joints include intra-articular (IA) antibiotic administration

[39,54,71,81], antibiotic-impregnated beads [82], and indwelling drains [31,46,68,83]. Initial studies [39,54] of IA administration of antibiotics have suggested that this therapy can produce a chemical synovitis, but the effect of this synovitis has been shown to be minimal [81,84], especially compared with the deleterious effects of the infection. IA administration results in significantly higher synovial fluid concentrations than systemic routes [84,85]. It can be performed whenever the joint is tapped to obtain synovial fluid or immediately after lavage or surgery. In addition, IA administration of antibiotics on a daily basis after lavage or surgery also can be beneficial [69]. For reasons previously mentioned, aminoglycosides such as amikacin or gentamicin (250–500 mg per joint) are used routinely. For more refractory cases, antibiotics such as gentamicin can be impregnated in polymethylmethacrylate (PMMA) beads to allow for a more controlled and periodic sustained release and can be temporarily placed in the joint [82,86]. The biggest disadvantage of PMMA beads in the joint is the need for another surgery to remove them. In addition, indwelling surgical drains or closed suction drains can be placed in the joint to allow for periodic flushing and continuous drainage [31,46,68,83]. Systemic antibiotics should be continued for 2 weeks after cessation of clinical signs, unless osteomyelitis also is present and then antibiotics should be continued for 2 to 3 months because bacteria can survive in the bone and physeal cartilage for a long time [37]. After the infection has been completely eliminated from the joint, hyaluronic acid can be administered either intravenously or intra-articularly to provide lubrication and aid in repair of the synovial membrane [69].

The prognosis for septic joints in the foal has been reported to range from poor to unfavorable for survival [51,68]. From 42% to 84% of foals have been reported to survive to discharge [26,27,40,47]. Early diagnosis and treatment through lavage and debridement have been shown to be the most important components of obtaining a successful outcome [26,27,40,47], even more so than the choice of antibiotics; in other words, early and aggressive treatment is paramount for success. One study [26] demonstrated that 71% of foals treated within 2 days of the onset of clinical signs survived, whereas only 4% survived when treated after 2 days. However, the potential for future athletic function may not be good for those foals that survive, because only 30% to 48% of Thoroughbred foals that had septic arthritis as a neonate started more than 1 race [26,38,40]. Other factors that affect the prognosis include the systemic status of the foal, the number of joints involved, and the extent of corresponding bony lesions. If a foal is septic and has septic arthritis or osteomyelitis, it has been reported that the prognosis for survival and future athletic performance is significantly less than for those septic foals that lack joint or bone infections [26,38,87]. The survival and long-term prognosis for athletic function also is less for those foals with multiple affected joints, but it does not matter which particular joints are affected [26,40]. The addition of osteomyelitis can complicate the determination of prognosis, especially if extensive debridement of the physis has been performed because this can lead to early closure of the physis and a resultant angular limb deformity [37,46]. Overall, the prognosis for survival and successful athletic performance in foals with septic joints or osteomyelitis is guarded but has the best chance for success if it is treated early and aggressively using any combination of the methods described above.

Hyperextension

Laxity in neonates often presents as weakness of the flexor tendons because of dysmaturity or prematurity, causing the foal to have a general lack of muscle tone [88], and partly because of the insufficient cross-linking of collagen fibrils in the flexor tendons [89]. However, it also is common for term foals to present with laxity immediately after parturition. With flexor tendon laxity, muscular abnormalities have not been identified with either electromyography or histology [90]. The fetlock joint usually is affected the most, with evidence of weakness in both forelimbs, both hindlimbs, or all four fetlocks [88,91]. The foals generally rock back onto the caudal portion of the hoof wall and heel bulbs such that the pastern hyperextends and the fetlock drops and the toe flips upward. Radiographs can be taken to demonstrate the abnormal bony alignment, but other bony abnormalities are rarely identified. Obtaining radiographs, therefore, is not imperative, unless the foal was born normal and then developed hyperextension. In these foals, the foot should be radiographed to rule out an avulsion fracture of the deep digital flexor tendon from its insertion on the third phalanx [92].

Most foals are only mildly to moderately affected and will spontaneously correct within the first few days of life as they start to move around and strengthen their musculotendinous unit [88,91]. Therefore, nothing needs to be done to these foals, unless they do not improve or they get worse. If the laxity does not improve over the first few days of life, corrective trimming and shoeing of the foot should be considered [88,92]. The heels should be lowered initially in an attempt to allow the foot to completely contact the ground. This also requires that the bedding be kept shallow so that the foot has the capability of completely contacting the surface of the ground. If lowering of the heels is not successful, then heel extension shoes should be placed on the foot so that the weight-bearing surface is extended caudally, thus providing more support for the fetlocks. This can be accomplished with commercially available shoes or with tongue depressors glued to the bottom of the foot. Most foals will obtain some degree of soft tissue trauma to their heel bulb region that can be protected by loosely applying an adherent bandage around the phalanges. Thicker bandages and splints should be avoided, if possible, because they will likely worsen the laxity. In fact, when normal foals are placed in splints or casts, they will generally develop laxity within 5 to 10 days, with younger foals developing worse deformities [93]. In those foals with severe hyperextension and sloughed skin with exposed tissues, euthanasia should be considered [88].

It also is important to note that foals with longstanding systemic illness can develop laxity from general nonuse of the limbs [92]. These foals will spontaneously correct as their systemic status improves and they have the ability to ambulate normally. It also is important to examine completely the foal's neurologic status, to make sure that there are no underlying central or peripheral nervous system defects that might lead to decreased tendon reflexes and weakness [94].

Contractural deformities

Contractural deformities often are referred to as "contracted" tendons, even though there is no evidence that the tendons are shorter or contracted with respect to the bone [91]. Contractural deformities are a common problem in foals that can be either bilateral or unilateral [17]. They are present at birth but can be acquired within 1 year of age [95]. Congenital deformities usually are the result of external environmental factors during gestation, bone or joint malformation, or from other physiologic causes such as intrauterine malpositioning [88,95,96]. The relative position of the fetus in the uterus with respect to the body wall and gastrointestinal tract can prevent the foal from extending its leg or legs resulting in a joint that cannot be straightened.

These deformities are described with reference to the joint that is affected, that is, the joint that cannot be straightened. The severity often is assessed in terms of degrees of the deformity from normal. For example, if the entire forelimb is considered a straight line, then a 30° deformity of the carpus would describe the angle of the limb distal to the carpus in the caudal direction. The carpus, fetlock, pastern, coffin, and tarsus can all be affected, with multiple joints occasionally affected at the same time [88]. Contractural deformities are relatively straightforward in terms of diagnosis because most of the foals have trouble standing right after birth. When manual straightening of the limb around the affected joint is attempted, it often is unsuccessful. Palpation of the flexor tendons when the limb is extended can identify which tendons are affected by determining which tendons become taught. Radiographs of the affected joints usually are normal, but changes can occur to the palmar aspect of the third carpal bone and radiocarpal bone [92].

For carpal, fetlock, and coffin joint contractural deformities, if the neonate is able to stand on the affected leg usually no therapy is required, and the foal will spontaneously improve over 4 to 5 days [88,97]. If the deformity is mild to moderate in cases in which the limb is manually reducible, then the combination of splinting and medical therapy often is successful. The combination of bandages and splints helps to apply a consistent pressure to the tendons so that the limb stays in a straightened position and helps the musculotendinous unit to become more lax. This relaxation occurs presumably because of a reflex inhibition of the respective muscles [88]. Either polyvinyl chloride (PVC) pipe or fiberglass cast material can be used successfully to create a splint. Generally, cast material is better for the more severe deformities because it allows for better molding of the splint to the leg. Care must be taken with any splint with regard to protecting the underlying soft tissues. The splints need to be replaced every day or every other day.

Medical therapy consists of symptomatic and supportive care through analgesia and controlled exercise as well as pharmaceutical intervention with oxytetracycline. Most foals with contractural deformities require assistance with standing and nursing. In addition, any source of pain in the limb, such as physitis, can lead to flexural deformities. Therefore, analgesics such as NSAIDs may be required to eliminate the source of pain. Oxytetracycline is a calcium channel blocker that allows the musculotendinous unit to become more lax, as demonstrated with marked alterations in the fetlock and coffin joint angles of mildly to moderately contracted and clinically normal foals, after intravenous administration [97–99]. Embertson [88] describes the use of oxytetracycline best by saying that its effects can be remarkable but not reliable.

The mechanism of action of oxytetracycline in flexural deformities is unknown. It was initially hypothesized that oxytetracycline may chelate calcium [96], thus affecting striated muscle contraction. This could potentially explain relaxation of the musculotendinous unit, but it does not explain relaxation of the deep digital flexor tendon distal to the inferior check ligament. Recent in vitro studies [100] have suggested that the chelation of calcium might inhibit the contraction of myofibroblasts within the flexor tendon itself. In addition, oxytetracycline may be responsible for inhibiting collagen remodeling during rapid growth of the myofibroblasts through down-regulation of matrix metalloproteinase-1 mRNA expression, making the check ligament and tendon more susceptible to creep [101]. This could explain why neonates respond more dramatically to oxytetracycline than adults do and why normal foals become more lax when they are given oxytetracycline [98,99,101]. The most commonly reported dose of oxytetracycline for flexural deformities is 3 g ($\sim$6–70 mg/kg intravenously in 500 mL of saline) regardless of body weight [97], which is much higher than the antimicrobial dose (5–20 mg/kg) [102]. However, 2 g ($\sim$40–50 mg/kg administered intravenously) has proven to have similar effects in neonates. It is important to note that foals that are candidates for treatment should undergo a complete hematologic examination before administration because acute renal failure can occur secondary to nephrotoxicosis, especially with pre-existing renal insufficiency [103]. However, the 3-g dose has been shown to be safe in foals with normal renal function [104]. Oxytetracycline appears to have a transient effect clinically [97], as well as in vitro [101]. Therefore, some foals require a second or third dose, given 24 hours apart. This tends to occur mostly with carpal deformities and those involving both the superficial and deep digital flexor tendons [97]. The only adverse affect noticed in foals that received two doses was soft feces 24 hours after the last administration [97]. Overcorrection secondary to oxytetracy-cline administration has been reported, and if it occurs, the foals tend to resolve spontaneously within 5 to 10 days [98].

If splinting and medical therapy do not significantly improve these foals after 2 to 4 days, either surgery or euthanasia should be considered. For foals with a flexural deformity of just the coffin joint, an inferior check ligament desmotomy may be performed with a reasonable chance for success. However, in more moderate cases involving the fetlock, both the inferior and superior check ligaments often need to transected; in the most severe cases, a suspensory ligament desmotomy also must be performed. For severe carpal deformities, the palmar carpal structures may need to be transected. Once surgery is performed, the foals usually are salvaged for breeding or light riding [91,96,105]. However, when the suspensory and both check ligaments are transected, the prognosis for an athlete is poor.

A common problem that has been related to flexor tendon contraction is rupture of the common digital extensor tendon [106–108]. This also can occur independently of the flexor tendon contracture [107]. The cause is unknown, but it has been postulated that the contraction of the flexor tendons places too much tension on the extensor tendon so that it eventually ruptures in its sheath [106]. These foals receive a relatively large nonpainful effusion of the common digital extensor tendon sheath on the dorsal lateral aspect of the carpus. The ruptured ends of the common digital extensor tendon often can be palpated within the sheath. The clinical picture varies depending on what other problems exist in the foal [106]. Some foals will have a buckled appearance to the carpus when standing that needs to be distinguished from contracture of the flexor tendons. Generally, most foals do not have much of a gait abnormality unless they move quickly and the fetlock buckles. There is no need for surgical intervention in these foals because the ends will reappose naturally over approximately 6 months, with minimal swelling [107,108]. Bandages and splints may be required for foals that continually buckle forward at the fetlock [106]; however, external coaptation generally is required only as long as flexor tendon contracture is present.

Dorsal subluxation of the proximal phalanx on the middle phalanx at the level of the pastern joint is rare but can occur bilaterally or unilaterally in the forelimbs. It usually is not manually reducible and often has soft tissue calcification or osseous changes present on radiographs. It is believed that this deformity is likely because of disruption of the distal sesamoidean ligaments [109]. The only treatments for this deformity are surgical realignment and arthrodesis of the pastern joint. The prognosis for soundness is fair but better if it is unilateral [92]. In addition, flexural deformities of the tarsus are rare because the deformity often causes a dystocia, leading to stillbirth. However there has been a report [110] of improvement in a foal with tarsal flexural deformity after a desmotomy of the peroneous tertius.

Angular limb deformities

Angular limb deformities (ALDs) are defined as conformational deviations in the frontal plane. These are axial deviations that are based on the relationship of the limb distal to a particular joint. For example, a carpal valgus deformity is defined as a lateral deviation of the limb distal to the carpus, compared with the limb proximal to the carpus, and a fetlock varus is a medial deviation of the limb distal to the fetlock joint, compared with the limb proximal to the fetlock. Angular limb deformities in foals are most often from congenital causes such as abnormal uterine positioning, in utero chemical insults, and hormonal or nutritional imbalances [111]. However, ALDs in foals also can result as a response to pathology. Foals that must bear an abnormal amount of weight on one limb because of injury of the contralateral limb are more prone to develop an ALD on the support limb. In addition, injuries or inflammation of the physis can result in an asymmetrical early closure of either the medial or the lateral aspect of the physis, resulting in an ALD. Angular limb deformities also can be a complicating component of prematurity or immaturity in foals. This usually is directly related to bone immaturity and delayed ossification of the cuboidal bones. The cuboidal bones of the carpus and tarsus undergo articular ossification during the last 2 to 3 weeks of gestation [112]. Therefore, if the foal was born premature or is weak and immature for its age, then some of the cuboidal bones may be incompletely ossified and will effectively be crushed when the foal bears weight across these bones, causing an ALD.

The most common angular limb deformities encountered in neonatal foals include carpal or tarsal valgus and fetlock varus. When examining foals for angular limb deformities, it is important to note that correct conformation for the foal is not the same as correct conformation for the adult [113–115]. In other words, the foal will undergo changes during growth and maturation that can rapidly change the conformation. For example, a normal carpal conformation for a newborn foal is considered to be 2° to 5° of carpal valgus [116], and this conformation should be maintained through the foal's weanling age [114]. The horse generally goes through a pronounced growth spurt at approximately 8 to 10 months of age, at which point the limb will straighten. Therefore, if the limb was manipulated in the first few months of life so that the limb was perfectly straight as a weanling, it would be likely that as the horse developed it would actually become slightly carpal varus, predisposing it to injury as an adult.

Generally, the examination of a foal for angular limb deformities should start as close to birth as possible and then every week until 1 one month of age, because this is a critical time in which many changes can occur in response to growth and exercise demands. The examinations should then be continued on a monthly basis until 6 months of age. A complete examination entails examination of the limb in a standing as well as a flexed position followed by exercise and radiographs. When examining the limb in a standing position, rotation of the limb can make the interpretation of the degree of angular limb deformities more difficult, especially those distal to the fetlock.

Rotation of the limb or torsion around the weight-bearing axis of the limb often is associated and coupled with angular limb deformities. Therefore, when examining a limb for ALD, it is very important to be directly lined up in front of the limb and not just in front of the foal. Being directly lined up in front of the limb will give a more accurate assessment of the ALD, especially when there is a rotational component to the limb as well. For example, for the novice that stands directly in front of the foal but not in front of the limb, the limb often appears as though it has a fetlock valgus. However, when the examiner looks directly in front of the limb, it often is noticed that the fetlock is actually straight or varus with an external rotation of the limb (toed out). This happens usually because the rotation originates up high in the limb, rotating the entire leg, making it pertinent to line up straight with the limb. Most foals have some degree of external (toed out) rotation that generally will improve with age, as the chest broadens and pushes the elbow outward.

Picking up and flexing the limb often will help alleviate some of the perceptual problems that can be encountered from rotation of the limb. Flexion of the limb around the joint of interest allows the examiner to compare the relative position of the distal limb to proximal limb by putting them in closer proximity to each other. In addition, it helps to distinguish some of the more complicated cases in which there are angular limb deformities involving both the carpus and fetlock [116]. Picking up and manipulating the limb in a medial to lateral direction also allows the examiner to determine whether the limb can be manually straightened. If the limb can be manually straightened, it is highly likely that the deformity is centered within the joint and is the result of delayed ossification of the cuboidal bones or laxity of the periarticular soft tissues. If the limb cannot be straightened, the deformity likely originates at the physeal region. Watching the foal walk is useful in distinguishing how much of the ALD is a component of ligamentous laxity. Ligamentous laxity will tend to show more exaggerated movements around the joints of interest, making the ALD more pronounced. In these foals, it is important to make note of the age and exercise level of the foal to know what the best treatment is for correcting the laxity so that a better evaluation of the ALD can be made. For example, neonates often are very lax and require more exercise, whereas older foals that have exercised rigorously need to be stall-confined for a few hours for the laxity to improve [117].

If foals are examined on a regular basis, radiographs are not required, unless radical changes have occurred between examinations. However, the first time the foal is examined for angular limb deformities, especially older foals, radiographs are useful in determining the cause. For angular limb deformities, only dorsopalmar and lateral radiographic views are required, unless there is evidence of problems within the joint, and then oblique views should be added. The radiographs should be centered over the joint of interest and include the mid-diaphysis of the proximal and distal long bones. These views allow identification of the "pivot point" of the angular limb deformity by drawing lines down the middle of the long bones on the dorsopalmar view [118]. Where the lines bisect is where the deformity originates. Radiographs are also useful in identifying any congenital abnormalities such as more distinct ulnas or fibulas, abnormal shapes to or fractures of the cuboidal bones, and infection of the physis.

The treatment of foals in which the ALD originates at the joint itself, such as with delayed ossification of the cuboidal bones or laxity of periarticular soft tissues, is different from the treatment of ALD that originate from the physeal region. For foals with laxity of the soft tissues but normal ossification, a gradual increase in exercise (5–10 minutes daily) is required to strengthen the muscles and soft tissues [118]. However, for those foals with delayed ossification, strict stall rest is required to prevent the development of osteoarthritis as well as further damage to the cuboidal bones. In fact, permanent deformation of the cuboidal bones will occur after 3 to 4 weeks of angulation [113]. Because the limb can be manually straightened at the level of the joint, these foals can be placed in splints. The type of splint used is not all that important, but the placement is. In other words, regardless of whether commercial splints or those made out of cast material or PVC pipe are used, the foot should not be incorporated in the splint. This allows the foal to strengthen the periarticular soft tissues while maintaining a correct vertical limb axis and limb loading [46]. The goal of the splint is to maintain the limb in the correct vertical limb axis so that normal ossification can proceed concentrically around the cartilaginous cuboidal bone. Radiographs should be taken every 10 to 14 days to determine the progress of the ossification.

It is important for the practitioner to know what treatment options are available for ALD of physeal origin and to understand how to determine when and if treatment needs to be performed [113]. Generally, allowing the foal to correct on its own with minimal intervention should be the most preferable method of therapy [113,119]. To do this, one needs to have an understanding of how the bone corrects on its own. When normal mechanical loads are applied to bone, it responds according to Wolff's law so that its structure is best able to resist the applied stress [120]. In other words, when bone is more heavily loaded on one side, it will grow faster, whereas the less loaded side will grow slower. Therefore, the concave side of the physeal region in ALD foals will grow faster than the convex surface, allowing the limb to straighten. For this to occur naturally there must first still be a period of growth available to the bone. Second, the load must be within physiologic limits and not be pathologic, so that the loading is dynamic rather than static [121]. This is why young foals can correct most angular limb deformities on their own, using only modification of their exercise. Trimming of the hoof is another way to attempt to balance the compressive forces across the physis so that the loads remain in physiologic limits and changes can occur naturally [122]. However, in more severe angular limb deformities, in which the loading has become static, the bone growth stops, and the angulation tends to get worse. In these cases, surgical intervention usually is required. Hemicircumferential periosteal transection and elevation (HPTE) is performed on the concave surface of the metaphysis to attempt to reduce the static compression, allowing bone growth to start again [123–125], whereas transphyseal bridging is performed on the convex surface to create a static compression so that bone growth is retarded on that side [126–129].

The management of physeal origin angular limb deformities in foals is controversial. Most of the discussion centers around whether HPTE, one of the most common equine elective surgical procedures, should be performed. Most investigators agree that in the severe ALD case, transphyseal bridging surgery still needs to be performed. The foal's potential future performance after HPTE has been described in many uncontrolled clinical retrospectives [130,131]. However, a controlled model of ALD has demonstrated no effect from HPTE surgery compared with controls, suggesting that most foals will correct on their own with minimal intervention [132]. Practices in which foals can be examined consistently have found that most foals will correct on their own with only changes in the exercise regimen [119]. However, many referral practices are at a disadvantage because they may only see a foal with ALD once. This becomes challenging for the practitioner to be able to determine adequately enough from the history where the ALD has been and where it is going. Also, the economics and management practices of the owner need to be taken into account [117].

General approaches to the management of angular limb deformity foals have been described previously [118]. No two foals will respond in exactly the same way, but if the concepts discussed earlier are used to determine how the growth potential can be manipulated at the physeal region, a reasonable plan can be established for each individual foal. With that said, there are still some basic concepts that are worth discussing here. If the ALD remains stagnant or becomes worse over a 2 to 3 week period, a change in the exercise protocol should be considered. For most foals, this will require exercise to become more restricted. However, for a few foals, an increase in exercise will actually provide appropriate loading to the bone so that the limb will begin to straighten. In addition, balancing of the foot at this time may also prove to be effective in balancing the forces across the growth plate. This is especially true for fetlock ALDs but also works for some carpal ALDs. Generally, to balance the hoof, the outside wall of the foot needs to be trimmed with valgus deformities, and the inside wall needs to be trimmed for varus deformities [133]. If trimming does not improve the foal within 2 weeks, foot extensions (medial extension for valgus and lateral extension for varus) can be applied to the foot in an attempt to increase the weight-bearing surface of the foot [133].

All improvements should be made within the time frame for maximal growth for each particular growth plate so that the bone can still respond. The maximal growth in the distal physes is over after 2 months for the metacarpal or metatarsal bones, 4 months for the tibia, and 6 months for the carpus [118]. HPTE should be considered during this time if the conservative management is not improving the foal in a timely fashion for the intended use of the horse or if the philosophy of the farm management dictates it. Transphyseal bridging should be considered for all severe ALDs foals less than 3 months of age and for those not responding at or near the end of the rapid growth phase for each particular physis [118].

Miscellaneous orthopedic problems

Physitis is inflammation of the physeal region of immature bone. The metaphysis provides much of the longitudinal growth in the foal and is therefore more prone to inflammation from repetitive loading than the epiphysis [134]. Generally, the physis at the distal metacarpus-metatarsus and the proximal physis on the proximal phalanx are most often affected because they have the most active growth in the first 3 months of life [135]. However, most of the time, physitis is not much of a clinical problem until most of the physes start to close, around 4 to 8 months of age [135,136]. In young foals, inflammation around the physis tends to occur when this newly forming bone is unable to withstand the load being placed on it [134]. This usually is because either the normally growing bone has loads placed on it that are too high, as a result of exercise, weight, or conformation, or because the bone itself is abnormal and cannot withstand normal loads [134]. When physitis is caused by the level of exercise or the amount of weight, the physitis is symmetrical (eg, involves medial and lateral aspect of physis), whereas for those that are caused by conformation or cartilage retention, the physitis is asymmetrical (eg, involves only part of the physis, either medial or lateral) [134]. The clinical signs in young foals are variable but usually include a stiff gait with a shortened cranial phase to the stride, an increased amount of time spent lying down, and trembling when standing, potentially buckling forward at the carpus or fetlock [134–136]. These clinical signs are directly related to pain at the physis and can therefore result in a progressive increase in muscle tension that can lead to contraction of the flexor tendons

[134,136]. The treatment of the physitis in young foals needs to incorporate treatment of the symptoms (eg, pain) and the source. In other words, if an ALD is present, this should be treated appropriately, or if the foal is getting too much exercise, this should be reduced but not eliminated [134]. In addition, one of the most common examples of and reasons why young foals get physitis is because of the lack of exercise caused by disease. If a foal spends the first few weeks of its life recumbent, the bone needs to adapt to the loads placed on it when the foal is standing. If the exercise level increases dramatically in this time frame, the adaptation of the bone will not occur quickly enough, resulting in some degree of clinical physitis [134]. Therefore, careful control of exercise is important in these particular foals.

It is relatively uncommon for neonates to sustain a fracture. When this occurs, often it is a direct result of trauma such as being stepped on or kicked by the mare or overzealous assistance during parturition. In young foals, the tendinous structures tend to be stronger than the bone. Therefore, the bone tends to fracture before injury occurs to the tendon or tendon-bone interface. The weakest area in a long bone generally is the physis because it is made has a cartilaginous portion that extends across the bone [122]. The most common physes that are fractured in foals involve the pressure physes or those that contribute to longitudinal growth and are subjected to compressive forces, as opposed to traction physes that are associated with muscle attachments [137]. The types of fractures that occur at the growth plate have been described previously and are based on the relationship of the fracture to the physis itself as well as the epiphysis and metaphysis [138]. It has been reported that 27% of physeal fractures in foals were less than 1 month of age [137]. The most common type of fracture to occur in young foals is a Salter-Harris type II fracture, in which the fracture goes through the physeal cartilage and part of the metaphysis; the second most common fracture is the Salter-Harris type I fracture, in which the fracture goes only through the physeal cartilage [137]. Each type of fracture, whether it is physeal or mid-diaphyseal, caused by trauma from the mare standing on the foal, should be assessed based on the clinical signs, severity of injury, degree of contamination, and economic value. Depending on this assessment, the initial management can include internal fixation, external coaptation, stall confinement, or euthanasia [139]. The prognosis for a straight, functional, pain-free limb is better with a lower Salter-Harris classification (ie, a type I fracture has a better prognosis than a type V) [139]. However, even though 54% of physeal fractures have been shown to heal, only 25% have resulted in a sound horse [139]. Repair of these physeal fractures often results in premature closure of the physis, which can result in an angular limb deformity, but obtaining healing overshadows this potential growth retardation [139].

Rupture of the gastrocnemius muscle at the level of its fossa in the femur has been observed in foals during parturition, especially in assisted deliveries [140,141]. Rupture may occur if the stifle is forced into extension during delivery while the hock is flexed [140,141]. The gastrocnemius, in combination with the superficial flexor tendon, supports the hock in a standing position and is the main extensor of the hock. Therefore, when the gastrocnemius muscle is ruptured, moderate hyperflexion of the hock occurs. The diagnosis of a ruptured gastrocnemius muscle can be confirmed based on palpation and flexion of the hock when the stifle is extended. Ultrasonography usually demonstrates a large amount of hemorrhage within the muscle belly of the gastrocnemius, along with fluid and edema at its fossa [141]. The gastrocnemius tendon usually is unaffected in these foals [140,141]. Most cases are unilateral, but the occasional bilateral rupture occurs [141]. The management of these ruptures has included complete stall rest or external coaptation [140,141]. Generally, if the foal can bear weight, then stall rest without any external support is recommended; however, if the hock is severely dropped, a full limb cast should be applied, with the leg in a normal weight-bearing position. Some foals can develop abscessation of the hematoma, presumably from hematogenous bacteria [141]. The prognosis is favorable for future athletic soundness [141].

Lateral luxation of the patella is another potentially heritable, congenital abnormality in foals [142–144]. The clinical presentation is of foal in a squatting position because the quadriceps act as flexors to the limb when the patella is displaced [116]. The foal can be either unilaterally or bilaterally affected, and the degree of squatting position obtained depends on the severity. Some of these foals can have hypoplasia of the lateral trochlear ridge of the femur, resulting in intermittent lateral luxation. This deformity can be identified radiographically. Surgery can be performed to reposition the patella by releasing the soft tissues on the lateral side, including part of the lateral patellar ligament, or by performing a medial imbrication [144,145]. For foals that have hypoplastic lateral trochlear ridges, a trochleoplasty may need to be performed to keep the patella in the trochlear grooves [146]. Regardless of the treatment, the prognosis for athletic soundness is guarded [116].

Summary

A wide variety of orthopedic disorders can be present in the neonatal foal. Rapid and accurate diagnoses of these conditions are imperative so that the best future athletic potential can be achieved.

References

[1] Huston R, Saperstein G, Leipold HW. Congenital defects in foals. Journal of Equine Medicine and Surgery 1977;1:146–61.
[2] Crowe MW, Swerczek TW. Equine congenital defects. Am J Vet Res 1985;46(2): 353–8.

[3] Riley CB, Yovich JV, Huxtable CR. A phalangeal fusion defect and osteochondrosis dissecans with subluxation of the distal interphalangeal joints in a foal. Aust Vet J 1990; 67(9):331–3.

[4] Frew DG, Wright IM. Supernumerary digits in the horse. Equine Practice 1990;12(5):21–6.

[5] Barber SM. Unusual polydactylism in a foal: a case report. Vet Surg 1990;19(3):203–7.

[6] Leipold HW, Dennis SM, Huston K. Polydactyly in cattle. Cornell Vet 1972;62(2): 337–45.

[7] Stanek C, Hantak E. Bilateral atavistic polydactyly in a colt and its dam. Equine Vet J 1986; 18(1):76–9.

[8] McGavin MD, Leipold HW. Attempted surgical correction of equine polydactylism. J Am Vet Med Assoc 1975;166(1):63–4.

[9] Evans LH, Jenny J, Raker CW. Surgical correction of polydactylism in the horse. J Am Vet Med Assoc 1965;146:1405–8.

[10] Modransky P, Thatcher CD, Welker FH, et al. Unilateral phalangeal dysgenesis and navicular bone agenesis in a foal. Equine Vet J 1987;19(4):347–9.

[11] Smith DR, Leach DH, Bell RJ. Phalangeal and navicular bone hypoplasia and hoof malformation in the hind limbs of a foal. Can Vet J 1986;27:28–34.

[12] Gaughan EM, DeBowes RM. Congenital diseases of the equine head. Vet Clin North Am Equine Pract 1993;9(1):93–110.

[13] Gift LJ, DeBowes RM, Clem MF, et al. Brachygnathia in horses: 20 cases (1979–1989). J Am Vet Med Assoc 1992;200(5):715–9.

[14] DeBowes RM. Brachygnathia. In: White NA, Moore JN, editors. Current practice of equine surgery. Philadelphia: JB Lippincott; 1990. p. 469–72.

[15] Valdez H, McMullan WC, Hobson HP, et al. Surgical correction of deviated nasal septum and premaxilla in a colt. J Am Vet Med Assoc 1978;173(8):1001–4.

[16] Vandeplassche M, Simoens P, Bouters R, et al. Aetiology and pathogenesis of congenital torticollis and head scoliosis in the equine foetus. Equine Vet J 1984;16(5):419–24.

[17] Rooney JR. Contracted foals. Cornell Vet 1966;56(2):172–87.

[18] Blikslager AT, Wilson DA, Constantinescu GM, et al. Atlantoaxial malformation in a half-Arabian colt. Cornell Vet 1991;81(1):67–75.

[19] Rosenstein DS, Schott HC II, Stickle RL. Imaging diagnosis: occipitoatlantoaxial malformation in a miniature horse foal. Vet Radiol Ultrasound 2000;41(3):218–9.

[20] Mayhew IG. Large animal neurology: a handbook for veterinary clinicians. Philadelphia: Lea & Febiger; 1989. p. 380.

[21] Giles RC, Donahue JM, Hong CB, et al. Causes of abortion, stillbirth, and perinatal death in horses: 3, 527 cases (1986–1991). J Am Vet Med Assoc 1993;203(8):1170–5.

[22] Fretz PB, Allen AL, Doige CE, et al. Clinical manifestations, management, treatment, prognosis, and follow-up of foals with congenital hypothyroidism dysmaturity syndrome. Veterinary Comparative Orthopaedics and Traumatology 1994;7(2):48.

[23] McLaughlin BG, Doige CE. Congenital musculoskeletal lesions and hyperplastic goitre in foals. Can Vet J 1981;22(5):130–3.

[24] Doige CE, McLaughlin BG. Hyperplastic goitre in newborn foals in Western Canada. Can Vet J 1981;22(2):42–5.

[25] Stoneham SJ, Digby NJ, Ricketts SW. Failure of passive transfer of colostral immunity in the foal: incidence, and the effect of stud management and plasma transfusions. Vet Rec 1991;128(18):416–9.

[26] Steel CM, Hunt AR, Adams PL, et al. Factors associated with prognosis for survival and athletic use in foals with septic arthritis: 93 cases (1987–1994). J Am Vet Med Assoc 1999; 215(7):973–7.

[27] Meijer MC, van Weeren PR, Rijkenhuizen AB. Clinical experiences of treating septic arthritis in the equine by repeated joint lavage: a series of 39 cases. J Vet Med A Physiol Pathol Clin Med 2000;47(6):351–65.

[28] Brewer BD. Neonatal infection. In: Koterba AM, Drummond WH, Kosch PC, editors. Equine clinical neonatology. Philadelphia: Lea & Febiger; 1990. p. 317–30.

[29] Koterba AM, Brewer BD, Tarplee FA. Clinical and clinicopathological characteristics of the septicaemic neonatal foal: review of 38 cases. Equine Vet J 1984;16(4):376–82.

[30] Raisis AL, Hodgson JL, Hodgson DR. Equine neonatal septicaemia: 24 cases. Aust Vet J 1996;73(4):137–40.

[31] Martens RJ, Auer JA. Hematogenous septic arthritis and osteomyelitis in the foal. In: Proceedings of the 26th Annual Convention of the American Association of Equine Practitioners, Anaheim, CA. 1981. p. 47–63.

[32] Bennett D. Pathological features of multiple bone infection in the foal. Vet Rec 1978; 103(22):482–5.

[33] Firth EC. Specific orthopedic infections. In: Auer JA, editor. Equine surgery. Philadelphia: WB Saunders; 1992. p. 932–46.

[34] Curtiss PH. The pathophysiology of joint infections. Clin Orthop 1973;96:129.

[35] Stoneham SJ. Septic arthritis in the foal: practical considerations on diagnosis and treatment. Equine Veterinary Education 1997;9(1):25–9.

[36] Leitch M. Diagnosis and treatment of septic arthritis in the horse. J Am Vet Med Assoc 1979;175:701–4.

[37] Martens RJ, Auer JA, Carter GK. Equine pediatrics: septic arthritis and osteomyelitis. J Am Vet Med Assoc 1986;188(6):582–5.

[38] Platt H. Joint-ill and other bacterial infections on thoroughbred studs. Equine Vet J 1977; 9(3):141–5.

[39] Firth EC. Current concepts of infectious polyarthritis in foals. Equine Vet J 1983;15(1):5–9.

[40] Smith LJ, Marr CM, Payne RJ, et al. What is the likelihood that Thoroughbred foals treated for septic arthritis will race? Equine Vet J 2004;36(5):452–6.

[41] Firth EC, Goedegebuure SA. The site of focal osteomyelitis lesions in foals. Vet Q 1988; 10(2):99–108.

[42] Reef VB, Reimer JM, Reid CF. Ultrasonographic findings in horses with osteomyelitis. In: Proceedings of the 37th Annual Convention of the American Association of Equine Practitioners. San Francisco: 1992. p. 381–91.

[43] Frederiksen B, Christiansen P, Knudsen FU. Acute osteomyelitis and septic arthritis in the neonate, risk factors and outcome. Eur J Pediatr 1993;152(7):577–80.

[44] Tulamo RM, Bramlage LR, Gabel AA. Sequential clinical and synovial fluid changes associated with acute infectious arthritis in the horse. Equine Vet J 1989; 21(5):325–31.

[45] Trotter GW, McIlwraith CW. Clinical features and diagnosis of equine joint disease. In: McIlwraith CW, Trotter GW, editors. joint disease in the horse. Philadelphia: WB Saunders; 1996. p. 120–45.

[46] Leitch M. Musculoskeletal disorders in neonatal foals. Vet Clin North Am Equine Pract 1985;1(1):189–207.

[47] Schneider RK, Bramlage LR, Moore RM, et al. A retrospective study of 192 horses affected with septic arthritis/tenosynovitis. Equine Vet J 1992;24(6):436–42.

[48] Madison JB, Sommer M, Spencer PA. Relations among synovial membrane histopathologic findings, synovial fluid cytologic findings, and bacterial culture results in horses with suspected infectious arthritis: 64 cases (1979–1987). J Am Vet Med Assoc 1991;198(9): 1655–61.

[49] Ross MW, Orsini JA, Richardson DW, et al. Closed suction drainage in the treatment of infectious arthritis of the equine tarsocrural joint. Vet Surg 1991;20(1):21–9.

[50] Bertone AL, McIlwraith CW, Jones RL, et al. Comparison of various treatments for experimentally induced equine infectious arthritis. Am J Vet Res 1987;48(3):519–29.

[51] Firth EC. Infectious arthritis in foals. In: White NA, Moore JN, editors. Current practice of equine surgery. Philadelphia: WB Saunders; 1990. p. 577–80.

[52] Brewer BD. Bacterial isolates and susceptibility patterns in foals in a neonatal intensive care unit. Comp Cont Educ Pract Vet 1990;12:1773–80.

[53] Barragry TB. Drug therapy of septic arthritis/osteomyelitis syndrome. Irish Veterinary Journal 1991;18:21–3.

[54] McIlwraith CW. Treatment of infectious arthritis. Vet Clin North Am Large Anim Pract 1983;5(2):363–79.

[55] Murphey ED, Santschi EM, Papich MG. Local antibiotic perfusion of the distal limb of horses. In: Proceedings of the 40th Annual Convention of the American Association of Equine Practitioners. Vancouver: 1994. p. 141–2.

[56] Wichtel ME, Buys E, DeLuca J, et al. Pharmacologic considerations in the treatment of neonatal septicemia and its complications. Vet Clin North Am Equine Pract 1999;15(3): 725–46.

[57] Ward TT, Steigbigel RT. Acidosis of synovial fluid correlates with synovial fluid leukocytosis. Am J Med 1978;64(6):933–6.

[58] Moore RM, Schneider RK, Kowalski J, et al. Antimicrobial susceptibility of bacterial isolates from 233 horses with musculoskeletal infection during 1979–1989. Equine Vet J 1992;24(6):450–6.

[59] Snyder JR, Pascoe JR, Hirsh DC. Antimicrobial susceptibility of microorganisms isolated from equine orthopedic patients. Vet Surg 1987;16(3):197–201.

[60] Sojka JE, Brown SA. Pharmacokinetic adjustment of gentamicin dosing in horses with sepsis. J Am Vet Med Assoc 1986;189(7):784–9.

[61] Adamson PJ, Wilson WD, Hirsh DC, et al. Susceptibility of equine bacterial isolates to antimicrobial agents. Am J Vet Res 1985;46(2):447–50.

[62] Orsini JA, Benson CE, Spencer PA, et al. Resistance to gentamicin and amikacin of gram-negative organisms isolated from horses. Am J Vet Res 1989;50(6):923–5.

[63] Palmer JL, Bertone AL. Joint biomechanics in the pathogenesis of traumatic arthritis. In: McIlwraith CW, Trotter GW, editors. Joint disease in the horse. Philadelphia: WB Saunders; 1996. p. 104–19.

[64] Traub JL, Gallina AM, Grant BD, et al. Phenylbutazone toxicosis in the foal. Am J Vet Res 1983;44(8):1410–8.

[65] Gunson DE. Renal papillary necrosis in horses. J Am Vet Med Assoc 1983;182(3): 263–6.

[66] Collins LG, Tyler DE. Phenylbutazone toxicosis in the horse: a clinical study. J Am Vet Med Assoc 1984;184(6):699–703.

[67] Snow DH, Bogan JA, Douglas TA, et al. Phenylbutazone toxicity in ponies. Vet Rec 1979; 105(2):26–30.

[68] Martens RJ. Pathogenesis, diagnosis and therapy of septic arthritis in foals. Journal of Veterinary Orthopaedics 1980;2:49–58.

[69] Schneider RK, Bramlage LR. Recommendations for the clinical management of septic arthritis in horses. In: Proceedings of the 36th Annual Convention of the American Association of Equine Practitioners. Lexington: 1991, p. 551–56.

[70] Schneider RK, Bramlage LR, Mecklenburg LM, et al. Open drainage, intra-articular and systemic antibiotics in the treatment of septic arthritis/tenosynovitis in horses. Equine Vet J 1992;24(6):443–9.

[71] Bertone AL, Davis DM, Cox HU, et al. Arthrotomy versus arthroscopy and partial synovectomy for treatment of experimentally induced infectious arthritis in horses. Am J Vet Res 1992;53(4):585–91.

[72] Scheuch BC, Van Hoogmoed LM, Wilson WD, et al. Comparison of intraosseous or intravenous infusion for delivery of amikacin sulfate to the tibiotarsal joint of horses. Am J Vet Res 2002;63(3):374–80.

[73] Murphey ED, Santschi EM, Papich MG. Regional intravenous perfusion of the distal limb of horses with amikacin sulfate. J Vet Pharmacol Ther 1999;22(1):68–71.

[74] Whitehair KJ, Adams SB, Parker JE, et al. Regional limb perfusion with antibiotics in three horses. Vet Surg 1992;21(4):286–92.

[75] Whitehair KJ, Blevins WE, Fessler JF, et al. Regional perfusion of the equine carpus for antibiotic delivery. Vet Surg 1992;21(4):279–85.

[76] Santschi EM, Adams SB, Murphey ED. How to perform equine intravenous digital perfusion. In: Proceedings of the 44th Annual Convention of the American Association of Equine Practitioners. Baltimore (MD): 1998. p. 198–201.

[77] Palmer SE, Hogan PM. How to perform regional limb perfusion in the standing horse. In: Proceedings of the 45th Annual Convention of the American Association of Equine Practitioners. Albuquerque (NM): 1999. p. 124–7.

[78] Butt TD, Bailey JV, Dowling PM, et al. Comparison of 2 techniques for regional antibiotic delivery to the equine forelimb: intraosseous perfusion vs. intravenous perfusion. Can Vet J 2001;42(8):617–22.

[79] Finsterbush A, Weinberg H. Venous perfusion of the limb with antibiotics for osteomyelitis and other chronic infections. J Bone Joint Surg [Am] 1972;54(6):1227–34.

[80] Scott WM, Butt TS, Fretz PB, et al. Daily intramedullary infusion: a practical treatment for orthopedic infections in horses. Veterinary Comparative Orthopaedics and Traumatology 2000;13(3):A9.

[81] Stover SM, Pool RR. Effect of intra-articular gentamicin sulfate on normal equine synovial membrane. Am J Vet Res 1985;46(12):2485–91.

[82] Butson RJ, Schramme MC, Garlick MH, et al. Treatment of intrasynovial infection with gentamicin-impregnated polymethylmethacrylate beads. Vet Rec 1996;138(19): 460–4.

[83] Morris PG. The clinical management of septic arthritis in the horse. Comp Cont Educ Pract Vet Suppl 1980;2:207–19.

[84] Lloyd KC, Stover SM, Pascoe JR, et al. Synovial fluid pH, cytologic characteristics, and gentamicin concentration after intra-articular administration of the drug in an experimental model of infectious arthritis in horses. Am J Vet Res 1990;51(9):1363–9.

[85] Lloyd KC, Stover SM, Pascoe JR, et al. Plasma and synovial fluid concentrations of gentamicin in horses after intra-articular administration of buffered and unbuffered gentamicin. Am J Vet Res 1988;49(5):644–9.

[86] Tobias KM, Schneider RK, Besser TE. Use of antimicrobial-impregnated polymethylmethacrylate. J Am Vet Med Assoc 1996;208(6):841–5.

[87] Paradis MR. Update on neonatal septicemia. Vet Clin North Am Equine Pract 1994;10(1): 109–35.

[88] Embertson RM. Congenital abnormalities of tendons and ligaments. Vet Clin North Am Equine Pract 1994;10(2):351–64.

[89] Barnard K, Leadon DP, Silver IA. Some aspects of tissue maturation in fetal and perinatal foals. J Reprod Fertil Suppl 1982;32:589–95.

[90] Fackelman GE, Clodius L. Surgical correction of the digital hyperextension deformity in foals. Vet Med Small Anim Clin 1972;67(10):1116–23.

[91] Wagner PC, Watrous BJ. Equine pediatric orthopedics: part 3. tendon laxity and rupture. Equine Practice 1990;12(6):19–22.

[92] von Matthiessen PW. Treating congenital limb deformities in the foal. Vet Med 1993; 88(10):989–94.

[93] Kelly NJ, Watrous BJ, Wagner PC. Comparison of splinting and casting on the degree of laxity induced in thoracic limbs in young horses. Equine Practice 1987;9(10):10–6.

[94] Adams R, Mayhew IG. Neurological examination of newborn foals. Equine Vet J 1984; 16(4):306–12.

[95] Rooney JR. Forelimb contracture in the young horse. Equine Communications 1977;1: 350–1.

[96] McIlwraith CW. Diseases of joints, tendons, ligaments, and related structures. In: Stashak TS, editor. Adams' lameness in horses. 4th edition. Philadelphia: Lea & Febiger; 1987. p. 453.

[97] Lokai MD, Meyer RJ. Preliminary observations on oxytetracycline treatment of congenital flexural deformities in foals. Mod Vet Pract 1985;66:237–9.
[98] Lokai MD. Case selection for medical management of congenital flexural deformities in foals. Equine Practice 1992;14:23–5.
[99] Madison JB, Garber JL, Rice B, et al. Effect of oxytetracycline on metacarpophalangeal and distal interphalangeal joint angles in newborn foals. J Am Vet Med Assoc 1994;204(2):246–9.
[100] Hartzel DK, Arnoczky SP, Kilfoyle SJ, et al. Myofibroblasts in the accessory ligament (distal check ligament) and the deep digital flexor tendon of foals. Am J Vet Res 2001;62(6):823–7.
[101] Arnoczky SP, Lavagnino M, Gardner KL, et al. In vitro effects of oxytetracycline on matrix metalloproteinase-1 mRNA expression and on collagen gel contraction by cultured myofibroblasts obtained from the accessory ligament of foals. Am J Vet Res 2004;65(4):491–6.
[102] Robinson NE. Table of drugs, approximate doses. In: Robinson NE, editor. Current therapy in equine medicine. 5th edition. Philadelphia: WB Saunders; 2003. p. 859–69.
[103] Vivrette S, Cowgill LD, Pascoe J, et al. Hemodialysis for treatment of oxytetracycline-induced acute renal failure in a neonatal foal. J Am Vet Med Assoc 1993;203(1):105–7.
[104] Wright AK, Petrie L, Papich MG, et al. Effect of high-dose oxytetracycline on renal parameters in neonatal foals. In: Proceedings of the 38th Annual Convention of the American Association of Equine Practitioners. Orlando (FL): 1993. p. 297–8.
[105] Auer JA. Flexural deformities. In: Auer JA, Stick JA, editors. Equine surgery. 2nd edition. Philadelphia: WB Saunders; 1999. p. 752–65.
[106] Yovich JV, Stashak TS, McIlwraith CW. Rupture of the common digital extensor tendon in foals. Comp Cont Educ Pract Vet 1984;6(7):S373–8.
[107] Myers VS, Gordon GW. Ruptured common digital extensor tendons associated with contracted flexor tendons in foals. In: Proceedings of the 21st Annual Convention of the American Association of Equine Practitioners. Boston: 1976. p. 67–74.
[108] Fackelman GE. Equine flexural deformities of developmental origin. In: Proceedings of the 26th Annual Convention of the American Association of Equine Practitioners. Anaheim: 1981. p. 97–105.
[109] Harrison LJ, May SA. Bilateral subluxation of the pastern joint in the forelimbs of a foal. Vet Rec 1992;131(4):68–70.
[110] Trout DR, Lohse CL. Anatomy and therapeutic resection of the peroneus tertius muscle in a foal. J Am Vet Med Assoc 1981;179(3):247–51.
[111] Caron JP. Angular limb deformities in foals. Equine Vet J 1988;20(3):225–8.
[112] Brown MP, MacCallum FJ. Observations on growth plates in limbs of foals. Vet Rec 1976;98(22):443–6.
[113] Bramlage LR, Embertson RM. Observations on the evaluation and selection of foal limb deformities for surgical treatment. In: Proceedings of the 36th Annual Convention of the American Association of Equine Practitioners. Lexington (KY): 1991. p. 273–9.
[114] Anderson TM, McIlwraith CW. Longitudinal development of equine conformation from weanling to age 3 years in the Thoroughbred. Equine Vet J 2004;36(7):563–70.
[115] Anderson TM, McIlwraith CW, Douay P. The role of conformation in musculoskeletal problems in the racing Thoroughbred. Equine Vet J 2004;36(7):571–5.
[116] Greet TRC. Managing flexural and angular limb deformities: the Newmarket perspective. In: Proceedings of the 46th Annual Convention of the American Association of Equine Practitioners. San Antonio (TX): 2000. p. 130–36.
[117] Hunt RJ. Management of angular limb deformities. In: Proceedings of the 46th Annual Convention of the American Association of Equine Practitioners. San Antonio (TX): 2000. p. 128–9.
[118] Auer JA. Angular limb deformities. In: Auer JA, Stick JA, editors. Equine surgery. 2nd edition. Philadelphia: WB Saunders; 1999. p. 736–52.

[119] Slone DE, Roberts CT, Hughes FE. Restricted exercise and transphyseal bridging for correction of angular limb deformities. In: Proceedings of the 46th Annual Convention of the American Association of Equine Practitioners. San Antonio (TX): 2000. p. 126–7.

[120] Frost HM. Structural adaptations to mechanical usage: a proposed three way rule for bone remodeling. Veterinary Comparative Orthopaedics and Traumatology 1988;2:80–5.

[121] Hueter C, Volkman R. Previous opinions concerning the reasons for the shape of bones. In: Wolf J, editor. The law of bone remodeling. Berlin: Verlag; 1982. p. 76–83.

[122] Adams R. Noninfectious orthopedic problems. In: Koterba AM, Drummond WH, Kosch PC, editors. Equine clinical neonatology. Philadelphia: Lea & Febiger; 1990. p. 333–66.

[123] Auer JA, Martens RJ. Angular limb deformities in young foals. In: Proceedings of the 26th Annual Convention of the American Association of Equine Practitioners. Anaheim (CA): 1981. p. 81–95.

[124] Auer JA, Martens RJ. Periosteal transection and periosteal stripping for correction of angular limb deformities in foals. Am J Vet Res 1982;43(9):1530–4.

[125] Auer JA, Martens RJ, Williams EH. Periosteal transection for correction of angular limb deformities in foals. J Am Vet Med Assoc 1982;181(5):459–66.

[126] Fackelman GE, Reid CF, Leitch MD, et al. Angular limb deformities in foals. In: Proceedings of the 21st Annual Convention of the American Association of Equine Practitioners. Boston: 1976. p. 161–6.

[127] Fackelman GE, Frolich D. The current status of ASIF techniques in large animals. In: Proceedings of the 18th Annual Convention of the American Association of Equine Practitioners. San Francisco: 1973. p. 325–42.

[128] Witte S, Thorpe PE, Hunt RJ, et al. A lag-screw technique for bridging of the medial aspect of the distal tibial physis in horses. J Am Vet Med Assoc 2004;225(10):1581–3.

[129] Campbell JR. Bone growth in foals and epiphyseal compression. Equine Vet J 1977;9(3):116–21.

[130] Bertone AL, Turner AS, Park RD. Periosteal transection and stripping for treatment of angular limb deformities in foals: clinical observations. J Am Vet Med Assoc 1985;187(2):145–52.

[131] Mitten LA, Bramlage LR, Embertson RM. Racing performance after hemicircumferential periosteal transection for angular limb deformities in thoroughbreds: 199 cases (1987–1989). J Am Vet Med Assoc 1995;207(6):746–50.

[132] Read EK, Read MR, Townsend HG, et al. Effect of hemi-circumferential periosteal transection and elevation in foals with experimentally induced angular limb deformities. J Am Vet Med Assoc 2002;221(4):536–40.

[133] Greet TR, Curtis SJ. Foot management in the foal and weanling. Vet Clin North Am Equine Pract 2003;19(2):501–17.

[134] Bramlage LR. Identification, examination, and treatment of physitis in the foal. In: Proceedings of the 39th Annual Convention of the American Association of Equine Practitioners. San Antonio (TX): 1993. p. 57–62.

[135] Williams JA, Collier MA, Ross MW. Physitis in the horse. Mod Vet Pract 1982;63(5):407–13.

[136] Wagner PC, Waltrous BJ. Equine pediatric orthopedics: part 4: physitis (epiphysitis). Equine Practice 1990;12(7):11–4.

[137] Embertson RM, Bramlage LR, Herring DS, et al. Physeal fractures in the horse I: classification and incidence. Vet Surg 1986;15(3):223–9.

[138] Salter RB, Harris WR. Injuries involving the epiphyseal plate. J Bone Joint Surg [Am] 1963;45:587–622.

[139] Embertson RM, Bramlage LR, Gabel AA. Physeal fractures in the horse II: management and outcome. Vet Surg 1986;15(3):230–6.

[140] Sprinkle FP, Swerczek TW, Crowe MW. Gastrocnemius muscle rupture and hemorrhage in foals: nine cases. Equine Practice 1985;7(5):10–7.

[141] Remier J. Atlas of equine ultrasonagraphy. St. Louis (MO): Mosby; 1998. p. 308.

[142] Rooney JR, Raker CW, Harmany KJ. Congenital lateral luxation of the patella in the horse. Cornell Vet 1971;61(4):670–3.

[143] Van Pelt RW, Keahev KK, Dalley JB. Congenital bilateral patellar ectopia in a foal. Vet Med Small Anim Clin 1972;66(5):445–7.

[144] Engelbert TA, Tate LP Jr, Richardson DC, et al. Lateral patellar luxation in miniature horses. Vet Surg 1993;22(4):293–7.

[145] Leitch M, Kotlikoff M. Surgical repair of congenital lateral luxation of the patella in the foal and calf. Vet Surg 1980;9:1–4.

[146] Kobluk CN. Correction of patellar luxation by recession sulcoplasty in three foals. Vet Surg 1993;22(4):298–300.

VETERINARY
CLINICS
Equine Practice

Vet Clin Equine 21 (2005) 387–406

Neurologic Disorders of Neonatal Foals

Robert J. MacKay, BVSc, PhD

Department of Large Animal Clinical Sciences, PO Box 100136,
University of Florida, Gainesville, FL 32610, USA

Normal neurologic development

Abnormal neurologic function of foals can only be appreciated if the examiner has a thorough understanding of the milestones of normal neurologic development, especially during the first few days of the foal's life [1–4]. Foals are minimally responsive during transit of the birth canal, but immediately after expulsion, they acquire righting reflexes and muscle tone [5]. Most foals are in sternal recumbency, with the head up, even before the umbilical cord separates, and certainly should become so within 15 minutes after birth. The head adopts a noticeably more flexed angle at the atlanto-occipital joint in newborn foals than it does in adults. Within 5 minutes of birth, the foal should look bright and alert and be responsive to tactile, visual, and auditory stimuli. Both the basic [6] and modified [2] Apgar scoring systems for foals include the evaluations of responses to stimulation by the examiner. Within 30 minutes, the foal should have vocalized, usually in response to the dam's nickering. Periods of limb extension and restlessness in sternal recumbency alternate with periods of sleep in lateral recumbency. Usually, beginning within 30 minutes of birth, the foal makes the first of several lurching attempts to stand [1]. Initially there is a base-wide swaying posture, and the foal rocks from side to side or back and forth. The foal may pitch to the ground several times before getting solidly to its feet. By the time it stands, the foal's head should follow movements of the mare around the stall. Once it stands solidly (approximately 1 hour after birth on average), the foal begins a series of increasingly accurate approaches to the mare's udder. This period often includes investigations of the chest between the mare's front legs and attempts to get to the udder by going between the back legs. Coarse bobbing of the head and rocking of the body during teat-seeking at this stage is considered normal. By 3 hours after birth (an average of 2 hours), the foal should begin suckling for periods of 1 to 5 minutes. Suckling is

---

E-mail address: mackayr@mail.vetmed.ufl.edu

followed typically by a period of obvious drowsiness. The head drops repeatedly, and the foal often collapses awkwardly to the ground and then may sleep in lateral recumbency before standing to suckle again a few minutes later. During the first 3 days of life, the foal becomes increasingly confident and coordinated and fully bonded with its dam. Although it usually stays close to the mare, the foal develops a growing interest in the environment away from the dam. At the walk, the gait is noticeably bouncy and hypermetric, but usually within a day, the foal is capable of trotting and galloping.

Neurologic examination

A detailed history-taking and a complete physical examination should precede any neurologic evaluation. Previous medical and reproductive conditions of the mare, a vaccination history, and environmental conditions all could point to risk factors for the development of neurologic disorders of the newborn foal [3,5].

To perform the passive part of the examination, have an assistant restrain the foal in a standing position by placing one arm around the front of the chest and another around the hindquarters. If the foal is recumbent, position it sternally to examine the head. The examiner must be flexible in the interpretation of the responses of the newborn foal. In comparison with the older foal, the responses of any neonate can seem random, demonstrably abnormal, unpredictable, and variable over time. For this reason, it is very important that results of neurologic examinations be recorded on a standardized form and repeated often to evaluate progress and solidify interpretations. The following list outlines a minimal examination protocol for the foal less than 3 days of age [1,2,4]:

1. Observe the foal while it moves around freely. Note particularly any interactions with the dam. This is the first opportunity to evaluate the foal's behavior and level of alertness. An evaluation of alertness and behavior should continue throughout the examination.
2. Assess the foal's overall conformation and muscle tone. The head should be above the horizontal plane in standing foals and the long axis (ie, from poll to nasal philtrum) should be in the median plane when viewed from the front. Note the direction of any head tilt or rotation. The skull may have a domed appearance in some foals with hydrocephalus or the nose may be deviated laterally in cases of "wrynose" (also known as "squiffy face"). Abnormal lateral, ventral, or dorsal curvatures of the spine are scoliosis, lordosis, or kyphosis, respectively.
3. Gently touch the inside of the ear canal and then touch the side of the nasal septum. These noxious stimuli should elicit avoidance responses

in which the foal moves its head away from the touched side. Compare the responses on either side.

4. Stand in front of the foal and evaluate facial expression, tone, and symmetry. Expression usually changes from "blank" to alert over the first few hours of life in normal foals. Unilateral facial paralysis is evident as drooping of the ear, eyelid, and lip on the affected side and deviation of the muzzle away from the affected side. Examine the flick reflexes on each side of the face, including the lip, palpebral, and ear reflexes. These reflexes are best elicited by gently touching the tip of a hemostat to the commisure of the lip, the medial and lateral canthi of the eye, and the pinna of the ear. Normal responses are a brisk lip retraction, eyelid closure, and ear flick, respectively. Remember that flick reflexes involve only the hindbrain and do not require any conscious reaction by the foal.

5. Examine the eyes. Use a light to check pupillary size, orientation, and diameter. A slight ventromedial rotation of the eyeballs is normal in neonatal foals compared with older foals. A strong light directed into the eye should elicit both a blink in the ipsilateral eye (dazzle reflex) and pupillary contraction in both eyes (direct and consensual pupillary light reflexes). These reflexes should be brisk and symmetric. As with older horses, the eyeballs should be oriented centrally within the orbits and should maintain their absolute positions when the chin is lifted (ie, they should appear to rotate ventrally relative to the long axis of the head). Look for rhythmic movements of the eyes when the head is held stationary in a normal position. Such spontaneous nystagmus is always abnormal. Next, move the head from side to side in a horizontal plane and look for normal physiologic nystagmus with the fast phase in the direction of head movement. Finally, in alert foals more than 24 hours old, try to elicit a visual avoidance response. Tap the face firmly to gain the foal's attention and then make a threatening gesture toward the eye. Although neonatal foals less than 1 to 2 weeks old do not have a menace response, many foals will move the whole head away in reaction to such a gesture.

6. Insert a clean (preferably gloved) finger into the mouth and assess the suckle reflex and jaw tone. The suckle reflex should be present within a few minutes of birth and should be strong within 1 hour. Allow the foal to suckle the mare and assess head and neck coordination as the foal seeks the teat; then, look for swallowing movements during suckling. Check after suckling for regurgitation of milk from the nose.

7. Check long spinal reflexes. First, test the cervicofacial reflex by prodding the skin over the brachiocephalicus muscle at intervals along the neck. Appropriate responses are simultaneous shrugging of the shoulder (brachiocephalicus contraction) and twitching of the face. Evaluate the cutaneous trunci reflex (also known as panniculus). Prod the skin over each intercostal space and look for twitching of the

cutaneous muscle. The reflex is present continuously from the back part of the triceps to the last intercostal space. If any deficits are found in the cervicofacial or cutaneous trunci reflexes, systematically evaluate cutaneous sensation by squeezing pinched skin with hemostats and looking for behavioral reaction by the foal. Next, run the tip of the hemostat briskly in a caudal direction along the skin over the longissimus muscle to test postural responses. The foal should extend then relax its lumbosacral spine without buckling or wobbling the pelvic limbs. Finally, run the hemostat caudally along the gluteal region. The normal response is brisk flexion then relaxation of the lumbosacral spine and pelvis. The "slap" test or laryngeal adductor reflex, which is commonly performed in adult horses, is too inconsistent in neonates to be of value.

8. Test limb strength with one hand by pushing downward over the withers and then over the pelvis; pull sideways steadily on the tail. The normal response by the foal to these tests is to give slightly to the pressure then firmly resist.

9. Check caudal structures. Lift the tail, and note its tone. Test the anal-tail clamp reflex by tapping the anus with the tip of a hemostat. The expected response is a contraction of the anal sphincter and flexion of the tail. If this reflex is abnormal, carefully check for perineal cutaneous sensation.

10. Evaluate the gait. This evaluation is necessary in a limited examination in neonates compared with older foals or adults. Watch the gait during spontaneous unconstrained movement and then lead the dam in lines and circles and watch the foal as it follows. In most cases, the walk is precise and symmetric and has a four-beat cadence. The foal alternates typically between walking and trotting to keep pace with the mare. The trunk and limbs should move smoothly around turns without toe dragging or circumduction. In some breeds, a two-beat lateral gait is considered normal for neonates. Compared with adults, the neonate trunk "bounces" when a foot contacts the ground, and the limbs are a little more stiff and hypermetric during protraction.

11. Place the foal in lateral recumbency. Test the tone of each limb during passive flexion and extension. With the hand against the sole of the hoof, keep the phalangeal joints extended while pushing the rest of the leg into a flexed position and watch for the limb to extend in response. This extensor thrust reflex is normal. Pinch the skin over the distal part of the limb in several areas and watch for reflex flexion of the ipsilateral limb (flexor or withdrawal reflex) and extension of the opposite limb (crossed extensor reflex). A brisk flexor reflex is expected in normal foals, and some normal foals also exhibit a crossed extensor reflex. Use a reversed hemostat or plexor to test additional reflexes in the upper limbs. The patella, sciatic, and gastrocnemius reflexes can be elicited reliably in the pelvic limb. The triceps and biceps reflexes can be obtained in the

thoracic limbs. If the results of reflex testing of the limbs are abnormal, evaluate the sensation over the limbs by pinch testing. "Autonomous zones," areas where the sensation to particular areas of skin are supplied by single nerves, have been described previously for the horse.

Neuroanatomic localization

Use the results of the neurologic examination in combination with anatomic information in Table 1 to localize the lesions and generate a list of possible differential diagnoses. The following section (including lists of differential diagnoses) includes the most common disorders.

Selected neurologic diseases of the neonatal period

Hypoxic-ischemic encephalopathy

Hypoxic-ischemic encephalopathy (HIE) refers to noninfectious syndromes of foals younger than 3 days of age that are characterized by signs of central nervous system (CNS) disease [3]. HIE excludes diseases caused directly by congenital and genetic defects or trauma involving the CNS. Synonyms for HIE include hypoxic-ischemic encephalomyelopathy, neonatal maladjustment syndrome, neonatal encephalopathy, dummy, wanderer, and perinatal asphyxia syndrome [7].

Etiology

Presumably, the final common pathway in all cases is hypoxia at the level of the neurons of the CNS [3,8]. A singular occurrence or a combination of hypoxemia, anemia, hypoglycemia, ischemia, hemorrhage, and reperfusion likely initiates the damage to the CNS. Cascades of injurious mediators, including excitatory amino acids and oxygen-free radicals, are released that cause neuronal necrosis, hemorrhage, and tissue edema [9–13]. Placental disease, premature placental separation, maternal illness, dystocia, caesarean section, birth "trauma," and pulmonary hypertension, airway obstruction, or other causes of neonatal asphyxia are thought to be risk factors for HIE [3,5].

Clinical signs

Within the continuum of clinical signs possible in foals with HIE, two major categories have been discerned [1,14]. Category-1 foals are born normally and then develop signs within the first 48 hours. Category-2 foals usually have risk factors for HIE and are abnormal from birth. Clinical signs are referable mostly to cerebral dysfunction, but some foals (usually category 2) show additional signs indicating involvement of the brain stem or spinal cord [4]. There are usually behavioral abnormalities,

Table 1
Neuroanatomic localization based on results of neurologic examination

Evaluation	Pathways	Major signs of Disorder
Behavior	Forebrain (mostly cerebrum)	Reduced affinity for dam, restlessness, head-pressing, compulsive walking
Alertness	All of brain	Lethargy, stupor, semicoma, coma
Avoidance, nasal	V[a], pons, cerebral cortex	Facial hypalgesia
Avoidance, visual	II, thalamus, cerebral cortex	Blindness
Head position	VIII, hindbrain	Head tilt, turn, body lean, walking in circles, ataxia, nystagmus
Eye position and movement	III,IV,VI,VIII, midbrain, hindbrain	Strabismus, nystagmus
Flick reflexes	V,VII, pons, hindbrain	Facial paralysis, facial hypalgesia, absent flick reflexes
Dazzle reflex	II, subcortex, midbrain, VII	Absent dazzle reflex
Pupillary light reflex	II, midbrain, III	Absent pupillary light reflex
Suckle	V,VII,XII, pons, hindbrain, cerebrum	Weak or absent suckle
Swallow	IX,X, hindbrain	Flow of milk from the nose
Cervicofacial reflex	Cervical spinal nerves and spinal cord, VII, (hindbrain)	Diminished cervicofacial reflex
Cutaneous trunci reflex	Thoracic spinal nerves and spinal cord, brachial plexus, lateral thoracic nerve	Diminished reflex caudal to spinal cord lesion
Cutaneous sensation	Peripheral nerves, spinal cord, cerebral cortex	Cutaneous hypalgesia/ anesthesia
Gait	VIII, cerebellum, hindbrain, spinal cord, peripheral nerves	Ataxia
Limb strength	Spinal cord, peripheral nerves	Limb weakness at or caudal to the level of the lesion
Flexor reflex (pelvic), patella, sciatic reflexes	Spinal cord, peripheral nerves (L3–S2)	Pelvic limb weakness, diminished or absent reflexes
Flexor reflex (thoracic), biceps, triceps reflexes	Spinal cord, peripheral nerves (C6–T2)	Weakness of thoracic with or without pelvic limbs, diminished or absent reflexes
Anal/tail clamp reflex	Spinal cord, cauda equine, peripheral nerves (S2-Co)	Reduced or absent anal/tail clamp reflex

Abbreviation: Co, coccygeal spinal cord segments.
[a] Roman numerals refer to cranial nerves.

including a lack of affinity for or interest in the mare, restlessness, hyper-responsiveness to handling, an abnormal posture, tongue protrusion, abnormal jaw and facial movements, "star-gazing," head-pressing, obsessive licking, and abnormal vocalization. Recurrent seizures are common; signs range from mild abnormal movements of the face and jaw to generalized seizures with recumbency and paddling of the limbs. In addition to behavioral abnormalities, there may be lethargy or stupor, head tilt, facial paralysis, abnormal breathing patterns and ataxia, and weakness of the limbs. Signs of multiple organ dysfunction involving pulmonary, renal, hemostatic, gastrointestinal, or hepatic systems may complicate the clinical picture of HIE [3,5].

Diagnosis

The diagnosis of HIE relies on a compatible history and clinical findings and the exclusion of competing diagnoses [1,4]. Normal complete blood count (CBC) and serum chemistry results usually are found, unless the presentation is complicated by sepsis or organ dysfunction. Cerebrospinal fluid may be normal or xanthochromic, with an increased concentration of red blood cells and protein [4,10]. CNS necrosis, edema, and hemorrhage are characteristic postmortem findings.

Treatment

The aims of therapy are (1) general support, (2) control of seizures, (3) prevention of sepsis, and (4) drug-based treatment of edema and hemorrhage of the CNS. Broad-spectrum antimicrobial coverage and general support are the cornerstones of management. Seizures should be controlled with one or two doses of diazepam (0.1–0.2 mg/kg, intravenously [IV]). If seizures persist, phenobarbital should be given (10–20 mg/kg, IV, over 15 min and then 5 mg/kg, orally [PO] twice daily) and continued for at least 7 days. Occasionally, in foals that have intractable seizures, a continuous infusion of midazolam (0.1–0.2 mg/kg/h) has been effective. Total intravenous anesthesia (eg, infusion of propofol) for several hours may be necessary if status epilepticus persists. The most uncertain part of therapy is the use of anti-inflammatory or antiedema drugs designed to treat or prevent CNS injury. The following therapies are used empirically in foals with HIE, but such uses have not yet been validated by the results of clinical trials (in humans or horses): flunixin meglumine (1.1–1.5 mg/kg IV, every 12 or 24 h); $MgSO_4$ (0.05 mg/kg/h loading dose and then 0.025 mg/kg/h) [5]; thiamine (5 mg/kg IV, slowly, or subcutaneously [SC] once daily); dimethyl sulfoxide (DMSO) (1 g/kg as a 10% solution IV, every 12 or 24 h); vitamin E (20 IU/kg SC or PO, once daily); vitamin C (10 mg/kg IV or PO, once daily); mannitol (0.5–2.0 g/kg IV, every 6 h); hypertonic saline (2 mL/kg 7.2% NaCl, every 4 h for 5 treatments); furosemide (1 mg/kg IV, every 12 to 24 hours). There is no role for corticosteroids in the treatment of HIE.

Differential diagnoses

Differential diagnoses include infection from bacterial meningitis and equine herpesvirus 1; metabolic causes, including hypoglycemia, hypoxemia, electrolyte or acid-base derangement, kernicterus, or hepatoencephalopathy; trauma to the skull or spine; birth defects such as lavender foal, hydrocephalus, hydranencephaly, or other brain anomalies; and non-neurologic causes, including severe sepsis, branching enzyme deficiency, and nutritional myodegeneration (white muscle disease).

Prognosis

Uncomplicated (category 1) HIE generally resolves completely within several days if treated appropriately. The survival rate for these foals is estimated to be at least 75% [4,15]. The spinal cord, brain stem, or multiple organ dysfunction typical of category 2 HIE dramatically worsens the prognosis.

Bacterial meningitis

Etiology

Bacterial meningitis is a rare complication of sepsis or cranial trauma. Multiple species of gram-positive and gram-negative bacteria have been implicated, in published reports [4,16–18].

Clinical signs

Hyperesthesia and rigidity of the neck in combination with signs of CNS disease are highly suggestive of bacterial meningitis. Degrees of obtundation may range from coma, opisthotonus, seizure activity, cranial nerve abnormalities, and ataxia and weakness of the limbs. An associated extradural abscess may cause additional localizing neurologic signs. Signs of extraneural sepsis such as fever, joint distension, pneumonia, or umbilical abscess are expected.

Diagnosis

CBC and serum chemistry results reflect systemic sepsis and organ failure. Serum IgG concentration typically is low (≤ 800 mg/dL) if there is a failure of passive transfer. The definitive diagnosis is obtained by cerebrospinal fluid (CSF) analysis; there is a neutrophilic pleocytosis (usually ≥ 500 cells/μL), with cellular degeneration and bacteria often seen on microscopic examination of CSF sediment.

Treatment

Intensive antimicrobial therapy should be guided by culture results, if available. In the absence of culture results, an effective broad-spectrum coverage can be provided by the third-generation cephalosporins cefotaxime (40 mg/kg IV, every 6 or 8 h) or ceftriaxone (25 mg/kg IV, every 12 h).

Although they are expensive, these drugs likely have excellent penetration into the CNS. Alternative antimicrobial regimens include ceftiofur (5 mg/kg IV, every 12 h), amikacin sulfate (25 mg/kg IV, every 24 h) plus ampicillin sodium (25 mg/kg IV, every 6 h), trimethoprim-sulfamethoxazole (30 mg/kg IV or PO, every 12 hours), or chloramphenicol sodium succinate (50 mg/kg IV or PO, every 12 h in foals less than 7 days old, then every 6 h). Dexamethasone has improved survival in some forms of bacterial meningitis in human beings, especially if it is administered early in the clinical course [19]. On the basis of recommendations for children, a reasonable regimen for foals with meningitis is dexamethasone sodium phosphate, 0.4 mg/kg IV, every 12 hours for 2 days, with the first dose given with or before the first dose of an antimicrobial agent.

Differential diagnoses

The differential diagnoses for bacterial meningitis are the same as those for tetanus (see below) in a foal older than 1 week of age. Otherwise, consider the same differential diagnoses as for HIE.

Prognosis

With neck stiffness and hyperesthesia only, the prognosis is fair ($\geq 50\%$), whereas in foals that are also obtunded or weak, the prognosis is guarded to poor.

Central nervous system trauma

Etiology

Brain trauma most commonly results from a blow to the head over the frontal or parietal bones. Such injuries often occur as a result of a kick from the dam or another horse. The brain also may be injured when a foal flips over backward (usually while being handled) and strikes the poll or temporal area [4]. Spinal trauma is usually seen in foals more than 1 week of age. Vertebrae are fractured or dislocated when galloping foals pitch into the ground or collide with an immobile object, accidents that often occur at night. In all cases of trauma to the CNS, neurologic signs result from both the immediate injury and the subsequent (secondary) tissue reaction to the injury [20].

Clinical signs

There may be skin abrasions, soft tissue swelling, sensitivity and resistance to palpation of affected areas, bleeding from the nostrils and external ears, or crepitus associated with skull or vertebral fractures. With any head injury, there often is a brief period of unconsciousness (concussion) after the trauma. After a blow to the front of the head, subsequent signs are suggestive of cerebral dysfunction, with disorientation, disinterest in the dam, head-pressing, lethargy or stupor, and a tendency to walk compulsively, often in circles. After an impact to the poll or temporal area, signs predominantly reflect injury to the brain stem. There often is profound obtundation, head tilt or facial paralysis, and ataxia and weakness of the limbs. Vertebral facture or dislocation causes paralysis or weakness and ataxia of the limbs at or caudal to the site of injury. With upper cervical involvement, a reluctance to move the head may be the only sign.

Diagnosis

Radiography, CT, or MRI is required to document fractures and dislocations. Skull fractures often are difficult to identify on radiographs because of the complex anatomy of the skull; in neonates, the interpretation is further complicated by the numerous suture lines and synchrondroses that are evident normally. Cross-sectional (CT and MRI) scans also may show brain or spinal cord morphology at the site of the injury. Contrast myelography is still commonly used to determine spinal cord compression, although MRI (and CT to a lesser extent) eventually will obviate the need for this procedure.

Treatment

In addition to general supportive therapy and attention to any skin wounds (including the use of broad-spectrum antimicrobials), the therapies outlined above for HIE may be used in an attempt to suppress the secondary phase of CNS injury. Evidence from a large prospective study in adult human beings suggests that corticosteroids are contraindicated in the treatment of traumatic brain injury [21]. By contrast, a slight benefit has been demonstrated for the treatment of spinal cord injury with high-dose methylprednisolone sodium succinate (30 mg/kg IV, over 30 minutes and then 5.4 mg/kg/h for the next 48 h) [22]. Surgery is indicated to elevate and stabilize bone fragments in depressed fractures of frontal or parietal bones [23]. Successful repair or decompression of atlantoaxial subluxation and dens fractures of foals has been described previously [24–26].

Differential diagnosis

The differential diagnosis for head trauma is the same as for HIE. For spinal trauma, the differential diagnoses include peripheral nerve injury, extradural abscess, equine degenerative myeloencephalopathy (EDM), bacterial meningitis, myelodysplasia or other congenital anomaly of the spine or spinal cord, and myopathy, including nutritional myodegeneration, and branching-enzyme deficiency.

Prognosis

Closed head injury with cerebral signs or upper cervical injury without limb weakness has a fair to good prognosis for survival. All other forms of CNS injury carry a serious prognosis.

Peripheral nerve injury

Etiology

Peripheral nerve and plexus injury can occur as a result of forced extraction of the fetus, secondary to injection, or because of soft tissue trauma or fractures. Type-1 injuries cause a loss of function (neurapraxia), but axonal continuity is not affected. Type-2 injuries result in disruption of the axon (axonotmesis) or the entire nerve (neurotmesis).

Clinical signs

There is weakness and hyporeflexia of the affected limb and there may be areas of cutaneous anesthesia [27]. Examples include signs of brachial plexus injury or femoral nerve paralysis after vigorous extraction of a foal from the birth canal and sciatic or tibial nerve paralysis after injections into the muscles of the rump or back of the leg, respectively. After approximately 2 weeks, there may be obvious muscle atrophy.

Diagnosis

The diagnosis is presumptive based on history and clinical signs. Electrodiagnostic studies, including nerve conduction and needle electro-myography (after 10–14 days), can be performed to support the diagnosis and define the nerves involved.

Treatment

Wounds associated with nerve injury must be cleaned and debrided, and fractured bones must be stabilized. If the nerve is severed, the ends should be identified. Anastomosis after epineurial alignment is technically possible, although rarely performed in horses. A support wrap or splint should be kept on the affected limb to prevent contracture and protect against further injury. Joints on the affected limb can be kept flexible by passive flexion and extension routines performed several times daily. The use of faradic or galvanic electrical stimulation of affected muscles may prevent denervation atrophy [28]; however, this therapy is controversial. Recent evidence suggests that the regeneration of muscle may be delayed after electrical stimulation [29]. Acutely, anti-inflammatory therapy should be provided with a cyclooxygenase inhibitor such as flunixin meglumine (1.1 mg/kg IV, once or twice daily) and DMSO (1 g/kg as a 10% solution, IV or by nasogastric tube). An additional anti-inflammatory effect can be provided locally by the use of skin-permeant drugs such as DMSO or diclofenac.

Differential diagnosis

The differential diagnoses of peripheral nerve injury include spinal cord trauma, epidural abscess, myelodysplasia or other congenital spinal cord anomaly, and myopathy.

Prognosis

The signs associated with type-1 nerve injuries and partial nerve tears should resolve in a period of days to several weeks. Regrowth by axonal sprouting from the proximal stump of a type-2–injured nerve should occur at the rate of about 1 inch per month. It has been suggested that the reinnervation of muscle is not likely after more than 12 months have passed [27], although recoveries after years have been recorded following nerve repair in humans.

Equine degenerative myeloencephalopathy

Etiology

EDM has been seen in horses of many different breeds [30–32]. It is speculated that the clinical expression of the disease involves an interaction between a vitamin E-deficient diet and an inherited predisposition to the disease.

Clinical signs

Symmetric weakness and ataxia are evident in all limbs that begin any time from birth to 2 years of age. Signs usually are progressive for several months and then level out. Cutaneous trunci and cervicofacial reflexes often are poor or absent.

Diagnosis

The disease may be suspected because of characteristic clinical signs and exclusion of other possible diagnoses. A supportive finding is the demonstration of a serum vitamin E concentration less than 1 μg/mL [33]. Characteristic postmortem findings are demyelination and axonal degeneration within white matter of the spinal cord.

Differential diagnosis

The differential diagnoses of EDM include cerebellar abiotrophy, spinal cord trauma, occipitoatlantoaxial malformation (OAAM) (see below), congenital spinal cord anomaly, epidural abscess, and myopathy.

Treatment and prognosis

EDM is incurable, although it is believed that large doses of vitamin E (eg, 6000 IU PO, daily) can prevent the progression of clinical signs or even effect some slight improvement [30]. Supplemental vitamin E likely can prevent EDM in genetically susceptible horses.

Narcolepsy and cataplexy

Etiology

"Fainting" attacks occur as transient events in all breeds of foals and as syndromes involving persistent and repeated episodes in some lines of

Shetland, Suffolk, Morgan, and American Miniature horses. Such attacks have been suggested to be an exaggerated version of the normal relaxation response that occurs when foals are restrained [4]. The cause is not known, but some narcoleptic syndromes in human beings have been traced to a deficiency in the production of arousal peptides (orexins and hypocretins) by the hypothalamus.

Clinical signs

Foals may collapse suddenly, usually during restraint, and then remain laterally recumbent for several minutes in a hypotonic, hyporeflexic state. Rapid eye movements may be obvious after collapse.

Diagnosis

The clinical signs are definitive. A physostigmine test has been used to provoke the signs in miniature foals [34].

Differential diagnosis

The differential diagnoses of narcolepsy and cataplexy are the same as for causes of seizures, including HIE and skull trauma.

Treatment and prognosis

Most foals have only a few episodes and then grow out of these conditions. In other foals, the signs persist for months or even for life. There is no treatment.

Cerebellar abiotrophy

Etiology

Cerebellar abiotrophy is an inherited disorder of certain lines of Arabian and Oldenburg horses and Gotland ponies [35–37]. The cerebellum undergoes full development and then degenerates before or shortly after birth.

Clinical signs

The signs of cerebellar abiotrophy usually are present at birth or begin within the first few months of life and progress for weeks or months. Affected foals may stand base wide and even sway back and forth at rest. Movements are jerky and dissymmetric, and foals are hyper-responsive to handling. Such foals are extremely difficult to train to accept a halter and be led. They are particularly likely to fall when they are handled or when they change direction at gaits above the walk. There usually is a coarse head bob that is exaggerated during teat-seeking activity. Although foals with cerebellar abiotrophy can see, they never develop a competent menace response.

Diagnosis

The breed association and signs of symmetric ataxia without weakness are highly suggestive of the diagnosis. Cross-sectional CT or MRI scans of the brain may demonstrate that the cerebellum is small. Reportedly, CSF protein concentration is increased in foals during the progressive stage of abiotrophy [36]. Postmortem examination reveals degeneration of Purkinje cells and thinning of the molecular and granular layers of the cerebellar cortex [37].

Differential diagnosis

The differential diagnoses of cerebellar abiotrophy include HIE, head trauma, cerebellar hypoplasia or other congenital anomalies of the brain, otitis media and interna, and spinal cord disorders.

Treatment and prognosis

Most foals are euthanized for humane reasons. Some mildly affected horses have had a normal lifespan.

Occipitoatlantoaxial malformation

Etiology

The OAAM syndrome occurs sporadically in all breeds but is an inherited disorder of Arabians [38]. Signs result from the instability and stenosis of the vertebral canal caused by anomalies of the occiput, atlas, and axis.

Clinical signs

Foals may be born dead or comatose. Typically, however, there is tetraparesis and ataxia of all four limbs. Signs range in severity from inapparent to quadriplegia. There may be a head tilt, or the head may be held extended or deviated to the side. Movements of the head and neck may elicit obvious clicking sounds.

Diagnosis

The diagnosis can be made on plain radiographs. Typically, a fusion of the atlas and occiput and hypoplasia of the dens are seen.

Differential diagnosis

The differential diagnoses include spinal cord trauma, congenital anomaly of the spine or spinal cord, EDM (see above), and myopathy.

Treatment and prognosis

Mildly affected foals may survive, but most foals are euthanized for humane reasons.

Botulism

Etiology

Botulism is caused by the actions of botulinum toxin, an exotoxin produced by the gram-positive spore-forming anaerobic bacillus *Clostridium botulinum*. Most equine cases are caused by *C botulinum* types B and C [39,40]. The toxin prevents the release of acetylcholine at neuromuscular junctions and results in signs of generalized flaccid paralysis. The disease occurs endemically in areas of the eastern US and sporadically elsewhere. Endemic cases in foals are known as "shaker foal" syndrome and are believed to be caused by the ingestion of the organism and subsequent colonization of the gastrointestinal tract by *C botulinum* type B. Botulism also may occur because of the ingestion of preformed toxin or the proliferation of the organism in a wound or abscess.

Clinical signs

Foals may be found dead. Usually, there is a sudden onset of weakness and a stilted gait in previously healthy foals [41,42]. An early sign is dribbling of milk from the nose and mouth after suckling. The facial expression is blank and pupillary dilatation and ptosis may be noted. Within hours of the first signs, trembling of the triceps and quadriceps muscles and progression to increasingly prolonged periods of recumbency occurs. Terminally, the neck is extended, and breathing is labored. Death occurs within 72 hours of the onset and is caused by respiratory paralysis.

Diagnosis

The diagnosis is presumptive based on clinical signs. Hypercapnia is found on blood gas analysis [42,43]. A definitive diagnosis additionally requires the demonstration of toxin in blood or feces by mouse inoculation or immunoassay [41]. The detection of toxin or spores in feed sources or a fecal culture of the organism is strongly supportive of the diagnosis of botulism.

Treatment

A polyvalent antitoxin made in horses is commercially available and effective, especially if given early in the course. It is recommended that 200 mL IV be given to foals. Foals that become recumbent because of botulism are unlikely to survive without mechanical ventilation [43]. Ventilation must be continued for a period of several days up to 2 weeks before foals are able to breathe on their own. Full recovery may take months.

Differential diagnoses

The differential diagnoses of botulism include spinal cord trauma, myopathy, and sepsis.

Prognosis

Without treatment, more than 90% of affected foals die within 72 hours [42]. Conversely, more than 80% of affected foals survive if given antitoxin within several hours of the onset of signs. The incidence of endemic botulism has been reduced by vaccinating mares during pregnancy with a type-B toxoid.

Tetanus

Etiology

Tetanus usually occurs in foals older than 7 days and is caused by the actions of exotoxins produced by the gram-positive, spore-forming anaerobic bacillus *Clostridium tetani*. Tetanospasmin is released from proliferating *C tetani*, circulates to peripheral nerve terminals, and then is transported centrally in axons to presynaptic inhibitory neurons. The toxin acts by blocking the release of the neurotransmitter γ-amino benzoic acid (GABA) [44]. A loss of motor neuron inhibition leads to the signs of muscle rigidity, muscle spasm, and autonomic overactivity. The disease has become rare because of the widespread use of vaccines containing tetanus toxoid.

Clinical signs

The disease is characterized by a rapidly progressive muscular rigidity and hyper-responsiveness to stimuli of any kind [45,46]. Affected foals may at first appear to have trouble suckling because of spasms of the masticatory muscles (trismus) and neck that are induced during teat-seeking. Even if the foal can drink milk, reflex pharyngeal spasms prevent swallowing, and milk is returned from the mouth and nose. Limb and back extension result in a "sawhorse" posture, with the elevation of the tail and rigid extension of the head and ears. Attempts to move or change direction or gait may provoke muscle spasms and cause the foal to fall. The face often has a wooden, anxious expression (risus sardonicus), and there may be an intermittent prolapse of the nictitans in response to external stimuli. Sympathetic overactivity may result in tachycardia, fluctuant heart rate, and profuse sweating. Eventually the foal becomes laterally recumbent in a rigidly extended position and is subject to rounds of severe tonic muscle contractions. Death is caused by respiratory failure or, possibly, by the cardiac effects of sympathetic overactivity.

Diagnosis

The diagnosis is based on clinical signs in the context of a history of poor vaccination of the dam against tetanus or the failure of passive transfer of immunity to the foal.

Treatment

Any wound or abscess should be cleaned, flushed, and debrided to remove the source of toxin. Circulating toxin can be neutralized by IV antitoxin (arbitrary dose of 5000 units IV). Metronidazole (10–25 mg/kg IV or PO, every 12 h) should be given to kill residual organisms [44]. Penicillin is no longer recommended because of potential GABA antagonism. The basis of therapy in horses is drug-induced sedation and muscle relaxation [4,46]. Diazepam and midazolam are effective for short-term control (eg, for the facilitation of procedures) but may be impractical for chronic use. Sodium pentobarbital (3–10 mg/kg IV, every 8 h or by continuous infusion), a GABA agonist, and chlorpromazine (0.04–0.08 mg/kg), an α-adrenergic antagonist, are used in combination. Intensive supportive therapy is essential. It is theoretically possible to paralyze and mechanically ventilate an affected foal for the several weeks required for toxin to be removed.

Recently, the use of magnesium as the sole therapy has been adopted for treatment of human neonatal tetanus in underdeveloped countries [44]. Magnesium has the advantage of blocking both neuromuscular transmission and sympathetic overactivity. Although not yet tested for this purpose in horses, the use of continuous infusion of $MgSO_4$ seems logical. As used by Wilkins [5] for treating HIE, a dosage of 0.05 mg/kg/h loading dose and then 0.025 mg/kg/h thereafter is recommended. The dose should be titrated to control clinical signs without causing respiratory depression.

Differential diagnosis
The differential diagnosis of tetanus includes meningitis and myopathy.

Prognosis
The fatality rate reported for horses of all ages has been 75% [46]. Thus, the prognosis is at best guarded for foals that are treated before they become recumbent and poor for foals that are unable to stand.

Hydrocephalus

Etiology
Foals are born with hydrocephalus caused by genetic defects in the cerebral ventricular system [1,4]. The condition also may be acquired as a result of inflammatory changes associated with meningitis. In all cases with clinical signs, there is attenuation of cerebral structures associated with abnormally distended ventricles.

Clinical signs
Most foals appear physically normal, although a few may have obvious doming of the skull. Signs vary greatly in severity but are referable to cerebral dysfunction. There may be dullness, poor bonding with the mare, head-pressing, compulsive walking, seizures, and the variable development of menace responses. Involvement of the brain stem is indicated by strabismus or limb ataxia and weakness.

Diagnosis

The diagnosis is presumptive, unless it is confirmed by cross-sectional imaging techniques (CT and MRI), which have replaced the older techniques of ventriculography.

Differential diagnoses

The differential diagnoses of hydrocephalus include HIE, hydranencephaly or other congenital brain anomalies, and sepsis.

Treatment and prognosis

There is no treatment. Foals with hydrocephalus are unlikely to ingest adequate colostrum and are therefore unusually susceptible to neonatal sepsis. Even if they are intensively supported, most foals remain ill-thrifty.

References

[1] Knottenbelt D, Holdstock N, Madigan JE. Equine neonatology: medicine and surgery. Edinburgh: WB Saunders; 2004.

[2] Vaala WE, House JK, Madigan JE. Initial management and physical examination of the neonate. In: Smith BP, editor. Large animal internal medicine. St Louis: Mosby; 2002. p. 277–93.

[3] Vaala WE, House JK. Perinatal adaptation, asphyxia, and resuscitation. In: Smith BP, editor. Large animal internal medicine. St Louis: Mosby; 2002. p. 266–76.

[4] Green SL, Mayhew IG. Neurologic disorders. In: Koterba AM, Drummond WH, Kosch PC, editors. Equine clinical neonatology. Philadelphia: Lea & Febiger; 1990. p. 496–530.

[5] Wilkins PA. Disorders of foals. In: Reed SM, Bayly WM, Sellon DC, editors. Equine internal medicine. St Louis: WB Saunders; 2004. p. 1381–431.

[6] Martens RJ. Pediatrics. In: Mansmann RA, McAllister ES, Pratt PW, editors. Equine medicine and surgery. Santa Barbara (CA): American Veterinary Publications; 1982.

[7] Vaala WE, House JK. Manifestations of disease in the neonate. In: Smith BP, editor. Large animal internal medicine. St Louis: Mosby; 2002. p. 319–86.

[8] Drummond WH. Neonatal maladjustment syndrome: its relationship to perinatal hypoxic-ischaemic insults. Equine Vet J Suppl 1988;5:41–3.

[9] Mayhew IG. Neurological and neuropathological observations on the equine neonate. Equine Vet J Suppl 1988;5:28–33.

[10] Mayhew IG. Observations on vascular accidents in the central nervous system of neonatal foals. J Reprod Fertil Suppl 1982;32:569–75.

[11] Palmer AC, Rossdale PD. Neuropathological changes associated with the neonatal maladjustment syndrome in the thoroughbred foal. Res Vet Sci 1976;20(3):267–75.

[12] Palmer AC, Rossdale PD. Neuropathology of the convulsive foal syndrome. J Reprod Fertil Suppl 1975;23:691–4.

[13] Palmer AC, Leadon DP, Rossdale PD, et al. Intracranial haemorrhage in pre-viable, premature and full term foals. Equine Vet J 1984;16(4):383–9.

[14] Hess-Dudan F, Rossdale PD. Neonatal maladjustment syndrome and other neurologic signs in the newborn foal. Equine Veterinary Education 1996;8:24–32.

[15] Baker SM, Drummond WH, Lane TJ, et al. Follow-up evaluation of horses after neonatal intensive care. J Am Vet Med Assoc 1986;189(11):1454–7.

[16] Koterba AM, Brewer BD, Tarplee FA. Clinical and clinicopathological characteristics of the septicaemic neonatal foal: review of 38 cases. Equine Vet J 1984;16(4):376–82.

[17] Stuart BP, Martin BR, Williams LP Jr, Von Byern H. Salmonella-induced meningoencephalitis in a foal. J Am Vet Med Assoc 1973;162(3):211–3.
[18] Morris DD, Rutkowski J, Lloyd KC. Therapy in two cases of neonatal foal septicaemia and meningitis with cefotaxime sodium. Equine Vet J 1987;19(2):151–4.
[19] Chaudhuri A. Adjunctive dexamethasone treatment in acute bacterial meningitis. Lancet Neurol 2004;3(1):54–62.
[20] MacKay RJ. Brain injury after head trauma: pathophysiology, diagnosis, and treatment. Vet Clin North Am Equine Pract 2004;20(1):199–216.
[21] Roberts I, Yates D, Sandercock P, et al. Effect of intravenous corticosteroids on death within 14 days in 10008 adults with clinically significant head injury (MRC CRASH trial): randomised placebo-controlled trial. Lancet 2004;364(9442):1321–8.
[22] Bracken MB, Shepard MJ, Holford TR, et al for the National Acute Spinal Cord Injury Study. Administration of methylprednisolone for 24 or 48 hours or tirilazad mesylate for 48 hours in the treatment of acute spinal cord injury: results of the Third National Acute Spinal Cord Injury Randomized Controlled Trial. JAMA 1997;277(20):1597–604.
[23] McIlwraith CW, Robertson JT. Surgical repair of depression fractures of the skull. In: McIlwraith and Turner's equine surgery: advanced techniques. Philadelphia: Lippincott Williams & Wilkins; 1998. p. 276–7.
[24] Owen R, Maxie LL. Repair of fractured dens of the axis in a foal. J Am Vet Med Assoc 1978; 173(7):854–6.
[25] Nixon AJ, Stashak TS. Laminectomy for relief of atlantoaxial subluxation in four horses. J Am Vet Med Assoc 1988;193(6):677–82.
[26] McCoy DJ, Shires PK, Beadle R. Ventral approach for stabilization of atlantoaxial subluxation secondary to odontoid fracture in a foal. J Am Vet Med Assoc 1984;185(5): 545–9.
[27] Mayhew IG. Large animal neurology: a handbook for veterinary clinicians. Philadelphia: Lea & Febiger; 1989.
[28] Eberstein A, Eberstein S. Electrical stimulation of denervated muscle: is it worthwhile? Med Sci Sports Exerc 1996;28(12):1463–9.
[29] Schimrigk K, McLaughlin J, Gruninger W. The effect of electrical stimulation on the experimentally denervated rat muscle. Scand J Rehabil Med 1977;9(2):55–60.
[30] Mayhew IG, Brown CM, Stowe HD, et al. Equine degenerative myeloencephalopathy: a vitamin E deficiency that may be familial. J Vet Intern Med 1987;1(1):45–50.
[31] Blythe LL, Hultgren BD, Craig AM, et al. Clinical, viral, and genetic evaluation of equine degenerative myeloencephalopathy in a family of Appaloosas. J Am Vet Med Assoc 1991; 198(6):1005–13.
[32] Gandini G, Fatzer R, Mariscoli M, et al. Equine degenerative myeloencephalopathy in five Quarter Horses: clinical and neuropathological findings. Equine Vet J 2004;36(1):83–5.
[33] Blythe LL, Craig AM, Lassen ED, et al. Serially determined plasma alpha-tocopherol concentrations and results of the oral vitamin E absorption test in clinically normal horses and in horses with degenerative myeloencephalopathy. Am J Vet Res 1991;52(6):908–11.
[34] Lunn DP, Cuddon PA, Shaftoe S, et al. Familial occurrence of narcolepsy in miniature horses. Equine Vet J 1993;25(6):483–7.
[35] Bjorck G, Everz KE, Hansen HJ, et al. Congenital cerebellar ataxia in the gotland pony breed. Zentralblatt fur Veterinarmedizin A 1973;20(4):341–54.
[36] DeBowes RM, Leipold HW, Turner-Beatty M. Cerebellar abiotrophy. Vet Clin North Am Equine Pract 1987;3(2):345–52.
[37] Palmer AC, Blakemore WF, Cook WR, et al. Cerebellar hypoplasia and degeneration in the young Arab horse: clinical and neuropathological features. Vet Rec 1973;93(3):62–6.
[38] Mayhew IG, Watson AG, Heissan JA. Congenital occipitoatlantoaxial malformations in the horse. Equine Vet J 1978;10(2):103–13.
[39] Haagsma J, Haesebrouck F, Devriese L, et al. An outbreak of botulism type B in horses. Vet Rec 1990;127(8):206.

[40] Kinde H, Bettey RL, Ardans A, et al. *Clostridium botulinum* type-C intoxication associated with consumption of processed alfalfa hay cubes in horses. J Am Vet Med Assoc 1991;199(6): 742–6.
[41] Whitlock RH, Buckley C. Botulism. Vet Clin North Am Equine Pract 1997;13(1):107–28.
[42] Wilkins PA, Palmer JE. Botulism in foals less than 6 months of age: 30 cases (1989–2002). J Vet Intern Med 2003;17(5):702–7.
[43] Wilkins PA, Palmer JE. Mechanical ventilation in foals with botulism: 9 cases (1989–2002). J Vet Intern Med 2003;17(5):708–12.
[44] Attygalle D, Rodrigo N. New trends in the management of tetanus. Expert Rev Anti Infect Ther 2004;2(1):73–84.
[45] Beroza GA. Tetanus in the horse. J Am Vet Med Assoc 1980;177(11):1152–4.
[46] Green SL, Little CB, Baird JD, et al. Tetanus in the horse: a review of 20 cases (1970 to 1990). J Vet Intern Med 1994;8(2):128–32.

ELSEVIER
SAUNDERS

Vet Clin Equine 21 (2005) 407–429

VETERINARY
CLINICS
Equine Practice

Equine Neonatal Thoracic and Abdominal Ultrasonography

Michael B. Porter, DVM, PhD[a],*, Sammy Ramirez, DVM, MS[b]

[a]*Department of Large Animal Clinical Sciences, College of Veterinary Medicine, University of Florida, 2015 SW 16th Avenue, PO Box 100136, Gainesville, FL 32610, USA*
[b]*College of Veterinary Medicine, Louisiana State University, Baton Rouge, LA, USA*

Ultrasonography has become a well-established imaging modality in the diagnostic workup of a wide variety of equine neonatal disorders. The small size of neonates compared with adult horses makes foals ideal patients for evaluation by this modality. Because ultrasonographic examination rarely requires patient sedation, there are no contraindications for its use.

Improved image quality, availability, and cost of portable machines have resulted in expanded use of this modality. The sonologist must have a good understanding of the machine, equine anatomy, and indications and limitations of ultrasonography to maximize its diagnostic potential, however. This article is intended to serve as a review of ultrasound technique, normal anatomy, and some disease processes affecting the equine neonatal thorax and abdomen.

General technique

As the name implies, ultrasound is characterized by high-frequency sound waves that are inaudible to the human ear. Although ultrasound frequencies can vary from 1 to 100 MHz, ultrasound waves commonly used in diagnostic veterinary examinations produce sound waves with a frequency range between 2 and 15 MHz.

Ultrasound machines generate sound waves in pulses by intermittently energizing piezoelectric crystals within transducers (probes or scan head). The same crystals then detect the returning echoes resulting from sound

---

* Corresponding author.
E-mail address: portermi@mail.vetmed.ufl.edu (M.B. Porter).

reflecting tissue interfaces. These returning echoes generate electrical impulses that are electronically manipulated and displayed on ultrasound machine monitors. Crystal thickness dictates the frequency of the transducer; thus, decreased crystal thickness produces shorter wavelengths and higher frequencies. Frequency is inversely related to the depth of sound beam penetration. Hence, low-frequency ultrasound waves (2–5 MHz) are able to penetrate deeper distances compared with higher frequency ultrasound waves (10–15 MHz).

Most equine neonatal examinations can be performed with a transducer frequency between 5 and 7.5 MHz. The highest frequency transducer providing adequate penetration should be chosen to maximize resolution. Newer multifrequency transducers have made clinical examinations easier and faster because they allow multiple organs to be evaluated without having to switch transducers.

Linear, curved (convex) linear, and sector transducers can be used. The sector and curved linear transducers are preferred to a linear array transducer because of the smaller contact area, allowing placement of the transducer in the intercostal spaces and under the sternum. Additionally, the wedge-shaped beam configuration of the sector and curved linear transducers allows deeper structures to be imaged and provides a wider field of view than that of linear arrays.

The foal can be examined standing or in lateral recumbency. Hair clipping of the ventral body wall from the xiphoid to the inguinal region and one third to one half of the way up the lateral body wall is recommended for optimum image resolution. Hair clipping may not be necessary if the hair coat is thin, however. Because of the acoustic impedance between air and soft tissue, the body wall should be moistened with aqueous ultrasound gel or isopropyl alcohol to facilitate transmission of the ultrasound beam into soft tissues.

Gastrointestinal tract

Normal structures

The stomach can be visualized from the left tenth intercostal space approximately one half of the way up the lateral body wall and from the ventral aspect of the cranial abdomen [1]. Its appearance varies depending on its size and intraluminal contents, but it typically appears as a curvilinear echo medial to the spleen and caudal to the liver (Fig. 1A). If it is filled with gas, reverberation artifact and acoustic shadowing obscure deep portions of the stomach. If it is filled with fluid, however, it is possible to examine a larger portion of the stomach (see Fig. 1B). Gastric wall thickness in adult horses can measure up to 7.5 mm and is usually thinner in foals [1]. The duodenum can be visualized from the right side of the abdomen at approximately the fifteenth intercostal space. It can be seen along the caudal

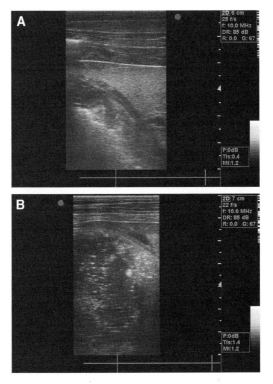

Fig. 1. (*A*) Sonogram of the left side of the abdomen in the tenth intercostal space obtained from a normal neonatal foal. A portion of the fluid- and gas-filled stomach is seen cranial to the spleen and deep to the intercostal musculature. The image was obtained with a 10-MHz linear transducer and 6-cm displayed depth. (*B*) Sonogram of the left side of the abdomen in the tenth intercostal space obtained from a neonatal foal with colic. A fluid-filled stomach is seen cranial to the spleen and deep to the intercostal musculature. The spleen is displaced caudally because of the overdistention of the stomach. The image was obtained with a 10-MHz linear transducer and 7-cm displayed depth.

medial margins of the liver and followed caudodorsally around the caudal pole of the right kidney. The ventral abdomen is usually occupied by the large colon and small bowel. Because of the poorly developed large colon in neonatal foals, sonographic evaluation of a large portion of the small intestine is possible [1,2]. In foals older than 4 months of age, sonographic visualization of the small intestine is limited to the inguinal region [3]. Sections of small bowel are viewed sagittally and transversely as the transducer is moved from left to right and cranial to caudal. The depth of field is set to visualize dorsally located bowel and is then decreased to visualize superficially located bowel. The small intestine is generally flaccid, characterized by little or transiently visible lumen contents [2,4], and usually has rhythmic contractions (Fig. 2) [3]. Using a high-frequency transducer, visualization of the hyperechoic mucosal surface, hypoechoic mucosa,

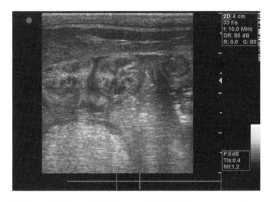

Fig. 2. Sonogram of the caudal ventral abdomen obtained from a normal neonatal foal. Several loops of normal small intestine can be seen immediately adjacent to the body wall in cross section. The image was obtained with a 10-MHz linear transducer and 4-cm displayed depth.

hyperechoic submucosa, hypoechoic muscularis propria, and hyperechoic serosa is possible. In the ileum, an additional thin hyperechoic layer, which represents connective tissue separating the longitudinal and circular muscular layers, can also be seen [1]. Excluding the ileum, which is slightly thicker (4–5 mm), the small and large bowel wall rarely exceeds 3 mm in thickness [1]. It should be noted that large quantities of gas within the gastrointestinal tract cause reverberation and shadowing artifacts, resulting in difficulties in bowel wall measurement.

When evaluating the neonatal gastrointestinal tract, one should evaluate bowel wall thickness and layering, uniformity in bowel diameter, luminal contents, and peristalsis. If disease is present, one should determine whether the disease is focal or generalized and which portion of the gastrointestinal tract is affected. Because fluid-filled or edematous bowel gravitates toward the dependent portion of the abdomen, it is imperative that the ventral-most portion of the abdomen of a standing foal or the dependent side of a laterally recumbent foal is closely evaluated [1,2].

Evaluation of the quantity and echogenic characteristics of peritoneal fluid should be performed during examination of a neonatal abdomen. Normally, there is a small amount of anechoic fluid visualized within the abdomen. The ultrasonographic appearance of peritoneal effusion can vary but typically becomes more echogenic as the cellularity increases (Fig. 3). Visualization of gas echoes or particulate matter within the peritoneum is indicative of a ruptured viscus. If abdominocentesis is warranted, the most favorable site can be determined with the use of ultrasonography.

Abnormal structures

The ultrasonographic appearance of small intestine abnormalities, including enteritis, intussusception, and mechanical obstruction, has been

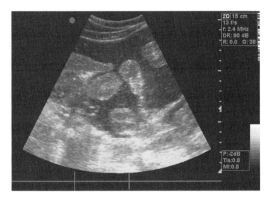

Fig. 3. Sonogram of the caudal ventral abdomen obtained from a depressed neonatal foal with colic. Several loops of small intestine in cross section can be seen suspended in anechoic fluid. Cellular debris can be seen diffusely throughout the fluid. The image was obtained with a 2.4-MHz sector transducer and 15-cm displayed depth.

reported. The most common ultrasonographic abnormality associated with enteritis is fluid-filled hypermotile bowel (Figs. 4 and 5) [1]. Hypomotile bowel may also be seen, however [4]. The intestinal wall may be normal or abnormally thickened, with normal wall layering. Multiple pinpoint gas echoes within the bowel wall and shreds of sloughed mucosa within bowel lumen, which appear as linear hyperechogenicities, may be seen in some foals affected with clostridial enteritis [1,2].

Intussusception is a commonly recognized cause of colic in foals [5]. Although jejunojejunal intussusception is the most common intussusception in foals, ileal-ileal, ileocecal, cecocolic, and cecocecal intussusceptions have also been described [6]. Ultrasonographically, intussusceptions appear as

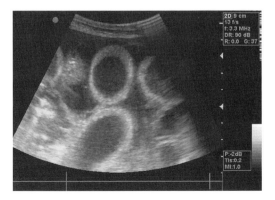

Fig. 4. Sonogram of the caudal ventral abdomen obtained from a depressed neonatal foal with colic. Several loops of hypomotile small intestine in cross section can be seen suspended in anechoic fluid. The intestinal wall appears thick, and the loops of intestine are distended. The image was obtained with a 3.3-MHz sector transducer and 9-cm displayed depth.

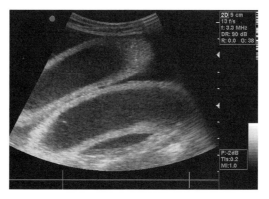

Fig. 5. Sonogram of the caudal ventral abdomen obtained from a depressed neonatal foal with colic. Several loops of hypomotile small intestine in longitudinal section can be seen suspended in anechoic fluid. The intestinal wall appears thick, and the loops of intestine are distended. The image was obtained with a 3.3-MHz sector transducer and 9-cm displayed depth.

symmetric and multiple concentric rings representing wall layers of the intussusceptum (inner bowel segment) and intussuscipiens (outer bowel segment) (Fig. 6). The intussusceptum usually appears as a central echogenic core representing normal bowel layering. Occasionally, invaginated mesenteric fat, fluid, or fibrin may be present between the intussusceptum and intussuscipiens. If the walls are compromised, they may appear hypoechoic because of edema. In most cases, excess peritoneal effusion is visible within the abdomen of foals affected with an intussusception [6]. With ileocecal intussusceptions, the sacculations of the outer segment of bowel (cecum) may not be easily imaged [1]. Cecocolic intussusceptions may

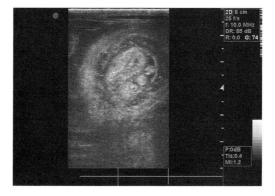

Fig. 6. Sonogram of the caudal ventral abdomen obtained from a neonatal foal with diarrhea and colic. Intussuscepted small intestines appear as multiple concentric rings (target lesions) representing the inner and outer layers of the intussuscepted bowel. The intestinal wall appears thick with edema and distended in cross section. The image was obtained with a 10-MHz sector transducer and 6-cm displayed depth.

be differentiated from cecocecal intussusceptions by visualization of the cecal tip of the intussuscepting cecum in cecocecal intussusceptions [6]. In cecocolic intussusceptions, the cecal tip enters the right ventral colon and may not be visualized [6]. Small intestinal intussusceptions may result in partial or complete distention of bowel proximal to the lesion. Jejunojejunal intussusceptions are usually imaged from the ventral abdomen, whereas ileal-ileal, cecocolic, and cecocecal intussusceptions are usually seen from the right flank and ventral abdominal region extending cranially toward the sternum [6].

Ultrasonographically, a strangulated section of small intestine caused by a hernia or congenital abnormality, such as Meckel's diverticulum, appears as turgid, fluid-filled, amotile or hypomotile small intestine (Fig. 7). The small intestine proximal to the lesion is distended, whereas normal loops of intestine are seen distal to the lesion. The affected intestinal wall is normal shortly after the volvulus occurs; however, the wall becomes thickened from congestion and edema, and the bowel distention becomes less noticeable as the bowel undergoes ischemic necrosis (Fig. 8) [7]. With a complete volvulus, the entire small intestine may be affected and congested mesenteric vessels surround the mesenteric root [1]. The quantity of peritoneal fluid may be increased, and fine linear echogenicities representing fibrin may be visualized in strangulating obstructions. Because mechanical obstruction can appear sonographically similar to enteritis, the sonographic findings should always be interpreted in conjunction with the physical examination findings, history, laboratory data, and abdominocentesis results. At times, the diagnosis may still be unclear despite the physical examination findings, history, laboratory data, and abdominocentesis results, and follow-up ultrasound may be warranted.

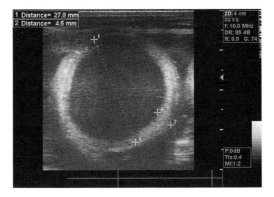

Fig. 7. Sonogram of the ventral abdomen obtained from a depressed neonatal foal with colic. A single loop of hypomotile small intestine in cross section can be seen. The intestinal wall is thick, and the loop of intestine is distended. The image was obtained with a 10-MHz sector transducer and 4-cm displayed depth.

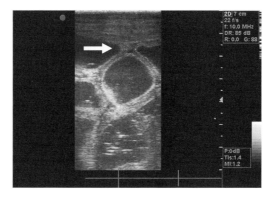

Fig. 8. Sonogram of the caudal ventral abdomen obtained from a refluxing neonatal foal. Several loops of hypomotile small intestine in cross section can be seen suspended in anechoic fluid. The intestinal wall appears thick, and the loops of intestine are distended. An adhesion is seen between the body wall and a loop of small intestine (*arrow*). The image was obtained with a 10-MHz sector transducer and 7-cm displayed depth.

Small intestinal adhesions and excessive peritoneal effusion may be seen in some foals with small intestinal volvulus, enteritis, intussusceptions, or viscus rupture (see Fig. 8). To identify adhesions, the transducer should be held still in one position while observing whether the intestines move independently between one another, adjacent organs, or peritoneum. Loops of bowel that are fixed in position, especially after abdominal surgery, suggest adhesions [3].

By far, one of the most common clinical complaints in equine neonates associated with colic is meconium impaction. Careful examination of the entire abdomen with an ultrasound transducer may provide information regarding the extent and severity of the impaction (Fig. 9).

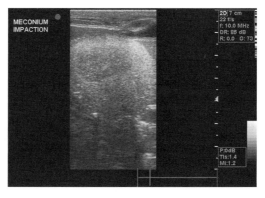

Fig. 9. Sonogram of the cranial ventral abdomen obtained from a newborn foal with colic. A hypoechoic structure that casts an acoustic shadow is noted within the lumen of the large colon, consistent with meconium impaction. The image was obtained with a 10-MHz sector transducer and 7-cm displayed depth.

Urogenital tract

Normal structures

In foals less than 4 weeks of age, the urinary bladder and umbilical remnants are located in the caudal ventral abdomen and easily examined sonographically. Between 4 and 8 weeks of age, these structures regress toward the pelvic brim and become difficult to visualize, especially when obscured by gas within the large colon [1]. The urinary bladder is visualized as an anechoic oblong structure with a thin echogenic wall (Fig. 10). At times, large blood clots caused by trauma during birth may be seen within the urinary bladder [3]. Because urinary bladder wall thickness varies with the degree of distention, the urinary bladder is best examined when moderately full. Ultrasonography has become the primary modality for evaluation of the umbilicus [1,2,8,9]. The umbilicus is formed by paired umbilical arteries, an umbilical vein, and the urachus and can be divided into external and internal parts. As the umbilicus atrophies, the external portion detaches from the skin, whereas the internal portion becomes normal ligaments that regress into the abdomen. The arteries become the left and right round ligaments of the urinary bladder, and the umbilical vein becomes the falciform ligament.

Abnormal structures

A diagnosis of uroperitoneum secondary to urinary bladder rupture may be easily and quickly assessed with the aid of ultrasonography. Typically, a ruptured urinary bladder is collapsed and floating within an anechoic peritoneal effusion. Urinary bladders with small tears can appear full and

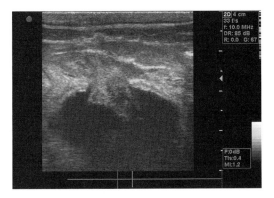

Fig. 10. Sonogram of the caudal ventral abdomen obtained from a normal neonatal foal. The urinary bladder appears as an irregularly shaped structure that is filled with anechoic fluid. A hyperechoic structure is seen protruding ventrally into the bladder, most likely consistent with a postfoaling blood clot. The image was obtained with a 10-MHz linear transducer and 4-cm displayed depth.

turgid, however [2]. The tear commonly occurs in the dorsal urinary bladder wall. The defect may not always be imaged during the sonographic examination because of infolding of the bladder wall. The infolding wall should not be mistaken for a recently voided small and contracted urinary bladder. During real-time examination, urine may be seen passing through the rent and into the peritoneum. Anechoic fluid is typically seen within the abdominal cavity in foals with uroperitoneum. Some foals may have echogenic fluid from peritonitis or urinary sediment, however [1]. In acute cases, the quantity of fluid within the peritoneum may be small. Therefore, the most dependent portion of the abdomen should be carefully evaluated [2].

Abnormalities associated with the external umbilical stump include infections, hernias, and a patent urachus. Pain, heat, discharge, and swelling of the external umbilicus can be seen on physical examination and may be indicative of an infection. Ultrasound helps to determine whether the swelling is associated with the vein, arteries, or urachus and differentiates whether edema, fibrosis, or intraluminal fluid is affecting these structures. In some foals with small defects in the body wall, leakage of peritoneal fluid can cause warm soft tissue swelling in the region of the umbilicus. In these cases, ultrasonography helps to differentiate between cellulitis and the dissection of peritoneal fluid into the subcutaneous tissues [2]. A hernia may be diagnosed with digital palpation alone; however, ultrasonography allows evaluation of the herniated contents (ie, omental fat, bowel) and, if bowel is present, the viability of its wall [2]. A moist external umbilicus consistent with a patent urachus may be seen on physical examination. Ultrasonography allows evaluation of the entire size and character of the urachus and periurachal tissues, however, assisting in differentiating between a simple patent urachus and an internal or external infectious process.

Evaluation of the internal umbilical remnants has been well described. The umbilical vein, which eventually forms the falciform ligament of the liver, is present on midline approximately 1 to 2 cm deep to the skin surface and extends cranially from the external umbilical stump to the liver (Fig. 11). Sonographically, it appears as a thin-walled ovoid structure with an anechoic center that measures from 0.5 to 1.0 cm in diameter [1]. The sections next to the liver and external umbilical stump are usually the largest in diameter [1]. The vein is easier to follow while orienting the transducer perpendicular to the spine. Transverse and sagittal measurements should be obtained. Normally, the transverse diameter is slightly larger than the sagittal diameter [1].

The umbilical arteries originate from the internal iliac arteries and descend ventrally along the urinary bladder, coursing past the apex toward the umbilicus along the urachus. Sonographically, they appear as thick-walled hyperechoic vessels that normally measure less than 1.3 cm in diameter (Figs. 12–16) [1]. They may be asymmetric in size, may be seen pulsating in foals less than 24 hours of age, and may contain an echogenic center if filled with clotted blood [1].

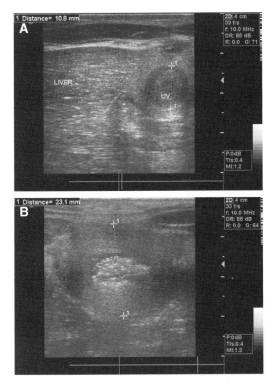

Fig. 11. (A) Sonogram of the cranial ventral abdomen obtained from a normal neonatal foal. The umbilical vein (UV) is seen adjacent to the liver and deep to the abdominal wall. The image was obtained with a 10-MHz linear transducer and 4-cm displayed depth. (B) Sonogram of the cranial ventral abdomen obtained from a neonatal foal with a persistent fever. The UV is seen in cross section and appears distended with hyperechoic material, consistent with abscessation of the vessel. The image was obtained with a 10-MHz linear transducer and 4-cm displayed depth.

The urachus extends from the external stump to the apex of the urinary bladder. It is a long tubular structure with a collapsed center that is normally difficult to view sonographically unless it is fluid-filled. Its communication with the apex of the urinary bladder is best seen with a sagittal view. At the apex of the bladder, a transverse view of the urachus and arteries normally measures less than 2.5 cm in diameter [1].

Infection is a common abnormality affecting the internal umbilical remnants. Intraluminal distention with fluid and thickening of surrounding tissue of any or all umbilical remnants is consistent with an infectious process. The echogenicity of the intraluminal fluid can be hypoechoic, anechoic, or echogenic (Fig. 17) [1,2,8]. The presence of small gas echoes may be indicative of anaerobic infection. An urachal infection may ascend proximally and result in concurrent cystitis in some foals [1]. Additionally, some foals with urachal infections may develop localized adhesions to the

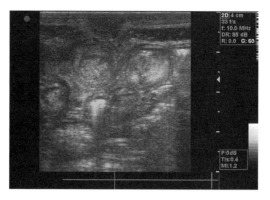

Fig. 12. Sonogram of the caudal ventral abdomen obtained from a normal neonatal foal. The ultrasound transducer is located immediately caudal to the external umbilical stump and perpendicular to the midline. The pair of umbilical arteries can be seen in cross section just deep to the body wall. The image was obtained with a 10-MHz linear transducer and 4-cm displayed depth.

adjacent gastrointestinal tract and spleen [1]. Thus, the surrounding tissues should be evaluated in all foals with colic and infected umbilical remnants. It should be noted that intraluminal fluid secondary to an infectious process could be indistinguishable from hemorrhage secondary to trauma during foaling (Fig. 18). For this reason, the ultrasonographic abnormalities should be correlated with the history, clinical signs, physical examination findings, and clinical laboratory data.

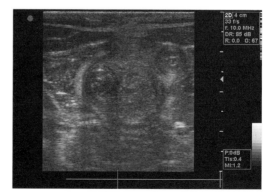

Fig. 13. Sonogram of the caudal ventral abdomen obtained from a normal neonatal foal. The ultrasound transducer is located slightly caudal to that in Fig. 12 and perpendicular to the midline. The pair of umbilical arteries can be seen in cross section, and the urachus is noted centered between the arteries. The image was obtained with a 10-MHz linear transducer and 4-cm displayed depth.

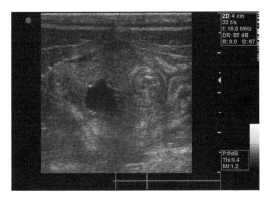

Fig. 14. Sonogram of the caudal ventral abdomen obtained from a normal neonatal foal. The ultrasound transducer is located slightly caudal to that in Fig. 13 and perpendicular to the midline. The pair of umbilical arteries can be seen in cross section moving further apart, and the tip of the urinary bladder is centered between the arteries. The image was obtained with a 10-MHz linear transducer and 4-cm displayed depth.

Renal

Normal structures

The right kidney is located high in the fourteenth to sixteenth intercostal space just ventral to the transverse processes and close to the lateral abdominal wall (Fig. 19) [1,8]. The left kidney is more variable in location but is commonly located in the seventeenth intercostal space or paralumbar fossa medial to the spleen and is more ventrally located than the right kidney (Fig. 20). Occasionally, it may be seen adjacent to the body wall.

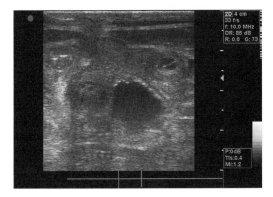

Fig. 15. Sonogram of the caudal ventral abdomen obtained from a normal neonatal foal. The ultrasound transducer is located slightly caudal to that in Fig. 14 and perpendicular to the midline. The pair of umbilical arteries can be seen in cross section, and a greater portion of the urinary bladder is visualized. The image was obtained with a 10-MHz linear transducer and 4-cm displayed depth.

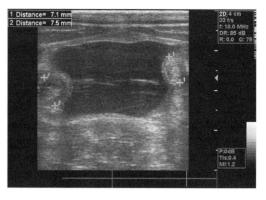

Fig. 16. Sonogram of the caudal ventral abdomen obtained from a normal neonatal foal. The ultrasound transducer is located slightly caudal to that in Fig. 15 and perpendicular to the midline. The pair of umbilical arteries can be seen in cross section on either side of the urinary bladder. The image was obtained with a 10-MHz linear transducer and 4-cm displayed depth.

Within the renal parenchyma, the renal medulla that contains the fluid-filled tubules is less echogenic than the cortex. The renal cortex is less echogenic than the liver and spleen. The normal ureters are not visible with ultrasonography [2].

Abnormal structures

Some renal abnormalities reported in foals include acute renal failure, embolic nephritis, and hydronephrosis [1,10]. Ultrasonography of a foal

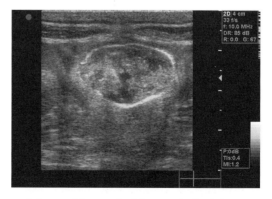

Fig. 17. Sonogram of the caudal ventral abdomen obtained from a neonatal foal with a persistent fever. The ultrasound transducer is located slightly caudal to the external umbilicus and perpendicular to the midline. The umbilical arteries are poorly visible because of the hyperechoic structure located in the center of the internal umbilicus. The variation in echogenicity and increased diameter are consistent with abscessation of the internal umbilicus. The image was obtained with a 10-MHz linear transducer and 4-cm displayed depth.

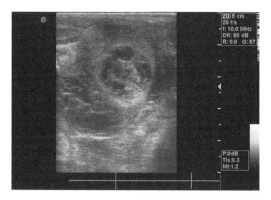

Fig. 18. Sonogram of the caudal ventral abdomen obtained from a normal 24-hour-old foal. The ultrasound transducer is located slightly caudal to the external umbilicus and perpendicular to the midline. The umbilical structures are poorly visible because of the apparent hematoma formation around both umbilical arteries. The image was obtained with a 10-MHz linear transducer and 5-cm displayed depth.

with acute renal failure may reveal no sonographic abnormalities, but some foals may have renomegaly, hypoechoic kidneys, and perirenal edema. Embolic nephritis, which has been reported in colostrum-deficient foals, may present as diffuse or multifocal parenchymal echogenicities [1,10]. Hydronephrosis typically occurs with urinary tract obstruction but has also been reported in one foal with ectopic ureters [1,11]. It should be noted that mild hydronephrosis might be seen in animals undergoing intravenous fluid administration [1,12].

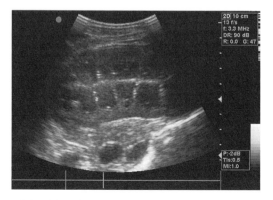

Fig. 19. Sonogram of the right side of the abdomen within the sixteenth intercostal space and just ventral to the transverse processes obtained from a normal neonatal foal. The right kidney is visualized in the long axis. The image was obtained with a 3.3-MHz sector transducer and 10-cm displayed depth.

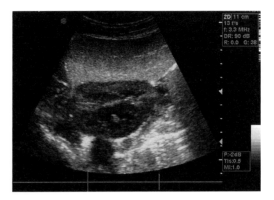

Fig. 20. Sonogram of the left side of the abdomen within the seventeenth intercostal space and cranial to the paralumbar fossa obtained from a normal neonatal foal. The left kidney is visualized in the partial long axis. The left kidney is immediately adjacent to the spleen and appears less echogenic when compared with the spleen. The image was obtained with a 3.3-MHz sector transducer and 11-cm displayed depth.

Hepatic

Normal structures

The liver can be seen from the right and left sides of the abdomen; however, a larger portion can be seen from the right side [1,8]. It can be seen ventral to the lung margins between the sixth and fifteenth intercostal spaces on the right and between the sixth and ninth intercostal spaces on the left. In foals less than 8 weeks of age, the cranial ventral portion of the liver is in contact with the abdomen and therefore can be imaged just caudal to the xiphoid. Normally, the hepatic parenchyma is uniformly of medium echogenicity (ie, hyperechoic to the kidneys, hypoechoic to the spleen), with the hepatic and portal veins interrupting the uniform echo pattern (Fig. 21). The biliary tracts and hepatic arteries are not normally visualized unless abnormal. The portal vasculature has echogenic walls and therefore can be differentiated from the hepatic veins, which lack echogenic walls. Because biliary tracts contain echogenic walls, Doppler ultrasonography is needed to differentiate abnormally dilated biliary tracts from portal veins.

Abnormal structures

Although determination of liver size is usually based on subjective assessment, it has been reported that approximately 4 to 8 cm of liver is visible from the lateral body wall [1]. Multiple factors, however, including size of the thoracic cavity and colonic distention, can influence the quantity of liver visualized in this manner. Subjectively, hepatomegaly should be suspected when there is rounding of the liver margins and an increased distance between the stomach and diaphragm and when liver margins

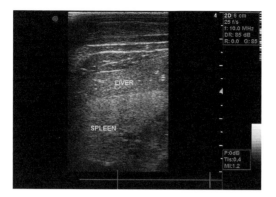

Fig. 21. Sonogram of the left side of the cranial ventral abdomen obtained from a normal neonatal foal. The spleen and liver are adjacent to each other, and the difference in echogenicity is apparent. The normal spleen is hyperechogenic compared with the normal liver. The image was obtained with a 10-MHz linear transducer and 6-cm displayed depth.

extend beyond the rib cage [13]. Conversely, a small liver should be suspected when there is a decreased distance between the stomach and diaphragm and poor visualization of the liver in the absence of pulmonary hyperinflation and gas within the stomach.

Suppurative hepatitis and cholangiohepatitis have been reported in foals. Bacterial infections of the liver, including *Bacillus piriformis* and *Actinobacillus*, occur in foals. A previous report of a foal diagnosed with acute hepatic disorder attributed to Tyzzer's disease revealed hepatomegaly and an increased vascular pattern noted on ultrasound examination [14]. A hypoechoic liver and collapse of the hepatic parenchyma may be seen in foals diagnosed with toxic hepatopathy or hepatocellular necrosis [1]. Cholangiohepatitis secondary to biliary reflux attributable to duodenitis or duodenal stricture may reveal thickened and distended biliary tracts and hyperechoic hepatic parenchyma [1].

Spleen

Normal structures

The spleen is the most echogenic organ within the abdomen. The parenchyma is primarily homogeneous, except for a few vessels derived from the splenic artery and vein. An echogenic capsule surrounds the spleen (see Figs. 1A and 21) [13]. The splenic vein is located medial to the spleen and is present around the 10 intercostal spaces [1]. The spleen is variable in location depending on gastric distention and the size of adjacent organs, such as the liver. Normally, it is seen from approximately the left sixth intercostal space to the paralumbar fossa. It is usually located lateral, caudal, and ventral to the left kidney and medial to the left lobe of the liver. It is variable in size and must be assessed subjectively.

Abnormal structures

When enlarged, it may extend caudally to the urinary bladder and cross midline. Although, splenic diseases are uncommon in foals, a hematoma from blunt trauma to the abdomen caused by a kick may occur [1]. A hematoma and a variable quantity of intra-abdominal hemorrhage may be seen. The hematoma may be within the parenchyma or subcapsular. Its ultrasound appearance may vary depending on its age. Initially, the hematoma may appear hyperechoic but gradually becomes hypoechoic over time.

Pulmonary

Scanning technique

It is typically not necessary to clip the thorax free of hair. Alternatively, rubbing alcohol can be used as a medium for generating adequate contact and providing a diagnostic image. Because of rapid evaporation, the alcohol is only applied immediately before placement of the ultrasound probe. Transthoracic ultrasound in equine neonates can be performed with ultrasound transducers ranging from 5.0 to 10.0 MHz and a depth setting of 5 to 10 cm. Thus, a 7.5-MHz transducer that is used for transrectal ultrasound is adequate in most cases. The author prefers to begin scanning at the dorsal-caudal border of the lung field located in the sixteenth intercostal space and level with the tuber coxae. The lung can be imaged from the right and left sides within the sixteenth to fourth intercostal spaces. In addition, the right apical lung lobe and cranial mediastinum can be imaged in the right third intercostal space by advancing the foal's right foreleg forward and pointing the transducer toward the point of the left shoulder [1,15,16]. Regardless of the type of ultrasound probe (sector versus linear), the probe orientation should not change from one intercostal space to the next. The operator should always scan in a dorsal-to-ventral direction through each intercostal space until visualizing the diaphragm and abdominal structures ventral to the diaphragm. In addition to documenting any abnormalities in the pulmonary tissues, as the operator scans each intercostal space, he or she should monitor for musculoskeletal problems, such as fractured ribs. These appear as "steps" producing acoustic shadowing (Fig. 22).

Normal structures

The normal visceral pleural surface of the lung appears as a straight hyperechoic line with equally spaced artifacts deep to the pleural surface (Fig. 23). These artifacts are attributable to the almost 100% reflection of ultrasound waves by the air– or gas–soft tissue interface. Therefore, if the lung is inflated or aerated, the image only yields information regarding the pleural surface of the lung. In the normal patient, the hyperechoic line

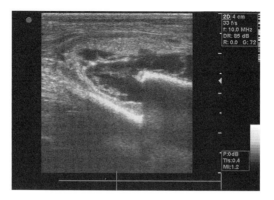

Fig. 22. Sonogram of the left side of the ventral thorax along the fifth rib obtained from a neonatal foal with neonatal maladjustment syndrome. The ultrasound transducer is positioned parallel to the rib, and a "step" is detected at the site of the fracture. A pocket of anechoic fluid is noted around the fracture site, most likely consistent with a hematoma. The image was obtained with a 10-MHz linear transducer and 4-cm displayed depth.

representing the pleural surface should be continuous with no aberrations (ie, comet tails) (Fig. 24). In addition, "the gliding sign" or back-and-forth movements of the pleural surface synchronous with respiration should be observed in normal patients with the transducer held motionless [1,16]. It is not normal to detect pleural fluid; however, a small volume of anechoic fluid may be considered normal just caudal to the heart in the most ventral portion of the thorax. Furthermore, the thymus may be visualized in the equine neonate from the right third intercostal space as a hypoechoic soft tissue mass located in the cranial mediastinum.

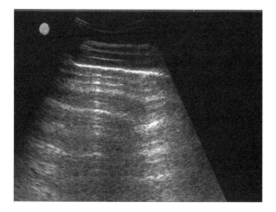

Fig. 23. Sonogram of the left side of the middle thorax along the sixth intercostal space obtained from a normal neonatal foal. The ultrasound transducer is located within the intercostal space and is parallel with the rib. The pleural surface appears as a hyperechoic line. The image was obtained with a 10-MHz linear transducer and 7-cm displayed depth.

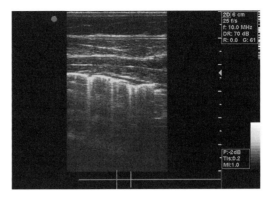

Fig. 24. Sonogram of the left side of the middle thorax along the sixth intercostal space obtained from a neonatal foal with mild pneumonia. The ultrasound transducer is located within the intercostal space and is parallel with the rib. The pleural surface appears as a hyperechoic line that is interrupted by "comet tails." These disruptions in the normal pleural surface correspond with thickening of the pleura. The image was obtained with a 10-MHz linear transducer and 6-cm displayed depth.

Abnormal structures

Pathologic conditions diagnosed by ultrasonography include pleuro-pneumonia, superficial pulmonary abscess, pulmonary consolidation, pneumothorax, and fractured ribs. The ultrasonographic appearance of pleural fluid in an equine neonate, although rare, is similar to that seen in adult horses. An area of anechoic space representing fluid is noted between the lung and the thoracic wall, diaphragm, or heart, depending on its location (Fig. 25). In adults, the presence of pleural fluid is commonly associated with infectious diseases of the lung. Additional differentials for pleural fluid in equine neonates include penetrating thoracic wounds, congenital abnormalities, hemothorax, and uroperitoneum resulting in the diffusion of urine from the abdomen into the pleural space. If pleural fluid is detected, it should be studied carefully to determine the presence of fibrin, cellular debris, and free gas. Thoracocentesis is required to assess the fluid accurately and should be performed where the largest pocket of loculated fluid is imaged with care to avoid causing trauma to the heart, diaphragm, or lung tissue. Ultrasonography can be used to monitor progress after pleural fluid drainage.

Consolidation of lung tissue or pulmonary parenchymal consolidation refers to the filling of alveolar tissue with fluid rather than air and can represent bronchopneumonia, pleural pneumonia, pulmonary edema, pulmonary necrosis, or neoplasia. Ultrasonographically, consolidated lung tissue is commonly wedge shaped, with areas of echogenicity ranging from anechoic to hyperechoic (Fig. 26) [1,16]. Lung tissue consolidation results in ultrasonographic visualization of normally unseen lung anatomy, including

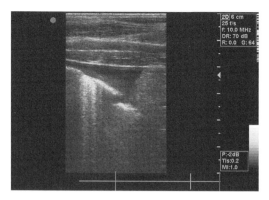

Fig. 25. Sonogram of the left side of the cranial ventral thorax along the fourth intercostal space obtained from a normal neonatal foal. The ultrasound transducer is located within the intercostal space and is parallel with the rib. A small amount of anechoic fluid is present in the cranial ventral aspect of the thorax immediately caudal to the heart. The image was obtained with a 10-MHz linear transducer and 6-cm displayed depth.

pulmonary vessels, air bronchograms, and fluid bronchograms [1,17]. In the most severe cases of lung consolidation, the tissue appears ultrasonographically similar to hepatic tissue and the branching pattern of fluid-filled bronchi (fluid bronchograms) can be noted. Sonographic air bronchograms appear as hyperechoic branching linear echoes within consolidated tissue and correspond to the interface between air-filled bronchi and consolidated pulmonary parenchyma [18]. Occasionally, multifocal hyperechoic gas echoes are detected in consolidated pulmonary parenchyma, indicating the

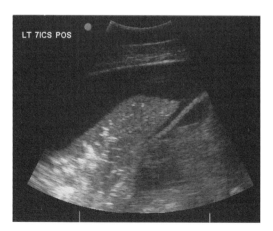

Fig. 26. Sonogram of the right side of the caudal ventral thorax along the seventh intercostal space obtained from a neonatal foal with severe aspiration pneumonia. The ultrasound transducer is located within the intercostal space and is parallel with the rib. The lung lobe appears as hepatic tissue because it is consolidated and suspended in anechoic fluid. The image was obtained with a 5.0-MHz sector transducer and 10-cm displayed depth.

presence of anaerobic bacteria. Ultrasonographic evidence of consolidation is often preceded by the development of comet tails that correspond to the accumulation of small amounts of exudate or cellular debris at the lung surface. Likewise, the resolution of consolidation is commonly associated with the appearance of comet tails in areas that were once without air (see Fig. 24). Meconium aspiration and sepsis are common causes of pulmonary parenchymal consolidation in equine neonates. In older foals, lung consolidation and pleural pulmonary abscesses are common findings in foals infected with *Rhodococcus equi*.

In contrast to pulmonary consolidation, a pulmonary abscess lacks any normal pulmonary architecture and appears as a cavitated lesion with an anechoic center and acoustic enhancement of the far wall indicative of a fluid-filled structure (Fig. 27) [1,8,16]. Pulmonary abscesses are not common in newborn foals; however, severe aspiration pneumonia may result in the development of an abscess. In addition, a pulmonary hematoma secondary to trauma during foaling may appear ultrasonographically as a fluid-filled structure. It is important to note that the absence of pulmonary abscesses on ultrasound examination does not preclude their existence; hence, radiographic evaluation of the thorax is required to evaluate the lung field fully.

A pneumothorax is difficult to detect via ultrasound, because the free gas within the pleural space and the air within the lung generate similar hyperechoic reflection and reverberation artifacts. Careful examination should reveal the absence of the gliding sign at the site of the pneumothorax, however, because the pneumothorax is hiding the respiratory excursions of the lung surface [1,8]. The detection of a pneumothorax in an equine neonate suggests the presence of a penetrating thoracic wound, such as

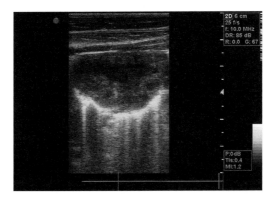

Fig. 27. Sonogram of the right side of the middle thorax along the fifth intercostal space obtained from a neonatal foal with severe aspiration pneumonia. The ultrasound transducer is located within the intercostal space and is parallel with the rib. The pulmonary abscess appears as a cavitated lesion with varying echogenicity. The image was obtained with a 10-MHz sector transducer and 6-cm displayed depth.

a fractured rib. Although rib fractures are relatively common in newborn foals, the incidence of pneumothorax associated with this condition is low.

Summary

Pathologic disorders of the equine neonate often develop shortly after foaling as a result of prematurity, dystocia, trauma, or septicemia. Recognition of these disorders requires routine patient assessment along with diagnostic aids, including abdominal and thoracic ultrasonography. Fortunately, modern technology affords today's equine practitioners the opportunity to use ultrasonography to advance their practice, and it is the authors' hope that this article might help in those efforts.

References

[1] Reef VB. Equine diagnostic ultrasound. Philadelphia: WB Saunders; 1998.
[2] Reimer JM, Bernard WV. Abdominal sonography of the foal. Baltimore, MD: Williams & Wilkins; 1998.
[3] Rantanen NW. Diseases of the abdomen. Vet Clin North Am Equine Pract 1986;2:7–88.
[4] Bernard WV. Assessment of abdominal pain in foals. Proc Am Assoc Equine Pract 2003;49: 22–6.
[5] Bernard WV, Reef VB, Reimer JM. Ultrasonographic diagnosis of small-intestinal intussusception in three foals. J Am Vet Med Assoc 1989;194:395–7.
[6] McGladdery AJ. Ultrasonographic diagnosis of intussusception in foals and yearlings. Proc Am Assoc Equine Pract 1996;40:239–40.
[7] Reimer JM. Sonographic evaluation of gastrointestinal disease in foals. Proc Am Assoc Equine Pract 1993;37:245–6.
[8] Reef VB. Equine pediatric ultrasonography. Compend Contin Educ Pract Vet 1991;13: 1277–85.
[9] Franklin RP, Ferrell EA. How to perform umbilical sonograms in the neonate. Proc Am Assoc Equine Pract 2002;48:261–5.
[10] Robinson JA, Allen GK, Green EM. A prospective study of septicemia in colostrum-deprived foals. Equine Vet J 1993;25:214–9.
[11] Blikslager AT, Green EM, MacFadden KE. Excretory urography and ultrasonography in the diagnosis of bilateral ectopic ureters in a foal. Vet Radiol Ultrasound 1992;33:41–7.
[12] Nyland TG, Mattoon JS, Herrgesell EJ, et al. Urinary tract In: Nyland TG, Mattoon JS, editors. Small animal diagnostic ultrasound. 2nd edition. Philadelphia: WB Saunders; 1995. p. 158–95.
[13] Cudd TA, Wilson JH. Diagnostic techniques for abdominal problems. In: Koterba AM, Drummond WH, Kosch PC, editors. Equine clinical neonatology. Malvern (PA): Lea & Febiger; 1990. p. 379–86.
[14] Peek SF, Byers TD, Rueve E. Neonatal hepatic failure in a Thoroughbred foal: successful treatment of a case of presumptive Tyzzer's disease. Equine Vet Educ 1994;6:307–9.
[15] Rantanen NW. Diseases of the thorax. Vet Clin North Am Equine Pract 1986;2:49–66.
[16] Reimer JM. Diagnostic ultrasonography of the equine thorax. Compend Contin Educ Pract Vet 1990;12:1321–7.
[17] Targhetta R, Chavagneux R, Bourgeois JM, et al. Sonographic approach to diagnosing pulmonary consolidation. J Ultrasound Med 1992;11:667–72.
[18] Weinberg B, Diakoumatis EE, Kass EG, et al. The air bronchogram: sonographic demonstration. AJR Am J Roentgenol 1986;147:593–5.

ELSEVIER
SAUNDERS

VETERINARY
CLINICS
Equine Practice

Vet Clin Equine 21 (2005) 431–455

Resuscitation and Emergency Management for Neonatal Foals

Kevin T.T. Corley, BVM&S, PhD, MRCVS[a,*],
Jane E. Axon, BVSc, MACVSc[b]

[a]Equine Referral Hospital, Royal Veterinary College, Hawkshead Lane,
North Mymms, Hertfordshire AL9 7TA, UK
[b]Clovelly Intensive Care Unit, Scone Veterinary Hospital,
Liverpool Street, Scone, NSW 2337, AUS

Neonatal foals deteriorate rapidly with disease and debilitation. A major contributing factor appears to be foals' physiologic adaptive response, which is poor compared with mature horses. Rapid deterioration demands early identification and treatment of compromised foals. This article outlines emergency resuscitation methods in the foal, including cardiopulmonary cerebral resuscitation, rapid restoration of circulating volume with emergency fluid therapy, respiratory support with oxygen therapy and nutritional support with glucose supplementation.

Cardiopulmonary cerebral resuscitation of the foal

Many procedures performed in equine medicine can be planned at the time they are required. This planning may involve careful selection of patients, gathering of personnel and equipment, reading references describing the procedure, and assigning jobs to the available personnel to carry out the procedure. Although cardiopulmonary cerebral resuscitation (CPCR) requires similar planning, it must be performed before or within a few seconds of the event. An arrest is often a high-intensity situation in which the veterinarian needs to calmly direct other people who may have only rudimentary or no knowledge of CPCR. Sometimes, this direction will be by telephone, because veterinarians are not present at many foalings. Veterinarians also can improve CPCR protocols on larger breeding operations by arranging training sessions for staff before the foaling season.

---

* Corresponding author.
E-mail address: kcorley@rvc.ac.uk (K.T.T. Corley).

0749-0739/05/$ - see front matter © 2005 Elsevier Inc. All rights reserved.
doi:10.1016/j.cveq.2005.04.010   *vetequine.theclinics.com*

Newborn foals can arrest as a result of the birthing process, without any specific underlying pathophysiology, which makes them good candidates for resuscitation, in contrast to critically ill foals and horses that arrest as a result of a disease process.

Recognition of respiratory or cardiac arrest

Normal stage two labor should take less than 20 minutes. Regular breathing should start within 30 seconds of birth. The heart rate should beat regularly at approximately 70 beats per minute (bpm). Foals have pain and sensory awareness at birth and develop a righting reflex within 5 minutes. Respiratory, rather than cardiac, arrest is virtually always primary in the newborn foal. The arrest is usually a result of asphyxia caused by premature placental separation, early severance or twisting of the umbilical cord, prolonged dystocia, or airway obstruction by fetal membranes. Some foals will not start breathing spontaneously without any apparent birthing misadventure.

Foals that require resuscitation gasp for longer than 30 seconds or have obvious dyspnea, or show no respiratory movements or no heartbeat, and have a heart rate less than 50 bpm. Foals at risk of arresting should be identified before foaling so that a veterinarian can be present. Risk factors include vaginal discharge during pregnancy, precocious udder development, placental thickening, illness of the dam during pregnancy, and delivery by caesarean (C)-section.

Equipment for cardiopulmonary cerebral resuscitation

Foals can occasionally be resuscitated successfully with little or no equipment, but a small amount of equipment greatly increases the chance of success. The basic list of equipment includes: clean towels; one 8-mm and one 10-mm (internal diameter) × 55-cm long nasotracheal tubes; a 5-mL syringe for nasotracheal tube cuff inflation; a self-inflating resuscitation bag (eg, Ambu SPUR adult disposable resuscitator with no mask; Ambu Inc., Glen Burnie, Maryland); a small flashlight; a bottle of 1 mg/mL epinephrine; five 2-mL sterile syringes; and one 20-ga × 1-in and one steel 14-ga × 1- to 1.5-in needles. Disposable resuscitation bags, which can be reused after a thorough cleaning, are considerably less expensive to purchase than reusable bags. An oxygen cylinder and flow meter should be available if at all possible. Although it is not strictly essential during resuscitation, many foals will benefit from supplemental oxygen immediately after resuscitation.

The following equipment also is useful during resuscitation: four 1-L bags of lactated Ringer's solution; a fluid administration set; a 14-ga intravenous (IV) catheter; a 6-F dog urinary catheter; a bulb syringe; an indirect arterial blood pressure monitor; a capnograph; and an electric defibrillator. Stud farms without resident veterinarians should consider purchasing a suitable facemask and a resuscitation bag or pump. The equipment for CPCR should be placed in a dedicated, single, easily carried container. Equipment should be thoroughly checked before the foaling season.

Outline of the plan for cardiopulmonary cerebral resuscitation

Preparation: the first 20 seconds

The first 20 seconds after birth are devoted to assessing the foal and preparing for CPCR (Fig. 1). The extent of action at this point depends on the likelihood that the foal will require resuscitation. In a foal born by C-section, these 20 seconds are spent vigorously drying the foal with clean towels (Fig. 2), manually clearing the mouth and nares of secretions, and positioning the foal in lateral recumbency on a firm dry surface. If the foal is covered in thick meconium, suctioning of the airways and trachea also may be attempted. In foals born normally within 20 minutes, these 20 seconds will consist of quiet observation to ensure that the foal's airway is clear and it is spontaneously breathing. If it is available, intranasal oxygen should be supplied during the initial assessment (see "Emergency oxygen therapy" below). CPCR should not be delayed to arrange oxygen supplementation.

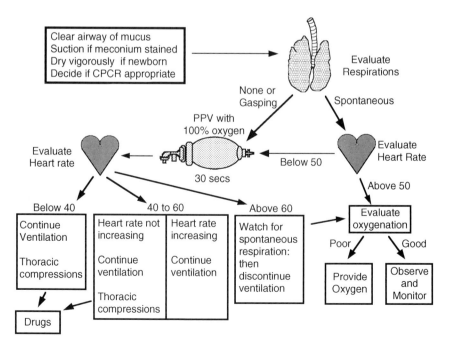

Fig. 1. Overview of resuscitation of the foal using a nasotracheal tube and a self-inflating resuscitation bag.

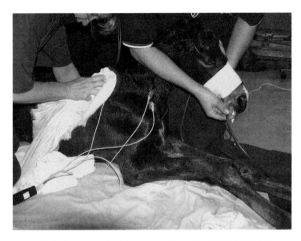

Fig. 2. Vigorous towel drying of a foal born by C-section. (© Kevin Corley and Jane Axon 2004.)

Airway

Foals that are not breathing, have an irregular respiratory pattern, are gasping for more than 30 seconds, or have a heart rate less than 50 bpm need respiratory support. The best way to ensure an adequate airway is to intubate the foal. Intubation through the nose is slightly preferred to intubation through the mouth, because there is less risk of tube damage as the foal regains consciousness. If two brief attempts at nasotracheal intubation are unsuccessful, further attempts should made to intubate be through the mouth. Ideally, intubation should be completed within less than 20 seconds.

For intubation, the foal can be in lateral or sternal recumbency. The head should be in a straight line with the neck. To pass a tube through the nose, the fingers of one hand should be used to push the tip of the tube medially and ventrally into the ventral meatus in the nares. The other hand is used to smoothly advance the tube until the adapter is at the level of the nares. To pass a tube through the mouth, the tongue should be gently pulled forward and to the side with one hand to help stabilize the larynx, and the finger of this hand is used to keep the mouth open. The tube is smoothly advanced over the tongue in a midline position. In both cases, rotation of the tube when the end is in the pharynx can be helpful. Once the tube is in place, the cuff should be gently inflated to ensure a seal with the trachea. If the cuff is insufficiently inflated, air leakage can be heard during application of positive pressure. Overinflating the cuff should be avoided because this may result in ischemia and necrosis of the tracheal epithelium.

It is vital to check that the tube has successfully passed into the trachea. If the tube has entered the esophagus, it can be felt in the cranial neck just dorsal to the larynx or proximal trachea. No resistance should be felt when negative pressure is applied to the tube. The thoracic wall should be seen to rise when the first breath is given.

It is possible to intubate a foal during the foaling process, allowing for the initiation of supported ventilation during foaling. This procedure is most appropriate when a dystocia occurs that cannot be corrected immediately. Providing that the foal's nares can be reached, a nasotracheal tube may be passed and attached to a self-inflating resuscitation bag. If it is available, a capnograph can be attached to the end of the nasotracheal tube to ensure correct placement into the trachea. Furthermore, an end-tidal carbon dioxide tension greater than 15 mm Hg (2 kPa) during this supported ventilation procedure suggests that the foal has adequate cardiac output [1]. It is then possible to provide respiratory support throughout the birthing process, except when manipulations require that the head be repulsed back into the uterus.

Breathing

The optimum rate of ventilation is unknown, but experience suggests that rates between 10 and 20 breaths per minute are appropriate. Studies in adult pigs [2] have shown that a rate of 30 breaths per minute results in dramatically lower survival rates than 12 breaths per minute. This difference in survival was associated with increased intrathoracic pressure and decreased coronary artery perfusion pressure. The relevance of these findings to the foal is, as yet, unknown. If it is available, 100% oxygen should be used for resuscitation. However, studies of human neonate CPCR [3] suggest that resuscitation with room air is equally effective. The best method of providing artificial respiration is with a self-inflating resuscitation bag connected to a nasotracheal or endotracheal tube (Fig. 3). This method allows for controlled ventilation and avoids the risk of aerophagia or forcing material (such as meconium or mucus) into the airways, which can occur with masks. Aerophagia can significantly constrain ventilation, because filling the stomach with gas can put pressure on the diaphragm and prevent the lungs from fully expanding.

When a resuscitation bag is used, the optimum method is to place the bag on the floor and kneel next to the bag with the shoulders over the bag. Ideally, the hands should be placed flat and together on the bag. This allows controlled use of body weight to help compress the bag. However, squeezing the bag in both hands also can provide adequate ventilation. Many resuscitation bags have a valve that limits the pressure to 30 to 40 cm H_2O, which is the maximum pressure that should be applied for the first breath. Subsequent breaths should require a pressure of only 15 to 20 cm H_2O. The foal should be kept initially in lateral recumbency, with the head on the floor, while the circulation is being assessed. Raising the head can reduce brain perfusion when the circulation is marginal. When good circulation in the foal has been established (by palpation of peripheral pulses or with

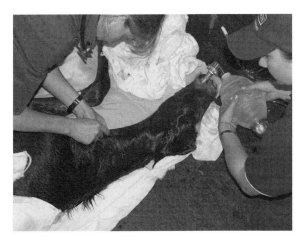

Fig. 3. Resuscitation of a foal after delivery by C-section. The foal has been intubated with an orotracheal tube and is receiving positive pressure ventilation with a self-inflating resuscitation bag. (© Kevin Corley and Jane Axon 2004.)

blood pressure measurements), the foal's position may be changed to sternal recumbency, to aid the ventilation of both lungs.

An alternative to a self-inflating resuscitation bag is a resuscitation pump (Fig. 4). The commercially available model (McCulloch Medical, Glenfield, Auckland, New Zealand) delivers a tidal volume of 780 mL and can be connected to a nasotracheal tube or to a mask. Anesthetic machines with a minimum reserve bag of 1 L and oxygen demand valves also may be used for resuscitation, but these devices carry a significant risk of volutrauma. Masks used with the resuscitation pump, rather than tracheal tubes,

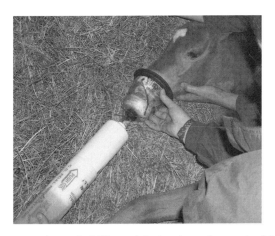

Fig. 4. Use of a pump mask on a foal. The mask is placed over the muzzle of the foal, and fixed ventilatory support is given with the pump. (© Kevin Corley 2004.)

probably represent the best option for the administration of CPCR by lay people. Aerophagia, a significant risk with masks, can be reduced by gentle occlusion of the esophagus over the larynx, but this may require an extra person.

Mouth-to-nose resuscitation also can be successful. With the foal in lateral recumbency, one hand should be used to cup the chin and occlude the downward nostril, and the fingers of this hand are used to open the upper nostril. The other hand can be placed on the back of the head to assist with dorsiflexion to straighten the airway, but the head should not be lifted. The esophagus should be occluded, if possible (Fig. 5).

Doxapram has been historically recommended for stimulating respiration at birth. The drug has been shown to reduce cerebral blood flow and to increase myocardial oxygen demands in experimental animals [4,5]. This class of drug also is ineffective in secondary apnea [6]; doxapram is therefore no longer recommended.

Circulation

Most human infants who require artificial ventilation at birth do not need chest compressions, and the same is probably true of foals. Thirty seconds after starting ventilation, the foal should be assessed to decide whether circulatory support is required. Thoracic compressions should be started if the heartbeat is absent or less than 40 bpm or is less than 60 bpm and does not increase after a further 60 seconds of positive pressure ventilation.

The optimum rate for thoracic compressions in the foal is unknown. A rate of 80 compressions per minute (cpm) has been shown to result in

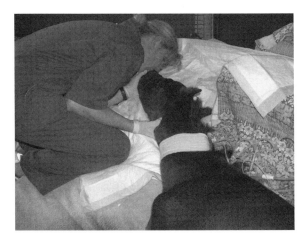

Fig. 5. Mouth-to-nose resuscitation in a foal. The mouth is placed over the uppermost nares. The lower nares is occluded with one hand. The other hand is used to gently occlude the esophagus and prevent aerophagia. (© Kevin Corley and Jane Axon 2004.)

significantly better circulation than 40 or 60 cpm in adult horses [7]. Rates between 80 and 120 cpm are therefore likely to be appropriate for foals. However, rates this high rapidly fatigue the resuscitator. Therefore, it is recommended to switch between the persons doing thoracic compressions every 2 to 5 minutes. Ventilation must continue during thoracic compressions. The recommended ratio is 2 breaths per 15 thoracic compressions [8]. It is not necessary to stop thoracic compressions during breaths.

The foal should be in lateral recumbency and moved to a firm dry surface, if that was not already done. The foal's rib cage should be quickly palpated and, if fractured ribs are suspected, the foal should be turned so these are on the side underneath. The person doing the thoracic compressions should kneel by the foal's spine with the hands placed on top of each other, just caudal to the foal's triceps, at the highest point of the thorax. The resuscitator's shoulders should be directly above the hands, enabling the use of body weight to help compress the thorax. This helps reduce resuscitator fatigue (Fig. 6).

Drugs

Drugs should be considered if the heart rate remains below 40 and is not increasing after 30 seconds of thoracic compressions and adequate ventilation. Thoracic compressions must continue after a drug has been given because all drugs require a circulation to reach the point of action, no matter by what route they are delivered. The preferred route of administration for drugs is intravenous. The jugular vein usually is obvious

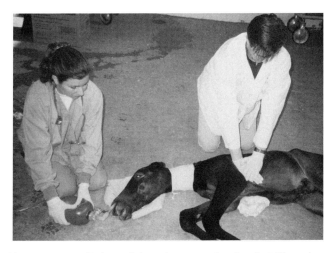

Fig. 6. Positive pressure ventilation and thoracic compressions in a foal. Thoracic compressions are delivered by kneeling with the shoulders over the hands. The hands are at the highest point of the foal's thorax, just behind the triceps mass. Thoracic compressions should not stop during delivery of breaths. (© Kevin Corley 2004.)

in foals and can be injected relatively easily, even when there is no circulation. If intravenous injection is not possible, drugs may be delivered either through the trachea or by intraosseous injection. For intratracheal administration, the needle of the syringe should be placed in the midline of the neck, through the skin and the ligament between two tracheal rings, below the level of the balloon of the nasotracheal tube, if present. An alternative method is to attach a dog urinary catheter to the syringe and pass the urinary catheter down the center of the nasotracheal tube so that the end is in the trachea. For intraosseous injection, a steel 14-ga needle is placed in the proximal medial one-third aspect of the tibia or the radius. The needle is harder to place in the radius. It is suggested that the intratracheal dose of drugs be higher than the intravenous dose, whereas the intraosseous dose is probably the same. Intracardiac injection should never be used because of the risk of lacerating a coronary artery or depositing the drug in the myocardium, resulting in fibrillation. Data from human infant resuscitation suggest that if drugs are required for resuscitation (following positive pressure ventilation and thoracic compressions) the prognosis is poor. The prognosis has been shown to be worse if multiple doses of drugs are used [9].

The primary drug for resuscitation is epinephrine [10]. Epinephrine increases vascular tone through α-adrenoreceptors. This action results in an increased aortic diastolic pressure, which increases blood flow through the coronary arteries and myocardium during the relaxation phase of thoracic compressions. The intravenous dose is 0.01 to 0.02 mg/kg, which is 0.5 to 1 mL of the 1 mg/mL (1:1000) solution for a 50-kg foal. The dose for the intratracheal administration of epinephrine is 0.1 to 0.2 mg/kg [11,12]. Epinephrine has a short half-life and therefore should be given every 3 minutes until the return of spontaneous circulation [10]. High-dose (0.1–0.2 mg/kg) intravenous epinephrine continues to be recommended for the resuscitation of foals [13]. However, this dose of epinephrine is now not recommended for human neonates. Increasing amounts of epinephrine used during CPCR in human adults has been shown to be an independent predictor of poor neurologic outcome. This effect persisted even when all confounders, such as the duration of resuscitation, had been taken into account [14]. Furthermore, high-dose epinephrine was recently shown to be associated with decreased survival at 24 hours in human pediatric resuscitation, compared with standard-dose epinephrine [15]. The high dose of epinephrine also has been associated with an increased risk of intracranial hemorrhage [11,16]. High-dose epinephrine has not been studied in foals.

Recent work in experimental animals has shown that the β-adrenergic effects of epinephrine during CPCR exacerbate postresuscitation myocardial dysfunction and that the concurrent administration of β-blockers improves survival [17,18]. This finding is supported with work by the same group of investigators in rats and pigs that shows that the α_2-adrenergic agonist α-methylnorepinephrine is an effective agent for CPCR and superior to either epinephrine and vasopressin [19,20]. Although this work cannot yet be translated directly to resuscitation of the foal, it is conceivable that an α_2 agonist such as xylazine or detomidine may be useful for CPCR if epinephrine is not available.

Volume expansion is recommended for foals with a poor response to resuscitative efforts, those with weak pulses with a good heart rate, or those that remain pale or cyanotic after oxygenation. The initial dose is 10 mL/kg balanced electrolyte solution (lactated Ringer's solution or Normosol-R) or 2 mL/kg hydroxyethyl starch (hetastarch 6% or pentastarch 10%). Care must be taken, however, to avoid the overzealous administration of fluids; thus, bolus administration rather than continuous high-flow rate is recommended. Fluids may be administered intravenously or intraosseously but not through the trachea. Inotrope and vasopressor agents such as dobutamine and norepinephrine should be considered if the patient continues to have a low mean arterial blood pressure (or weak pulses) after fluid resuscitation. The use of these drugs in the foal has been reviewed recently [21]. Drugs other than epinephrine and fluids should be used only in the case of documented cardiac dysrhythmias. Confirmation of this condition requires an ECG machine, which is unlikely to be readily available in the field. Moreover, most human infants with serious dysrhythmias have sustained overwhelming cerebral as well as cardiac injury, suggesting that newborn foals that develop dysrhythmias may be unlikely to survive. Atrial fibrillation occurs occasionally in the immediate postnatal period [22]. Atrial fibrillation may be identified by auscultation as an irregularly irregular rhythm. These foals do not usually require specific treatment and revert to sinus rhythm within a few hours of birth. Many normal foals may show arrhythmias for up to 15 minutes after birth, including wandering pacemaker, atrial premature contraction, and ventricular premature contractions [23]. In this circumstance, these dysrhythmias do not require specific treatment.

Asystole, which is recognized by the absence of cardiac electrical activity, should be treated with epinephrine as described above. Ventricular fibrillation, which is recognized by rapidly undulating electrical activity with no discernable complexes, is treated most effectively with an electrical defibrillator. The dose is 1 to 4 J/kg (50–200 J for a 50-kg foal), increasing the energy by 50% at each defibrillation attempt [24]. The electric defibrillator is potentially dangerous to personnel and thus should be used only by an experienced operator.

The use of sodium bicarbonate is highly controversial. There are conflicting data on its effectiveness in experimental cardiac arrest [25,26], and it may be counterproductive by initially decreasing the intracellular pH level [27,28].

Atropine and calcium should not be used in CPCR of newborn foals. Atropine has little effect if the bradycardia is not vagally mediated; it increases myocardial oxygen consumption, and it and may precipitate tachycardia [29]. The most common cause of bradycardia in the foal is hypoxia; thus, the recommended treatment for bradydysrhythmias is artificial ventilation and thoracic compressions [11]. Although calcium improves the contractility of the normal heart, during cardiac arrest, calcium leads to an increased cytosolic calcium concentration, which results in the disruption of myocardial function [30].

Monitoring the effectiveness of cardiopulmonary cerebral resuscitation

During CPCR, monitoring the effectiveness of the resuscitative efforts can help adjust the technique to the individual patient so that the rate of ventilation and the rate and pressure of thoracic compressions can be varied. The pulse, if palpable, is the best way of monitoring thoracic compressions, although this is often difficult in a patient undergoing CPCR. CPCR also can be monitored by the pupillary light reflex, which is an indirect indication of cerebral perfusion. If the person performing the thoracic compressions holds a flashlight in his or her mouth, the pupil response and size can be assessed without interrupting the resuscitation efforts. The pupil is widely dilated and fixed in the case of inadequate resuscitation and cerebral perfusion, whereas an adequate circulation results in a more normal pupil, which responds to light. The progress of CPCR can be monitored by the heartbeat, if present, which is used to decide when to stop thoracic compressions. Although an ECG is useful for monitoring the heart rhythm, it is not adequate for monitoring CPCR because electrical activity in the heart can continue without effective contractions (pulseless electrical activity). If the equipment is available, an end-tidal carbon dioxide monitor (capnograph) is extremely useful to assess the effectiveness of CPCR. Higher expired carbon dioxide tensions indicate more effective resuscitation efforts because more carbon dioxide is being transported to the lungs and ventilated. End-tidal carbon dioxide tensions greater than 15 mm Hg indicate good perfusion and portend a good prognosis, whereas tensions persistently lower than 10 mm Hg indicate ineffective CPCR and a poor prognosis [1,31].

When to stop

Ventilation should be stopped when the heart rate is above 60 and spontaneous breathing is well established. Spontaneous breathing should be assessed by stopping the ventilation and disconnecting the bag or pump for 30 seconds and checking for a respiratory rate above 16 bpm, a regular respiratory pattern, and normal respiratory effort. The first few breaths may be gasping but should be followed by a normal respiratory rate and pattern. Premature withdrawal of ventilation is reported to be the most common mistake in human neonatal CPCR [32].

If thoracic compressions have been started, they should be continued until a regular heartbeat of over 60 has been established. There should be no lag period between the stopping of support and the onset of a spontaneous heartbeat. Therefore, CPCR should not be stopped for longer than 10 seconds to assess the circulation. Clinical experience suggests that if spontaneous circulation and respiration are not present after 15 minutes, then survival is unlikely.

Care for foals after resuscitation

Foals that have been resuscitated continue to require support and should be intensively monitored for at least 30 minutes. Supplemental oxygen should be provided, either by facemask or by nasal cannula. A careful physical examination should be performed, and if possible, the heart should be monitored with an electrocardiogram.

The consequences of the period of asphyxia during arrest and resuscitation can be serious and may not be apparent for 24 to 48 hours after the arrest. Perinatal asphyxia can result in a syndrome, which may result in any or all of the following: altered neurologic status, seizures and impaired gastrointestinal, renal, and cardiovascular function. This syndrome was previously called hypoxic ischemic encephalopathy or neonatal maladjustment syndrome. There is no way to prevent the effects of asphyxia. Vitamin E, selenium, and dimethyl sulfoxide may possibly reduce damage caused by hypoxia-ischemia and reperfusion [33].

Many resuscitated foals are referred to intensive care units for further treatment. The decision whether to refer a foal for critical care is based on many factors, including availability and the costs versus the economic worth of the foal. Success rates also vary but are on the order of 70% to 80% for most units. Foals that have been successfully resuscitated are at high risk of complications, and referral should be strongly considered if circumstances allow.

New directions in human cardiopulmonary cerebral resuscitation

Research in CPCR is very active in human medicine. Many innovations have led to a greater percentage of successful CPCR (return of spontaneous circulation) but no change in hospital discharge rates. Recently, however, two treatments have been shown to increase hospital survival in human adult patients. Mild hypothermia (89.6°–93.2°F [32°–34°C]) induced for 12 to 24 hours after an arrest resulted in better neurologic outcome and 6-month survival than conventional treatment did [34,35]. It is important to note that shivering was controlled by the administration of pancuronium or vecuronium. These intriguing results may provide a way to limit hypoxic ischemic injury in resuscitated foals, but the use of muscle relaxants would necessitate mechanical ventilation, and results in neonates may be different from the adults studied. There is limited work investigating selective head cooling in experimental animals and neonatal humans, which may overcome the problems of whole-body cooling and shivering. The evidence to date is insufficient to make positive recommendations for the treatment of human infants [36], let alone foals. Amiodarone (5 mg/kg IV) has largely replaced lidocaine as the drug of choice for ventricular tachydysrhythmias in human adult patients [37]. These dysrhythmias are rare in the foal. A further innovation in human CPCR has been the introduction of vasopressin (0.4–0.8 U/kg IV) as a replacement or an adjunct to epinephrine, although large-scale clinical trial results have been equivocal [38,39]. However, the one experimental situation in which epinephrine was shown to be superior to vasopressin was in asphyxiated neonatal pigs [40]; therefore, pending further work, epinephrine remains the drug of choice for neonatal foals.

Emergency fluid resuscitation

Prompt, adequate fluid therapy is one of the easiest and most effective ways to maximize a foal's chance of survival. However, determining which foals require emergency fluids can be difficult because many of the clinical signs of hypovolemia that are familiar in the mature horse are inconsistently present in the foal. The clinical signs of hypovolemia in the mature horse are: tachycardia, weak pulses, poor filling of the jugular vein, tachypnea, and cold extremities [41]. Whenever any of these clinical signs occur in the foal, hypovolemia should be suspected.

Hypovolemic foals may have heart rates above, below, or within the normal range [42,43]. An increased heart rate is a physiologic defense against the decreased cardiac stroke volume associated with hypovolemia and helps to maintain cardiac output. Hypovolemic foals that fail to increase their heart rate are likely to have reduced oxygen supply to the tissues, resulting in organ damage and eventually failure. The lack of this defensive physiologic response in some foals may explain, at least in part, the very rapid deterioration seen in some foals. Unfortunately, other clinical signs of hypovolemia seen in mature horses are also not consistently present in neonatal foals. Cold extremities may arise as a result of another physiologic defense mechanism, in which vasoconstriction in the distal limbs and ears attempts to divert the remaining circulating volume to the central circulation and therefore the vital organs. This response also appears to be inconsistently present in foals, and cold extremities may represent a completely failing circulation, with no perfusion to any tissues. Weak pulses represent a decreased difference between systolic and diastolic pressure. This difference may be maintained, even when the foal is hypotensive (Fig. 7). Tachypnea occurs with hypovolemia as a respiratory compensation for lactic acidosis [44], another physiologic response that often does not occur in the debilitated foal.

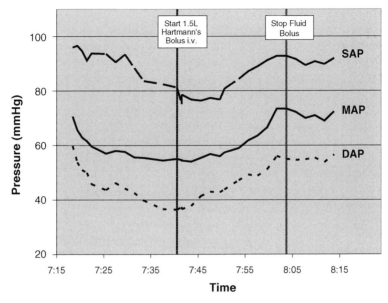

Fig. 7. Blood pressure changes in the first hours after hospital admission in a 2-hour old, 47-kg Thoroughbred colt. Blood pressure was measured indirectly using a tail cuff and an automated oscillometric sphygmomanometer (DS 7141, Fukuda Denshi, Japan). The foal was admitted at 7:12 AM, and the first blood pressure measurement was taken at 7:16 AM. Blood pressure was measured every 1 to 2 minutes, and each point represents the mean of the preceding five measurements. Although apparently normotensive after admission, the foal became hypotensive (MAP < 60 mm Hg) within 10 minutes. Hypotension was successfully reversed in the short term by bolus fluid therapy. The foal required inotropic therapy for 5 days and vasopressor support for 3 days to maintain blood pressure; it ultimately survived to leave the hospital. DAP, diastolic arterial pressure; MAP, mean arterial pressure; SAP, systolic arterial pressure. (© Kevin Corley 2004.)

Because the clinical signs of hypovolemia can be vague in the foal, more reliance must be placed on the history than in mature horses. Foals become dehydrated very rapidly when they do not nurse. Hypovolemia must be suspected in any foal that has not nursed for the previous four hours. Foals born by C-section may be clinically hypovolemic immediately after birth. This may be the result of a lack of transfer of blood from the placenta during the birthing process [45,46] or, in the case of foals taken from mares undergoing colic surgery, caused by the effects of endotoxemia.

In hospitalized foals, blood pressure also can be used to detect hypovolemia. Indirect blood pressure can be easily and quickly measured using a tail cuff and an automatic oscillometric sphygmomanometer, a method that is accurate in neonatal foals for mean and diastolic arterial pressure [47]. Low blood pressure on initial examination most often reflects hypovolemia. The first response is to administer fluid boluses, as outlined below. If an adequate blood pressure is not restored, inotrope and vasopressor therapy may be required (these treatment modalities have been reviewed recently [21]). It is important to realize that a normal blood pressure does not rule out hypovolemia because the maintenance of blood pressure is a primary physiologic response to hypovolemia, mediated by both the reduction of urine output and by arteriolar vasoconstriction. Normal blood pressure does not guarantee adequate tissue perfusion, thus other indirect methods of assessing tissue perfusion such as blood lactate concentration and urine output should be used [43]. Furthermore, hypovolemic foals may briefly have normal blood pressures at hospital admission but then develop hypotension (see Fig. 7). This initial blood pressure presumably is caused by endogenous catecholamine release associated with transport to the hospital.

Blood lactate concentrations also may be useful to detect hypovolemia in foals. Lactate is an end product of anaerobic metabolism and accumulates in the tissues when there is insufficient oxygen for aerobic respiration. Increased blood lactate concentrations in foals primarily reflect inadequate tissue perfusion, which in turn, occurs with hypovolemia. However, lactate concentration also has been reported to be increased in sepsis, systemic inflammatory response syndrome, trauma, and after seizures and during periods of increased circulating catecholamines [48–53]. Although age-specific normal values have been determined for the foal [54], using an upper limit for the normal value of 2.5 mmol/L appears to be sufficiently accurate for clinical use [53]. As for all laboratory information, lactate concentrations should be assessed in the context of the entire clinical picture. However, foals with high lactate concentrations (≥ 5 mmol/L) on initial examination are highly likely to benefit from fluid therapy.

In mature horses, increased creatinine concentrations reflect inadequate perfusion to the kidney, in the absence of nephropathy or postrenal problems such as ruptured bladders. The most common cause of inadequate perfusion to the kidneys is hypovolemia. In foals in the first 36 hours of life, increased creatinine concentrations may reflect compromised placental function in utero and therefore cannot be relied on to indicate hypovolemia. Foals with ruptured bladders also may have increased plasma creatinine concentrations [55]. Urine specific gravity can be used as an indicator of hydration in the foal without renal disease. The specific gravity should be less than 1.008; higher values would indicate hypovolemia.

Packed cell volume is a poor indicator of circulatory status in the neonatal foal [53]. It is uncommon to find increased packed cell volumes in severely hypovolemic foals, in contrast to their adult counterparts. The normal range for packed cell volume in foals in the first week of life (28%–46%; 0.26–0.46 L/L) [56] is slightly lower than in adult horses. Commonly, critically ill foals have packed cell volumes of 22% to 26%, possibly as a result of a combination of fluid therapy and bone marrow suppression with illness. Total solids concentration (total protein measured by a refractometer) also is an unreliable guide to hypovolemia in the foal. Total solids may be decreased by the failure of passive transfer or by loss through the gastrointestinal tract or kidney, and there is no correlation between total solids concentration and either packed cell volume or other signs of circulatory status such as lactate concentration in the foal (K.T.T. Corley, unpublished observations, 2004). The normal range for total solids in the foal (5.1–8.0 g/dL or 51–80 g/L) also is lower than that of the adult horse [56].

Fluid therapy for hypovolemia

Balanced electrolyte formulas designed for resuscitation, such as Hartmann's solution, lactated Ringer's solution, or Normosol-R, are the best fluids to use for reversing hypovolemia. These fluids contain approximately the same concentration of electrolytes as plasma. They are therefore the safest fluids to use if electrolytes cannot be measured. If blood electrolyte concentrations are available before beginning fluid therapy, the most common choice of fluid should still be balanced electrolyte solutions. It is inadvisable to attempt major electrolyte replacement before restoring a circulating volume. Exceptions to this rule are conditions of hyperkalemia, hyponatremia, and hypochloremia, which are seen in a percentage of cases of ruptured bladder [55]. For these foals, 0.9% or 1.8% sodium chloride solution is often the best resuscitation fluid.

Sodium chloride has traditionally been used as a resuscitation fluid in human medicine. Sodium chloride is an acidifying fluid [57,58] and therefore may not be the best choice for acute resuscitation in foals because most of these foals are acidotic as a result of lactic acid accumulation. Hypertonic saline (7.0% to 7.5% sodium chloride) has no role in resuscitation of neonates. Hypertonic saline may cause a rapid change in plasma osmolarity, resulting in brain shrinkage and subsequent vascular rupture with cerebral bleeding, subarachnoid hemorrhage, and permanent neurologic damage or death, to which neonates are particularly susceptible. The change in plasma osmolarity is more severe in animals with renal insufficiency, a common finding in critically ill foals.

Colloids are solutions that contain large protein or starch molecules, as opposed to crystalloids, which contain only electrolytes and water or glucose and water. The role of colloid solutions such as modified gelatins (Haemaccel and Gelofusine) and hydroxyethyl starches (pentastarch and hetastarch) for acute resuscitation of the foal is unclear. The theoretical advantage of these compounds is that they expand the plasma volume by a greater amount than the balanced electrolyte formulas and persist in the circulation longer, prolonging their positive effect. They also increase the plasma oncotic pressure, in contrast to crystalloids, which decrease it. However, there are no clear benefits of colloids in clinical practice, and research in human medicine has failed to find a benefit of colloids over crystalloids [59,60]. The total daily dose of hetastarch should not exceed 10 mL/kg and should not exceed 15 mL/kg for pentastarch. At higher doses, these hydroxyethyl starches interfere with coagulation and may cause clinical bleeding. Hydroxyethyl starches probably are indicated for resuscitation in foals with a plasma total solids concentration of less than 3.5 g/dL (35 g/L). The initial plasma expansion is greater with lower molecular weight colloids, and higher molecular weight colloids persist longer in the circulation. The average molecular weight of modified gelatins is small (30–35 kD) compared with albumin (69 kD), pentastarch (200 kD), and hetastarch (450 kD) [41]. Modified gelatins solutions are therefore preferred for the initial re-suscitation of markedly hypovolemic foals, and hydroxyethyl starches may be better for the long-term maintenance of plasma colloidal oncotic pressure. Plasma is a colloid solution often used for supplementing passive immunity in foals. Plasma needs to be defrosted (if stored) or collected from a donor and is therefore rarely available for acute fluid resuscitation. Furthermore, because some foals may have anaphylactoid reactions to plasma trans-fusions, it is good practice to initially infuse plasma slowly and check for a reaction. Again, this detracts from the use of plasma for fluid resuscitation.

Fluid rate

There are two ways to think about the treatment of hypovolemia, which both result in similar treatment patterns. Hypovolemic foals typically require 20 to 80 mL/kg of crystalloid fluids acutely.

Shock Dose

The "shock dose" concept is borrowed from small animal medicine and so is familiar to many practitioners. The shock dose for a neonatal foal is 50 to 80 mL/kg crystalloid fluids. Depending on the perceived degree of hypovolemia, 25% to 50% of the shock dose is given as rapidly as possible (over less than 20 minutes), and the foal is reassessed. If the foal requires further fluid, another 25% of the shock dose is given, and again the foal is reassessed. The final 25% of the shock dose is given only to severely hypovolemic foals.

Fluid boluses

The incremental "fluid bolus" concept is borrowed from human medicine. It is actually a much more practical method, except when an electronic infusion pump is available. The caveat is that this method assumes a similar body weight between all patients, and for this reason it has not been adopted in small animal medicine.

The bolus method simply is to give a bolus of 1 L of crystalloids (ie, approximately 20 mL/kg bodyweight (bwt) for a 50-kg foal), and reassess the foal. Up to three additional boluses may be given, reassessing the foal after each bolus. Most obviously hypovolemic foals require at least two boluses.

In foals in which body weight obviously varies from 50 kg, the method needs to be adjusted so that the bolus is approximately 20 mL/kg bwt. In pony foals and very premature thoroughbred foals, boluses of 500 mL are usually appropriate. In large draft foals, the first bolus should be 2 L.

How much to give

Whether the shock dose or the fluid bolus method is used, the animal is reassessed during acute fluid therapy to judge whether further fluids are required. A foal with a strong pulse, improved mentation, and that is urinating probably does not require any further resuscitation fluids. These foals are likely to still require fluids to correct dehydration and electrolyte imbalances and to provide for maintenance and ongoing losses (see below). Foals with continued weak pulses (or low blood pressure), depressed mentation, and those that have not urinated may require further acute fluids, up to the maximum of 80 mL/kg or 4 L.

It is advisable to auscultate the lungs and trachea before and during aggressive fluid therapy because pulmonary edema is an important theoretical complication. Fortunately, pulmonary edema appears to be extremely rare in critically ill foals that are aggressively resuscitated with crystalloids. Crackles, classically associated with pulmonary edema, are more likely to represent opening and closing of collapsed alveoli, rather than edema, in foals. Severe pulmonary edema will result in wet sounds in the trachea and a frothy pink fluid from the nares or mouth. If edema does occur, furosemide (0.25–1 mg/kg IV) should be administered and further fluid therapy carefully titrated, preferably by means of central venous pressure or pulmonary pressures.

The treatment of hypovolemia takes precedence over any concerns about possibly causing cerebral edema and thus worsening perinatal asphyxia syndrome. Inadequate cerebral perfusion, resulting from hypovolemia, prolongs the ischemic event and is thus extremely detrimental to these foals. This is far more important than theoretical concerns over cerebral edema.

Important exception to aggressive fluid therapy

Aggressive fluid therapy should be avoided in uncontrolled hemorrhage because it may increase bleeding. This is uncommon in neonatal foals but may occur with trauma, resulting in internal abdominal bleeds or rupture of an inaccessible artery. In humans and experimental animals, aggressive fluid therapy in uncontrolled hemorrhage has been demonstrated to increase mortality [61–63]. This and other evidence suggests that, if blood pressure can be measured, fluid therapy should be titrated to maintain the mean arterial pressure as close to 60 mm Hg as possible, without increasing the systolic pressure over 90 mm Hg. If blood pressure cannot be measured, then a fluid rate of 2 to 3 mL/kg/hr should be used until the hemorrhage can be stopped.

Foals with neonatal isoerythrolysis are not commonly hypovolemic, unless they have become so debilitated that they have stopped nursing for 4 or more hours. In foals with isoerythrolysis and hypovolemia, aggressive fluid therapy is not contraindicated. Although it will decrease the hematocrit level, fluid therapy will not decrease the number of circulating erythrocytes and may improve their distribution to the tissues. However, in foals with low packed cell volumes, restoring the blood oxygen-carrying capacity is a priority, and donor blood, washed mare's blood or hemoglobin substitutes (Oxyglobin), should be given as soon as possible.

Emergency glucose support

Intravenous glucose therapy often is part of emergency treatment in foals. This is because the glycogen stores at birth are sufficient only for approximately 2 hours of energy requirements in the unfed foal, and fat stores are also very low at birth [64]. Therefore, foals that are not nursing are very prone to hypoglycemia. Septicemia also may result in hypoglycemia [65,66], possibly as a result of the lack of glycogen reserves and poor nursing in septic foals [67]. However, foals also may be hyperglycemic at hospital admission, presumably as part of the physiologic response to cortisol release or associated with unregulated glucose metabolism with disease processes [68]. In a series of 221 referred foals at hospital admission, 84 (38%) foals were hypoglycemic (blood glucose < 80 mg/dL [4.4 mmol/L]) and 43 (19.5%) were severely hypoglycemic (<50 mg/dL [2.8 mmol/L]). Ninety-three foals (42%) were hyperglycemic (>110 mg/dL [6.1 mmol/L]), but only 20 (9.5%) foals were severely hyperglycemic (>180 mg/dL [10 mmol/L]) (K.T.T. Corley, J.E. Axon, unpublished observations, 2004).

Both hypoglycemia and hyperglycemia may be harmful. After cerebral hypoperfusion (a feature of both hypovolemia and perinatal asphyxia syndrome), hyperglycemia may be more detrimental than hypoglycemia [69]. For this reason, it is advisable to frequently monitor the serum glucose concentration in foals.

There is good evidence from human critical care that keeping serum glucose concentrations within a narrow range (80–110 mg/dL [4.4–6.1 mmol/L]) is associated with better outcomes [70,71]. For this reason, it may be advisable to measure glucose hourly in the initial stages of foal care and use insulin to control serum glucose concentrations if necessary. However, it is important to note that these data were generated in human adult patients, and no equivalent information exists for the foal, to date.

Fluids for supporting glucose concentration

5% dextrose and 5% glucose solutions

One liter of 5% dextrose provides approximately 170 kcal (712 kJ) of energy, and 1 L of 5% glucose provides approximately 190 kcal (796 kJ).

These 5% solutions are not a great source of energy for the foal. To meet the resting energy requirement (44 kcal/kg/day [184 kJ/kg/day] [72]) of a 50-kg foal, 11.5 (5% glucose) to 13 (5% dextrose) L per day would be required. This amount is more than double the foal's maintenance fluid requirements and would cause considerable electrolyte disturbances. Five percent dextrose has been suggested as a resuscitation fluid for foals because it provides both volume and energy. However, it is not a good fluid for treating hypovolemia. After 30 minutes, only 10% of volume given is left in the circulation [73], and each liter of 5% dextrose will drop the plasma sodium concentration by 4 to 5 mmol/L in a 50-kg foal.

50% dextrose and 50% glucose solutions

These fluids may be preferable to the 5% solution. Each mL of 50% dextrose is equivalent to 1.7 kcal (7.1 kJ), and each mL of 50% glucose is equivalent to 1.9 kcal (8 kJ). It may be used in two ways. In the hospital setting, the solution should be administered through an electric pump, separately from the resuscitation fluids. The starting rate will depend on the degree of hypoglycemia. As a rule of thumb, a starting rate of 20 mL/hour is appropriate for mild hypoglycemia (50–72 mg/dL [2.8–4 mmol/L]) and 50 mL/hour for severe hypoglycemia ($\leq$50 mg/dL [$\leq$2.8 mmol/L]). In the field, it is probably best to add the 50% dextrose solution to the resuscitation fluids. In this situation, 10 to 20 mL of the 50% solution should be added per liter of resuscitation fluid. If blood glucose concentration can be measured, the amount of 50% solution added to the resuscitation fluids should be varied based on the measured blood glucose to deliver approximately 20 mL/hour for mild hypoglycemia and 50 mL/hour for severe hypoglycemia. Glucose is not suitable as a long-term nutritional support for foals, and if enteral feeding is not possible or desirable after the first 12 hours of therapy, parenteral nutrition with solutions containing dextrose or glucose, amino acids, vitamins and trace minerals, and, in many foals, lipids, should be instituted.

Emergency oxygen therapy

Oxygen therapy is extremely useful for support of foals [74]. It should be considered in all foals following resuscitation and dystocia. Other foals that are likely to benefit from oxygen are those that are dyspneic, cyanotic, meconium-stained after birth, or recumbent. In the hospital setting, oxygen therapy should be based on the oxygen tension (Pao_2) in an arterial blood sample. Oxygen should be supplemented if the arterial tension is less than 65 to 70 mm Hg (8.7–9.3 kPa). The most convenient places for sampling arterial blood in the foal are the dorsal metatarsal artery and the median artery.

Small-bore flexible rubber feeding tubes are useful as oxygen cannulas for intranasal oxygen therapy in the foal. The length to be inserted into the nares should be measured as the distance from the nares to the medial canthus of the eye. The tube is then inserted into the ventral meatus of the nose. There are a variety of ways of fixing the tube in place. One method is to attach the tube to a tongue depressor that has been previously wrapped in tape. The oxygen tube is taped along one edge of the tongue depressor and then curled around one end so that it heads back in the direction from which it is coming. It is not taped to the bottom edge of the depressor. The tube and depressor are then attached to the foal's muzzle using tape or elastikon (Elastoplast) (Fig. 8), taking care not to prevent the foal from opening its mouth. An alternative method is to stitch the cannula to the foal's skin, at the point it enters the nares. Oxygen also may be delivered in the short-term by face mask.

If given for extended periods (greater than 1 hour), oxygen should be humidified before delivery to the foal. The simplest way of achieving this is to bubble it through sterile water. Easily sterilized bottles designed for humidification are available commercially. Oxygen therapy should be started at 9 to 10 L/min and titrated according to the response of the patient and, if available, arterial oxygen tensions. If arterial oxygen tension is being measured, the oxygen flow rate should be decreased if the tension is greater than 120 mm Hg (16k Pa).

Oxygen is not a completely benign therapy. Oxygen fractions of greater than 60% inspired for more than 48 hours result in pulmonary pathology, which results in tracheobronchitis, leading to acute respiratory distress syndrome and, subsequently, to pulmonary interstitial fibrosis. This is probably mediated through oxygen free-radical formation (increased free-

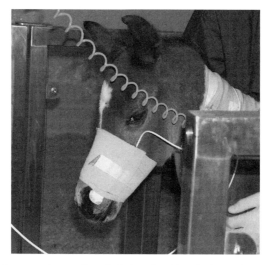

Fig. 8. Intranasal oxygen therapy in a foal. A soft rubber feeding tube is being used as the oxygen cannula. The tube has been fixed to a tongue depressor, which has been fixed to the muzzle of the foal. (© Kevin Corley 2004.)

radical formation with increased inspired oxygen overwhelms scavenging). There also may be non–free-radical-mediated injury through cellular metabolic alteration or by enzyme inhibition [75]. Fortunately, it is almost impossible to generate inspired oxygen fractions of greater than 60% with intranasal oxygen therapy.

Summary

The early recognition of foals that require emergency support is the key to success. This is achieved through an assessment of the history to anticipate which foals are likely to require intervention, rapid clinical assessment of foals, and a high index of suspicion. Cardiopulmonary cerebral resuscitation, fluid resuscitation, and glucose and oxygen supplementation, applied judiciously, can reduce both mortality and morbidity.

Early intervention can dramatically alter outcome in foals. Cardiopulmonary cerebral resuscitation can be successful and clinically worthwhile when applied to foals that arrest as part of the birthing process. Readily available equipment and an ordered plan starting with addressing the respiratory system (airway and breathing) followed by the circulatory system (circulation and drugs) are the keys to success. Hypovolemia can be clinically difficult to detect in foals because the physiologic adaptive responses to hypovolemia, such as tachycardia, are not uniformly present in foals. For most clinical situations, balanced electrolyte solutions (such as lactated Ringer's solution or Normosol-R) represent the best fluids to reverse hypovolemia. Up to four 1-L boluses (for a 50-kg foal) of this fluid of balanced electrolyte solution should be used, with most obviously hypovolemic foals requiring at least 2 L. Hypoglycemia is common in foals that are not nursing and in septic foals. Support of serum glucose can be an important emergency treatment. However, hyperglycemia should be avoided because it is likely that this also is detrimental, especially in foals with hypoxia-ischemia– induced encephalopathy. Respiratory support with oxygen therapy should be considered in all foals following resuscitation and dystocia. Other foals that are likely to benefit from oxygen are those that are dyspneic, cyanotic, meconium-stained after birth, or recumbent. Oxygen usually is supplied through an indwelling nasal cannula, at an initial rate of 9 to 10 L/min. These emergency therapies, applied correctly, are expected to result in decreased mortality and morbidity.

References

[1] Cantineau JP, Lambert Y, Merck P, et al. End-tidal carbon dioxide during cardiopulmonary resuscitation in humans presenting mostly with asystole: a predictor of outcome. Crit Care Med 1996;24(5):791–6.
[2] Aufderheide TP, Lurie KG. Death by hyperventilation: a common and life-threatening problem during cardiopulmonary resuscitation. Crit Care Med 2004;32(Suppl 9):S345–51.

[3] Saugstad OD, Rootwelt T, Aalen O. Resuscitation of asphyxiated newborn infants with room air or oxygen: an international controlled trial: the Resair 2 study. Pediatrics 1998; 102(1):e1.

[4] Miletich DJ, Ivankovich AD, Albrecht RF, et al. The effects of doxapram on cerebral blood flow and peripheral hemodynamics in the anesthetized and unanesthetized goat. Anesth Analg 1976;55(2):279–85.

[5] Kim SI, Winnie AP, Carey JS, et al. Use of doxapram in the critically ill patient: does increased oxygen consumption reflect an oxygen dividend or an oxygen debt? Crit Care Med 1973;1(5):252–6.

[6] Daniel SS, Dawes GS, James LS, et al. Analeptics and the resuscitation of asphyxiated monkeys. BMJ 1966;2(513):562–3.

[7] Hubbell JA, Muir WW, Gaynor JS. Cardiovascular effects of thoracic compression in horses subjected to euthanasia. Equine Vet J 1993;25(4):282–4.

[8] Dunkley CJ, Thomas AN, Taylor RJ, et al. A comparison of standard and a modified method of two resuscitator adult cardiopulmonary resuscitation: description of a new system for research into advanced life support skills. Resuscitation 1998;38(1):7–12.

[9] Sims DG, Heal CA, Bartle SM. Use of adrenaline and atropine in neonatal resuscitation. Arch Dis Child 1994;70(1):F3–10.

[10] Woodhouse SP, Cox S, Boyd P, et al. High dose and standard dose adrenaline do not alter survival, compared with placebo, in cardiac arrest. Resuscitation 1995;30:243–9.

[11] Neonatal Resuscitation Program Steering Committee. Textbook of neonatal resuscitation. 3rd edition. Dallas (TX): American Academy of Pediatrics/American Heart Association; 1994.

[12] Kleinman ME, Oh W, Stonestreet BS. Comparison of intravenous and endotracheal epinephrine during cardiopulmonary resuscitation in newborn piglets. Crit Care Med 1999; 27(12):2748–54.

[13] Palmer JE. Foal cardiopulmonary resuscitation. In: Orsini JA, Divers TJ, editors. Manual of equine emergencies. 2nd edition. Philadelphia: WB Saunders; 2003. p. 581–614.

[14] Behringer W, Kittler H, Sterz F, et al. Cumulative epinephrine dose during cardiopulmonary resuscitation and neurological outcome. Ann Intern Med 1998;129(6):450–6.

[15] Perondi MBM, Reis AG, Paiva EF, et al. A comparison of high-dose and standard-dose epinephrine in children with cardiac arrest. N Engl J Med 2004;350:1722–30.

[16] Burchfield DJ. Medication use in neonatal resuscitation. Clin Perinatol 1999;26(3): 683–91.

[17] Cammarata G, Weil MH, Sun S, et al. beta-1 Adrenergic blockade during cardiopulmonary resuscitation improves survival. Crit Care Med 2004;32(Suppl 9):S440–3.

[18] Huang L, Weil MH, Cammarata G, et al. Nonselective beta-blocking agent improves the outcome of cardiopulmonary resuscitation in a rat model. Crit Care Med 2004;32(Suppl 9): S378–80.

[19] Klouche K, Weil MH, Tang W, et al. A selective alpha(2)-adrenergic agonist for cardiac resuscitation. J Lab Clin Med 2002;140(1):27–34.

[20] Klouche K, Weil MH, Sun S, et al. A comparison of alpha-methylnorepinephrine, vasopressin and epinephrine for cardiac resuscitation. Resuscitation 2003;57(1):93–100.

[21] Corley KTT. Inotropes and vasopressors in adults and foals. Vet Clin North Am Equine Pract 2004;20(1):77–106.

[22] Machida N, Yasuda J, Too K. Three cases of paroxysmal atrial fibrillation in the Thoroughbred newborn foal. Equine Vet J 1989;21(1):66–8.

[23] Yamamoto K, Yasuda J, Too K. Arrhythmias in newborn thoroughbred foals. Equine Vet J 1992;24(3):169–73.

[24] Wechsler SB, Werknovsky G. Cardiac disorders. In: Cloherty JP, Stark AR, editors. Manual of neonatal care. 4th edition. Philadelphia: Lippincott-Raven; 1998. p. 393–451.

[25] Graf H, Leach W, Arieff AI. Evidence for a detrimental effect of bicarbonate therapy in hypoxic lactic acidosis. Science 1985;227:754–6.

[26] Bar-Joseph G, Weinberger T, Castel T, et al. Comparison of sodium bicarbonate, Carbicarb, and THAM during cardiopulmonary resuscitation in dogs. Crit Care Med 1998;26(8): 1397–408.

[27] Li Y-C, Wiklund L, Bjerneroth G. Influence of alkaline buffers on cytoplasmic pH in myocardial cells exposed to hypoxia. Resuscitation 1997;34:71–7.

[28] Bjerneroth G, Sammeli O, Li Y-C, et al. Effects of alkaline buffers on cytoplasmic pH in lymphocytes. Crit Care Med 1994;22(10):1550–6.

[29] Leuthner SR, Jansen RD, Hageman JR. Cardiopulmonary resuscitation of the newborn: an update. Pediatr Clin North Am 1994;41(5):893–907.

[30] Stempien A, Katz AM, Messineo FC. Calcium and cardiac arrest. Ann Intern Med 1986; 105(4):603–6.

[31] Callaham M, Barton C. Prediction of outcome of cardiopulmonary resuscitation from end-tidal carbon dioxide concentration. Crit Care Med 1990;18(4):358–62.

[32] Oriot D, Boussemart T, Cardona J, et al. Medical errors during cardiopulmonary resuscitation of neonates. Eur J Pediatr 1993;152:781.

[33] Shimizu S, Simon RP, Graham SH. Dimethylsulfoxide (DMSO) treatment reduces infarction volume after permanent focal cerebral ischemia in rats. Neurosci Lett 1997; 239(2–3):125–7.

[34] Holzer M, Cerchiari E, Martens P, et al. Mild therapeutic hypothermia to improve the neurologic outcome after cardiac arrest. N Engl J Med 2002;346(8):549–56.

[35] Bernard SA, Gray TW, Buist MD, et al. Treatment of comatose survivors of out-of-hospital cardiac arrest with induced hypothermia. N Engl J Med 2002;346(8):557–63.

[36] Jacobs S, Hunt R, Tarnow-Mordi W, et al. Cooling for newborns with hypoxic ischaemic encephalopathy. Cochrane Database Syst Rev 2003;(4):CD003311.

[37] Kudenchuk PJ, Cobb LA, Copass MK, et al. Amiodarone for resuscitation after out-of-hospital cardiac arrest due to ventricular fibrillation. N Engl J Med 1999;341(12):871–8.

[38] Stiell IG, Hebert PC, Wells GA, et al. Vasopressin versus epinephrine for inhospital cardiac arrest: a randomised controlled trial. Lancet 2001;358:105–9.

[39] Wenzel V, Krismer AC, Arntz HR, et al. A comparison of vasopressin and epinephrine for out-of-hospital cardiopulmonary resuscitation. N Engl J Med 2004;350(2):105–13.

[40] Voelckel WG, Lurie KG, McKnite S, et al. Comparison of epinephrine and vasopressin in a pediatric porcine model of asphyxial cardiac arrest. Crit Care Med 2000;28(12):3777–83.

[41] Corley KTT. Fluid therapy. In: Bertone JJ, Horspool LL, editors. Equine clinical pharmacology. London: WB Saunders; 2004. p. 327–64.

[42] Corley KTT. Monitoring and treating haemodynamic disturbances in critically ill neonatal foals. Part II. assessment and treatment. Equine Veterinary Education 2002;14(6):328–36.

[43] Corley KTT. Monitoring and treating haemodynamic disturbances in critically ill neonatal foals. Part I. haemodynamic monitoring. Equine Vet Educ 2002;14(5):270–9.

[44] Corley KTT, Marr CM. Pathophysiology, assessment and treatment of acid-base disturbances in the horse. Equine Vet Educ 1998;10(5):255–65.

[45] Rossdale PD. Clinical studies on the newborn thoroughbred foal. I. perinatal behaviour. Br Vet J 1967;123(11):470–81.

[46] Doarn RT, Threlfall WR, Kline R. Umbilical blood flow and the effects of premature severance in the neonatal horse. Theriogenology 1987;28(6):789–800.

[47] Nout YS, Corley KTT, Donaldson LL, et al. Indirect oscillometric and direct blood pressure measurement in anesthetized and conscious neonatal foals. Journal of Veterinary Emergency Critical Care 2002;12(2):75–80.

[48] Gore DC, Jahoor F, Hibbert JM, et al. Lactic acidosis during sepsis is related to increased pyruvate production, not deficits in tissue oxygen availability. Ann Surg 1996;224(1):97–102.

[49] Chrusch C, Bands C, Bose D, et al. Impaired hepatic extraction and increased splanchnic production contribute to lactic acidosis in canine sepsis. Am J Respir Crit Care Med 2000; 161(2 Pt 1):517–26.

[50] Magdesian KG, Madigan JE. Volume replacement in the neonatal ICU: colloids and crystalloids. Clinical Techniques in Equine Practice 2003;2(1):20–30.

[51] James JH, Luchette FA, McCarter FD, et al. Lactate is an unreliable indicator of tissue hypoxia in injury or sepsis. Lancet 1999;354(9177):505–8.

[52] De Backer D. Lactic acidosis. Intensive Care Med 2003;29(5):699–702.

[53] Corley KTT, Donaldson LL, Furr MO. Arterial lactate concentration, hospital survival, sepsis and SIRS in critically ill neonatal foals. Equine Vet J 2005;37:53–9.

[54] Magdesian KG. Blood lactate levels in neonatal foals: normal values and temporal effects in the post-partum period [abstract]. J Vet Emerg Crit Care 2003;13(3):174.

[55] Kablack KA, Embertson RM, Bernard WV, et al. Uroperitoneum in the hospitalised equine neonate: retrospective study of 31 cases, 1988–1997. Equine Vet J 2000;32(6):505–8.

[56] Harvey JW. Normal hematological values. In: Koterba AM, Drummond WH, Kosch PC, editors. Equine clinical neonatology. Philadelphia: Lea & Febiger; 1990. p. 561–70.

[57] Gossett KA, French DD, Cleghorn B, et al. Effect of acute acidemia on blood biochemical variables in healthy ponies. Am J Vet Res 1990;51(9):1375–9.

[58] Scheingraber S, Rehm M, Sehmisch C, et al. Rapid saline infusion produces hyperchloremic acidosis in patients undergoing gynecologic surgery. Anesthesiology 1999;90(5):1265–70.

[59] Finfer S, Bellomo R, Boyce N, et al. A comparison of albumin and saline for fluid resuscitation in the intensive care unit. N Engl J Med 2004;350(22):2247–56.

[60] Choi PT, Yip G, Quinonez LG, et al. Crystalloids vs. colloids in fluid resuscitation: a systematic review. Crit Care Med 1999;27(1):200–10.

[61] Bickell WH, Wall MJ, Pepe PE, et al. Immediate versus delayed fluid resuscitation for hypotensive patients with penetrating torso injuries. N Engl J Med 1994;331(17):1105–9.

[62] Soucy DM, Rudé M, Hsia WC, et al. The effects of varying fluid volume and rate of resuscitation during uncontrolled hemorrhage. J Trauma 1999;46(2):209–15.

[63] Burris D, Rhee P, Kaufmann C, et al. Controlled resuscitation for uncontrolled hemorrhagic shock. J Trauma 1999;46(2):216–23.

[64] Fowden AL, Mundy L, Ousey JC, et al. Tissue glycogen and glucose 6-phosphatase levels in fetal and newborn foals. J Reprod Fertil 1991;(Suppl 44):S537–42.

[65] Koterba AM, Brewer BD, Tarplee FA. Clinical and clinicopathological characteristics of the septicaemic neonatal foal: review of 38 cases. Equine Vet J 1984;16(4):376–83.

[66] Corley KTT, Furr MO. Evaluation of a score designed to predict sepsis in foals. J Vet Emerg Crit Care 2003;13(3):149–55.

[67] Paradis MR. Update on neonatal septicemia. Vet Clin North Am Equine Pract 1994;10(1):109–35.

[68] Gentz JC, Cornblath M. Transient diabetes of the newborn. Adv Pediatr 1969;16:345–63.

[69] Park WS, Chang YS, Lee M. Effects of hyperglycemia or hypoglycemia on brain cell membrane function and energy metabolism during the immediate reoxygenation-reperfusion period after acute transient global hypoxia-ischemia in the newborn piglet. Brain Res 2001;901(1–2):102–8.

[70] Van den Berghe G, Wouters P, Weekers F, et al. Intensive insulin therapy in critically ill patients. N Engl J Med 2001;345(19):1359–67.

[71] Van den Berghe G, Wouters P, Bouillon R, et al. Outcome benefit of intensive insulin therapy in the critically ill: insulin dose versus glycemic control. Crit Care Med 2003;31(2):359–66.

[72] Paradis MR. Caloric needs of the sick foal: determined by the use of indirect calorimetry. Available at http://www.havemeyerfoundation.org/NSW/III-13-Paradis.htm. Accessed June 13, 2005.

[73] Spalding HK, Goodwin SR. Fluid and electrolyte disorders in the critically ill. Seminars Anesthesia Perioperative Medicine and Pain 1999;18(1):15–26.

[74] Webb AI, Coons TJ, Koterba AM, et al. Developments in management of the newborn foal in respiratory distress. 2. treatment. Equine Vet J 1984;16(4):319–23.

[75] Carraway MS, Piantadosi CA. Oxygen toxicity. Respir Care Clin N Am 1999;5(2):265–95.

ELSEVIER
SAUNDERS

Vet Clin Equine 21 (2005) 457–486

VETERINARY
CLINICS
Equine Practice

Ventilatory Support of the Critically Ill Foal

Jonathan E. Palmer, VMD[a,b],*

[a]*New Bolton Center, School of Veterinary Medicine, University of Pennsylvania,
Kennett Square, PA 19348, USA*
[b]*Neonatal Intensive Care Service, Graham French Neonatal Section,
Connelly Intensive Care Unit, The George D. Widener Hospital, New Bolton Center,
382 West Street Road, Kennett Square, PA 19348, USA*

The first attempt to assist ventilation through intermittent positive pressure was performed by Vesalius in 1555 when he blew into a reed inserted into the trachea of animals. The first use of mechanical ventilation was recorded in 1667 by Hooke, who used bellows to inflate a dog's lungs. In the middle of the nineteenth century, negative-pressure ventilation was introduced in devices like the iron lung. In 1907, Heinrich Drager introduced the first positive-pressure mechanical ventilator. In 1963, the first human neonate was successfully ventilated. By the 1970s, mechanical ventilation was in widespread use [1,2]. Today, it is the second most frequently performed therapeutic intervention after treatment for cardiac abnormalities in human intensive care units (ICUs) [3]. Currently in the United States, an estimated 1 to 3 million human patients receive mechanical ventilatory support annually supplied by an installed base of approximately 50,000 positive-pressure ventilators [4]. We who practice equine neonatology have benefited from the maturation of this therapeutic modality. Respiratory support, including mechanical ventilation, has been used successfully in neonatal foals for more than a quarter of a century [5,6]. Using modern mechanical ventilators and principles learned in human medicine, ventilating foals without respiratory failure, such as those suffering from botulism or neonatal encephalopathy–associated central hypercapnia, has become successful, with 80% of such patients surviving to be discharged [5,7] and many becoming productive athletes (Fig. 1) [8].

* New Bolton Center, University of Pennsylvania, 382 West Street Road, Kennett Square, PA, 19348, USA.
E-mail address: jepalmer@vet.upenn.edu

0749-0739/05/$ - see front matter © 2005 Elsevier Inc. All rights reserved.
doi:10.1016/j.cveq.2005.04.002   *vetequine.theclinics.com*

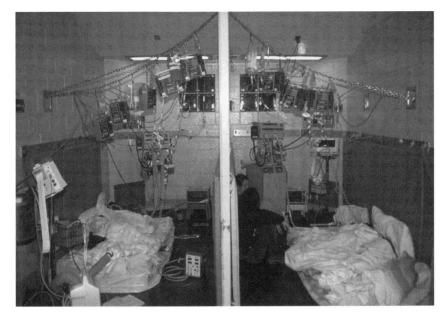

Fig. 1. Two foals suffering from neonatal encephalopathy being ventilated in adjacent stalls.

Those with secondary respiratory failure as with severe sepsis or acute respiratory failure associated with multiorgan dysfunction syndrome remain a major challenge, and successful outcomes in these cases are only achieved using all the accumulated knowledge and skills available. This article describes clinical principles currently used in the respiratory support of foals, with an emphasis on mechanical ventilation.

Oxygen therapy

The most useful drug in intensive care may be oxygen. The most dangerous drug in intensive care may be oxygen. Because of this duality, oxygen therapy should not be universally applied, but based on careful monitoring. Although many clinicians are satisfied monitoring Pao_2, I find monitoring oxygen saturation (Sao_2) and oxygen content equally as helpful. It is especially useful when the blood gas analyzer measures saturation directly instead of calculating it from the Pao_2. Although there is no fetal hemoglobin in the horse, there is a slightly lower level of 2,3-diphosphoglycerate (2,3-DPG) in fetal foal erythrocytes, which persists into the early neonatal period. This enhances erythrocyte loading at a lower Pao_2, aiding in pulmonary gas transport. There may be other organic phosphates or other substances that modify neonatal foal hemoglobin oxygen affinity, even in the absence of fetal hemoglobin [9]. In either case, the presence of these substances may make calculated saturations inaccurate. Increased oxygen affinity of the hemoglobin allows the neonate to load hemoglobin and transport enough oxygen to tissues with a Pao_2 that would be considered hypoxemic in an adult. Of course, enhanced erythrocyte loading at the lungs has the corollary of poor erythrocyte unloading at the tissues. This means that the neonate's tissues may have to exist at a lower Pao_2 to drive unloading. Neonates are uniquely suited to this because of hypoxic preconditioning as a fetus, however. There are clinical conditions in which there are changes in hemoglobin affinity that may affect oxygen delivery. In some circumstances, the affinity is enhanced enough that low Pao_2 is adequate for complete loading of hemoglobin in the lungs as may be seen with alkalosis or hypothermia. In other situations, such as with acidosis or hyperthermia, the affinity is decreased, resulting in poor oxygen loading but enhanced unloading at the tissues. Thus, it becomes valuable to monitor Sao_2 [9].

Oxygen therapy is indicated in any neonate with a Pao_2 less than 60 mm Hg or a Sao_2 less than 90%. The goal of oxygen therapy is to maintain the Pao_2 from 80 to 110 mm Hg and a Sao_2 greater than 92%. Oxygen content should also be monitored, but care must be taken that calculations are based on measured saturation and the patient's hemoglobin level. Many blood gas analyzers use standard hemoglobin levels and calculated saturations when calculating oxygen content in limited analysis modes, which results in erroneous reassurance. It is important to understand the relation between Pao_2, Sao_2, and oxygen content. It is the interaction of these three variables plus the oxygen affinity of the hemoglobin (which cannot be measured in a clinical setting) that determines oxygen loading and unloading. It is the gradient between blood and cellular Po_2 that powers blood oxygen unloading, making diffusion rapid and efficient. As long as the unloading occurs on the steep part of the oxygen-hemoglobin dissociation curve (a function of affinity and Sao_2), large quantities of oxygen can be moved to the tissues with minimal change in this gradient. Some neonates with a high resting packed cell volume (PCV) may have enough oxygen-carrying capacity that delivery is adequate despite a low Pao_2 and poor Sao_2. Oxygen delivery occurs at the expense of a lower tissue Po_2 and slower hemoglobin unloading. Neonates with mild anemia, which decreases oxygen content, still have enough reserve content to meet tissue needs as long as lung loading is normal and Pao_2 and Sao_2 are normal, allowing for more complete hemoglobin unloading at the tissues. The combination of marginal anemia and poor lung loading, which produces low Pao_2 and Sao_2, results in failure to deliver enough oxygen for tissue needs because of the limitation of hemoglobin unloaded, which is attributable to the small Pao_2 gradient between blood and tissues and movement to a less steep part of the oxygen-hemoglobin dissociation curve. Because neonates frequently have pulmonary problems that lead to periods of hypoxemia, in the face of marginal anemia, when the PCV drops below 24%, it is important to consider a blood transfusion as an important therapeutic option.

Ensuring adequate cardiac output is not only important in oxygen delivery to the tissues but in providing pulmonary perfusion allowing for adequate ventilation-perfusion (V/Q) matching, which is necessary for effective gas transport in the lungs. This often means the use of inopressor therapy [10]. Recent experience also suggests that vasopressin therapy can be quite helpful in maintaining perfusion [10,11]. This is probably because of a combination of autonomic failure and endocrine failure, because the levels used are expected to return vasopressin to a physiologic level and not to maintain a pharmacologic level. Another key to maintaining V/Q matching is maintaining the neonate in sternal recumbency. Maintaining sternal recumbency usually increases the Pao_2 at least 10 mm Hg and sometimes as much as 20 mm Hg when compared with maintaining the same foal in latter recumbency when the foal is weak and has poor inspiratory excursion and marginal perfusion [6,11].

The usual technique for delivering oxygen insufflation involves the use of a nasal cannula with the tip at the level of the medial cantus of the eye and several auxiliary openings closer to the external nares, because nasal discharge often occludes the openings. The nasal line can be secured to the nose using tape and a tongue depressor to act as a brace and to direct the line so that the foal has difficulty in displacing it. The oxygen should travel through a water-filled humidifier (do not use saline) controlled by a flowmeter. The usual flows necessary to maintain an adequate Pao_2 range from 2 to 15 L/min, with common flows between 6 and 10 L/min. The fraction of inspired oxygen (Fio_2) resulting from intranasal oxygen cannot be predicted easily because it varies with placement of the nasal cannula, patency of the cannula openings, tidal volume, minute volume, and size of the foal's nares.

Complications of intranasal oxygen insufflation include oxygen toxicity, nasal irritation and rhinitis, and airway drying, resulting in excessive tracheal and nasal discharge. Nasal irritation resulting in a rhinitis is the most common complication. This is manifested by teeth grinding, upper airway moisture, and the development of an occasionally profuse nasal discharge. This nasal irritation is attributable in part to the physical presence of the cannula and in part to the drying effect of the oxygen flow despite its humidification. Nasal drying results in nasal mucosa irritation, production of excessive goblet cells, and development of nasal discharge. Similar changes may occur in the trachea, resulting in excessive tracheal discharge. Preconditioning of medical gases through humidification and heating is an important medical practice. The most common device used to humidify intranasal oxygen is the bubble humidifier, in which gas bubbles through water, increasing the absolute humidity of the gas. The efficacy of the humidification depends on the contact time, which is inversely related to the flow rate, the bubble size (smaller bubbles with increased surface contact are more efficient), and the temperature of the water and gas [12]. With the high flow rates used in neonatal foals, a diffuser should be used to produce smaller bubbles to increase efficiency. This technique fails to humidify gases used at high flow rates in neonatal foals adequately, in part because most of the insufflated gas completely bypasses the nasal passages. The higher the flow rate, the more prominent are the complications. Some clinicians, out of desperation in treating severely hypoxemic neonates, have used bilateral nasal cannulas with combined flow rates up to 30 L/min. The beneficial effect of such an approach is questionable, and the adverse effect of this increased flow rate can be seen in the production of a copious nasal and tracheal discharge. It also occasionally significantly retards exhalation, leading to the production of auto–positive end-expiratory pressure (PEEP) and carbon dioxide (CO_2) retention. When high oxygen flow rates are indicated, new approaches to conditioning the medical gas, such as the Vapotherm system (Vapotherm, Stevensville, Maryland), which fully heats and humidifies gases at flow rates up to 40 L/min, could be useful.

Chemical adjuncts

Although mechanically assisted ventilation is the definitive treatment for hypoventilation, if the hypoventilation is secondary to blunted central CO_2 receptor sensitivity as often occurs with neonatal encephalopathy, the use of caffeine as a pharmacologic respiratory stimulant is indicated. Caffeine is the safest and most effective methylxanthine for use in foals with central respiratory center depression. It can be given orally or if there is gastrointestinal intolerance such as with necrotizing enterocolitis. It is also effective when given rectally. It is only effective in lowering the Pa_{CO_2} when there is a primary respiratory acidosis. When the Pa_{CO_2} is increased in an attempt to balance the pH secondary to a metabolic alkalosis, the caffeine has less effect. The usual dose is 10 mg/kg administered orally or per rectum once daily or more frequently based on arterial blood gas results. The full effect of a dose is usually evident within 2 hours. This drug seems to be safe [6]. It does act as a general central nervous system (CNS) stimulant, however, and transforms a somnolent and poorly responsive neonate into a more active patient [11]. Many hypercapnic foals that otherwise would require mechanical ventilation respond to caffeine, simplifying their treatment considerably.

Several conditions of neonates can lead to the development of pulmonary hypertension. Pulmonary hypertension has added significance in the neonate; as pulmonary pressure rises, right-to-left shunting often occurs through the foramen ovale and ductus arteriosus because these structures are not permanently closed for up to 3 weeks or more after birth. Actually, there is an adaptive advantage in the ability of the neonate to regress to the fetal circulatory pattern. If pulmonary hypertension is excessive, the only way to achieve adequate systemic cardiac output is shunted blood. The neonate's unique ability to exist in a hypoxemic state and its ability to regain cardiac output with pulmonary hypertension by shunting allow compensation and the ability to survive pulmonary hypertension without generalized systemic ischemic episodes.

Pulmonary hypertension may be present because of failure to make the birth transition, which is associated with an imbalance of pulmonary vasodilators and vasoconstrictors, such as nitric oxide (NO) and endothelin, or failure to arise from regression to fetal circulation because of perinatal hypoxemia or cytokine showers; alternatively, it can be secondary to pulmonary disease, septic shock, or development of acute respiratory distress syndrome (ARDS). The usual approach to treating pulmonary hypertension is to maximize pulmonary exposure to oxygen through ventilation with 100% oxygen, to alkalinize the arterial pH with mild hyperventilation or treatment with bases, and to maintain systemic blood pressure to counterbalance the increasing pulmonary pressure. The advent of inhaled NO therapy has revolutionized the treatment of neonatal pulmonary hypertension and seems to be effective in large animal species [13,14]. Inhaled NO at rates as low as 5 to 10 ppm of norepinephrine can effect a dramatic reversal of pulmonary hypertension. One problem with NO is that it can cause significant pulmonary toxicity through the production of free radicals in the presence of high oxygen concentrations; however, at low concentrations, this seems to be a rare complication [15]. NO causes pulmonary vasodilation by increasing cyclic guanosine monophosphate (cGMP) levels, which causes relaxation of the smooth muscles of the pulmonary vasculature. Recently, type V phosphodiesterase inhibitors that selectively prevent cGMP destruction have been developed [16,17]. Thus, endogenous NO or pulses of exogenous NO can be used to increase cGMP levels, resulting in vasodilation, and the phosphodiesterase inhibitors can be used to maintain vasodilation for a prolonged period. This results in a decrease in exposure to NO and simplification of therapy, because continuous NO delivery is no longer necessary. Although there are a number of phosphodiesterase inhibitors available with more or less pulmonary selectivity, we have had some success using sildenafil and a dose rate of 0.5 to 2.5 mg/kg [6]. Although it is too early to predict the success or anticipate the complications of this therapy, limited anecdotal experience is promising.

Mechanical ventilation

Mechanical positive-pressure ventilation supports and allows manipulation of pulmonary gas exchange; increases lung volume, returning normal functional residual capacity (FRC); decreases the work of breathing, allowing ventilatory muscles to rest when fatigued; and decreases the oxygen and energy use and perfusion that would be required to support the work of breathing. The main clinical indications for mechanical ventilation in the neonate are persistent pulmonary hypertension, acute respiratory failure, neonatal encephalopathy–associated weakness or central respiratory center failure, weakness associated with prematurity or intrauterine growth restriction (IUGR), central or sepsis-induced hypotension, septic shock, and neuromuscular disorders like botulism. Acute respiratory failure includes ARDS, organ dysfunction secondary to sepsis, infectious pneumonia (viral, bacterial, or aspiration pneumonia), noninfectious pneumonia (meconium aspiration, interstitial pneumonia, or aspiration pneumonia), and trauma secondary to fractured ribs. Typically, the goal is to provide respiratory support while therapies for underlying causes of the acute event are initiated [2,18,19].

The benefits of mechanical ventilation in improving gas exchange by increasing ventilation, improving V/Q matching, and decreasing intra-pulmonary shunting are well appreciated. Less well appreciated are the benefits of decreasing the work of breathing in cases of pulmonary failure and septic shock. With normal quiet breathing, inhalation is an active process requiring energy, using 3% to 5% of the oxygen the patient consumes. Exhalation is a passive process that requires no energy. When patients experience respiratory distress, as occurs with primary lung disease or septic shock, oxygen consumption required for the work of breathing increases up to 50% of the available oxygen and diverts perfusion resources as accessory muscles are recruited. Relieving this work of breathing allows redistribution of these oxygen and perfusion resources to support vital organ function. Respiratory support through mechanical ventilation is an important therapeutic modality in treating septic shock [3,20].

Ventilator modes

Only the generic modes that form the basis of modern conventional ventilation are discussed here (Table 1). Many modern conventional ventilators have proprietary modes, often confusing the uninitiated. The best source of information about these special modes is literature from the manufacturer. Most of these proprietary modes remain unproven, being supported only by a physiologic rational or, occasionally, with small and poorly powered studies.

Positive-pressure ventilation is classified according to the parameter that is used to terminate inspiration. Common cycling parameters include volume, pressure, flow, and time. With volume-cycled ventilation, inspiration is terminated after delivery of a preset tidal volume, irrespective of inspiratory time or the airway pressure during delivery. As the peak pressures in the patient's lungs increase, however, a greater proportion of the preset tidal volume is left behind in the ventilator's circuit. With pressure-cycled ventilation, inspiration ceases when a preset maximum airway pressure is reached, irrespective of the volume delivered, inspiratory time, or inspiratory flow rate. The delivered volume and inspiratory time vary with alterations in lung mechanics; thus, minute ventilation is not

Table 1
Ventilator modes

Mode	Description	Advantages	Disadvantages
Controlled mandatory ventilation	Machine-triggered mandatory breaths only	Ventilator has complete control of timing and amount of ventilation	Spontaneous breaths not allowed; patients often fight this mode; no synchrony with patient's efforts; only appropriate if foal is unconscious
Assist/control ventilation	Patient-triggered or machine-triggered mandatory breaths	Responds to patient respiratory efforts	Delivered breath is fixed and unvarying in tidal volume, inspiratory time, and flow rate, even in response to patient effort; may be poorly tolerated leading to dyssynchrony
Synchronized intermittent mandatory ventilation (SIMV)	Assist/control ventilation synchronized with additional patient breaths	Breaths beyond machine rate are spontaneous and under complete control of patient (timing, volume, and flow rate); synchrony prevents breath stacking; ensures a minimum rate and fosters better patient cooperation	Combination of spontaneous breaths and machine breaths results in erratic pressures and volumes; spontaneous breaths require a strong respiratory effort because of the resistance of the respiratory circuit (unless combined with PSV)
Pressure support ventilation (PSV)	Supported spontaneous breaths	Augmented inspiratory time, inspiratory flow rate, and tidal volume; decreases work of breathing; spontaneous breathing ensures patient cooperation	With severe dyspnea, there is an increased risk of alveolar collapse; poorly tolerated in patients that have high airway resistance
Continuous positive airway pressure (CPAP)	Maintenance of positive airway pressure during inhalation and exhalation and between breaths during spontaneous breathing	Increases functional residual capacity, stabilizes the chest wall, improves ventilation-perfusion ratios, and optimizes lung compliance and airway resistance	If inappropriate, results in low compliance, abnormal ventilation-perfusion ratios, detrimental effect on cardiac output, increased pulmonary resistance, and increased cerebral pressure; spontaneous breaths require a strong respiratory effort because of the resistance of the respiratory circuit (unless combined with PSV)

assured and may vary with time. With flow-cycled ventilation, inspiration is terminated when a particular flow rate is reached. Pressure support ventilation (PSV) is an example of flow-cycled mechanical ventilation. Here, a preset airway pressure is applied once the machine is triggered and is cycled off after the inspiratory flow decreases to a predetermined percentage of its peak value. Finally, with time-cycled ventilation, inspiration is terminated after a preset inspiratory time. The volume of gas delivered and the resulting airway pressure vary from breath to breath as a function of changes in lung mechanics. Many modern conventional ventilators incorporate several of these ventilator types in one machine [21].

The most important of the clinically available ventilator modes that can be found on pressure-cycled or volume-cycled ventilators are controlled mandatory ventilation, assist/control ventilation, and synchronized intermittent mandatory ventilation (SIMV), all with PEEP. Other clinically important modes found on pressure-cycled ventilators are PSV and continuous positive airway pressure (CPAP) (Fig. 2) [21].

With controlled mandatory ventilation, the ventilator delivers breaths at a preset interval, regardless of any ventilatory effort made by the patient. The patient cannot trigger a ventilator breath or take a spontaneous breath through the ventilator circuit. The delivered breath is a result of the preset volume or pressure and is no larger and no smaller. This mode is not

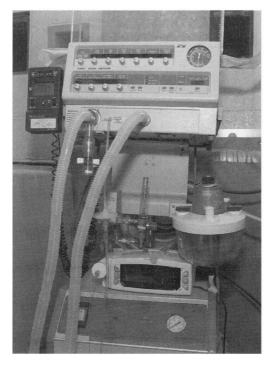

Fig. 2. Typical volume ventilator with control, assist/control, synchronized intermittent mandatory ventilation, and continuous positive airway pressure modes and also able to deliver pressure support ventilation. Note the black flowmeter attached to the left side and the capnograph on top of an air compressor.

appropriate for any conscious foal, because without extremely heavy sedation, the foal fights this mode and there is an absence of synchrony. In general, foals do not require any sedation for successful ventilation as long as they are in synchrony with the ventilatory mode. It is important to avoid sedation with its inherent complications. Sedation is not an acceptable substitute for choosing an appropriate mode and ventilator settings.

In the assist/control mode, respiratory efforts by the patient trigger a breath at the full preset volume or pressure. In the absence of any respiratory effort, the ventilator automatically cycles at a preset minimum background rate. For example, if the ventilator is set for 12 breaths per minute, the machine delivers a breath every 5 seconds in the absence of spontaneous inspiratory effort. If the patient's inspiratory effort triggers an assisted breath, the ventilator's timer resets for another 5 seconds. The patient is guaranteed at least the set breath rate but can breathe at a higher rate depending on the frequency of effective inspiratory efforts. The initiation of breaths synchronized with spontaneous efforts is welcomed by most foals, but the imposition of a preset breath at a fixed and unforgiving volume or pressure is poorly tolerated.

SIMV is a combination of spontaneous ventilation and assist/control ventilation. The delivery of the mechanical breath is synchronized to support the patient's spontaneous breaths at a preset rate, thus preventing the patient from stacking breaths (a mechanical breath being delivered at the same time as a spontaneous breath). Stacking may result in hyperinflation and volutrauma or barotrauma. If spontaneous breathing occurs at a rate faster than the ventilator's set SIMV rate, the patient breathes gas from the ventilator circuit. These spontaneous extra breaths consist of warmed, humidified, oxygen-enriched gas supplied from the ventilator's circuit but with no preset volume or pressure. If the patient's spontaneous efforts slow or stop, the ventilator breathes by default at the SIMV rate. SIMV is better tolerated, especially because breaths above the preset rate are completely controlled by the patient (timing, depth, and duration). The preset breaths are still at a fixed and unforgiving volume or pressure.

PSV is a partial ventilatory support flow-cycled mode in which breathing is controlled by the foal and peak pressures are controlled by the ventilator. The primary goal of PSV is to support the foal's spontaneous breathing effort while providing satisfactory oxygenation. PSV attempts to attain a preset peak inspiratory airway pressure each time the foal initiates inspiratory effort. If the foal's inspiratory effort is strong, the preset airway pressure may never be attained, because the inspiratory effort keeps the airway pressure below the pressure goal until the ventilator cycles off. Still, the inspiratory time, inspiratory flow rate, and tidal volume are augmented, whereas the inspiratory work of breathing is reduced. The machine senses the end of inspiration by first measuring the peak inspiratory flow and then waiting until that flow falls to a preset "off-switch" value (typically 25% of the peak flow or some fixed low-inspiratory flow rate); at that time, exhalation is allowed to proceed spontaneously. As a result, a PSV breath is delivered when the ventilator senses a respiratory effort by opening a demand valve at a preset pressure. Gases are forced into the ventilator circuit in an attempt to raise the airway pressure to the preset value, decreasing the work of inspiration. As the foal decides the tidal volume is sufficient, inspiratory flow slows and the demand valve shuts, ending inspiration and allowing expiration. Increasing levels of PSV decrease the work of breathing. Because the foal has complete control of initiation of breaths, inspiratory time, and tidal volume, it readily cooperates with the ventilator; however, because respiratory rate and tidal volume are not controlled, careful monitoring is required. Some new ventilators allow the clinician to set a target tidal volume. These ventilators titrate the delivered airway pressure based on feedback from past breaths. Frequently, SIMV and PSV are used together so that spontaneous breaths in SIMV are supported, helping to overcome the inherent resistance of the ventilator circuit, and when the predominant mode is PSV, the SIMV rate acts as a fail-safe breath rate [22,23].

There are situations in which PSV can be detrimental. When a foal is severely dyspneic despite ventilation, unless the pressure support is set high, there is an increased risk of alveolar collapse. PSV also may be poorly tolerated in patients that have high airway resistance with long time constants and may not provide sufficient minute ventilation because of the preset high initial flow and terminal inspiratory flow algorithms that are standard on most critical care ventilators [24]. In patients that have long inspiratory demands, the breath may be terminated too early if the flow rate slows before completion of inspiration. Conversely, the breath may terminate too late in patients that have obstructive airway disease. This can result in a short expiratory time, exacerbating air trapping. New ventilators attempt to solve these problems by using a pressure-targeted time-cycled breath, allowing for control of inspiratory time or control of the pressure slope, with a rapid peak resulting in a higher peak flow, and thus a shorter inspiratory time, and a slow peak initial flow resulting in a longer inspiratory time. A more direct approach used in some ventilators is to allow adjustment of the flow criteria, which causes the inspiratory assist to cycle off [23].

PEEP refers to the maintenance of positive pressure in the airways between ventilator-induced positive-pressure inspiration (during exhalation and between breaths) so that the airway pressure never falls below the set PEEP value. CPAP refers to maintaining positive airway pressure throughout spontaneous respiration (during inspiration and exhalation and between breaths). The terms are usually used synonymously, but strictly speaking, there is the possibility of subatmospheric pressure during inspiration, with PEEP depending on the ventilator inspiratory mode. PEEP may be added to any of the ventilation modes discussed previously. The primary physiologic effect of PEEP is to increase FRC by maintaining patency of alveoli at the end of exhalation.

PEEP or CPAP is often effective in treating hypoxemia by decreasing intrapulmonary shunting and V/Q mismatch. Beneficial physiologic affects of PEEP or CPAP are created by an increased transpulmonary pressure, resulting in an increased FRC, stabilization of an unstable chest wall, and improvement in V/Q ratios.

PEEP or CPAP affects pulmonary mechanics, cardiovascular stability, and pulmonary vascular resistance. FRC is the volume of gas remaining in the lungs at the end of a normal expiration. At a low FRC (low volumes [eg, diseased lungs]), compliance is low. At a higher FRC (volume), compliance increases. At a high FRC (overdistention), compliance again decreases. Optimum FRC, which is also normal FRC, results in optimum compliance and the lowest work of breathing. Lung volume is also related to airway resistance. At low lung volumes, airway resistance is high; because atelectasis is not resolved, the work of breathing is high. At optimum lung volumes, airway resistance is low. PEEP or CPAP can improve distribution of ventilation to optimize FRC, and thus lung compliance and airway resistance. High PEEP or CPAP can have a detrimental effect on the cardiovascular system, compressing right-sided vessels and decreasing cardiac return, which results in decreased cardiac output. The amount of PEEP or CPAP that is excessive and produces this effect depends on the lung compliance. If the lung compliance is low, less intra-airway pressure is transmitted to the plural space and cardiac compromise is less. Hypovolemia exacerbates the negative effect of high PEEP or CPAP. Overdistention of the lung may cause direct pressure on pulmonary arterials and capillaries, increasing pulmonary vascular resistance and pulmonary artery pressure. Low levels of PEEP or CPAP do not resolve atelectasis. Atelectasis results in shunting of blood away from collapsed alveoli and a regional increase in pulmonary vascular resistance. Optimal PEEP or CPAP optimizes the V/Q ratio. The effects of PEEP or CPAP on cerebral pressure are directly related to the level of positive pressure applied to the airway and the lung compliance affecting blood flow. If the pressure is transmitted to the pleural space and the anterior vena cava, it may result in increased cerebral pressure.

In healthy individuals, the FRC is maintained so that almost all alveoli are open and ventilated. In foals that are weak or fatigued, the FRC can be significantly reduced, resulting in poor ventilatory function. The lungs began to collapse to a volume at which alveoli collapse during expiration and must be opened on each breath to receive ventilation. Alveoli that repeatedly close in this manner increase the risk of injury from the shear stress and tend to break down surfactant [25,26]. As the amount of surfactant decreases, it becomes more difficult to open these alveoli on inspiration; eventually, atelectasis results. This further decreases the compliance of the lungs and further tends to cause collapse of more alveoli. The sum affect of this is progressive atelectasis. Even in those alveoli that are being ventilated, the ventilation is less evenly distributed because alveoli not already open do not open until part way through inspiration. Other alveoli that are already opened accept gas throughout inspiration. This results in maldistribution of ventilation and perfusion. Also, alveoli that close during expiration only participate in gas exchange during inspiration. Decreased FRC is most effectively treated through initiation of PEEP or CPAP. By increasing the airway pressure during expiration, alveoli tend to stay open, and more alveoli may be recruited on each new inspiration. Full recruitment using PEEP or CPAP requires 15 to 20 minutes. Optimal PEEP or CPAP can be estimated by producing a PEEP or CPAP grid. By adjusting PEEP or CPAP to 1 cm above and 1 cm below current levels and then allowing maximal recruitment after 10 to 15 minutes, obtaining a Pao_2 measurement or measuring effective compliance, the optimum PEEP or CPAP can be identified. Because alveolar injury is often quite heterogeneous, PEEP that is appropriate in one region may not be appropriate in another, being suboptimal or excessive. Optimizing PEEP is thus a balance between enrolling the recruitable alveoli in diseased regions without overdistending already recruited alveoli in healthier regions. Another potential detrimental effect of PEEP is that it raises mean and peak airway pressure, potentially contributing to barotrauma or volutrauma [3,27].

Typical ventilator settings

Initial ventilator settings depend on the ventilator make and model, ventilator mode, goal of the ventilatory intervention, and underlying cause of respiratory failure. The basic parameters to be set in volume-cycled ventilators in an assist/control or SIMV mode are Fio_2, tidal volume, rate, peak flow that in combination with rate determines the inspiratory-expiratory (I/E) ratio, trigger sensitivity, and PEEP (Table 2). Many ventilator models also allow setting an inspiratory pause (a brief hold at peak inspiration) and a fail-safe ventilatory rate that is activated if apnea occurs or a preset minute volume is not achieved. On ventilators offering a PSV mode, the pressure support level can also be set as well as other pressure support parameters in some ventilators [2,3].

Setting the tidal volume is important for successful mechanical ventilation. It is one parameter that has recently been shown to be important in determining the likelihood of ventilator-induced acute lung injury in human medicine. The recently published National Institutes of Health ARDS Network study showed that the use of 6-mL/kg tidal volume resulted in a significantly lower fatality rate than 12 mL/kg [28]. The interpretation of these results, that a tidal volume of 6 mL/kg is ideal in ARDS patients, has been debated [29]. The study shows that 12-mL/kg tidal volumes are not as successful as 6-mL/kg tidal volumes, but the ideal tidal volume may depend on the individual patient and could be 7 to 9 mL/kg or less than 6 mL/kg [29–33]. Indeed, clinicians have not fully embraced the use of these low tidal volumes in ARDS [33,34]. Recently, the use of high tidal volumes in ventilated patients who have no evidence of lung disease at the

Table 2
Typical initial ventilator settings

Parameter	Setting	Comments
FIO_2	0.5 (0.3–1.0)	Initial setting based on preventilatory response to oxygen therapy; titrated by pulse oximetry and ABG
Tidal volume	6–10 mL/kg	Goal is low airway pressure; set lower with preexisting lung injury
Breath rate	20–30 bpm	Adjust with capnography and ABG
Peak flow	60–90 L/min	Highly dependent on breath rate; set for an I/E ratio of approximately 1:2
Trigger sensitivity	2–3 cm H_2O	Do not set low enough that auto-triggering might occur
PEEP	4–5 cm H_2O	Should be adjusted based on compliance and Pao_2 values
Pressure support	8–12 cm H_2O	Set higher with low compliance; increase if tidal volume is too small (tidal volume may not respond to pressure support level)

Abbreviations: ABG, arterial blood gas; bpm, beats per minute.

onset of ventilation has been shown to predispose to ventilatory-associated acute lung injury [35]. We should also be careful not to overinterpret these data when choosing a tidal volume in ventilated foals. It could be dangerous to extrapolate the critical volume based on body weight from one species to another when the ratio of lung volume to body weight differs. High tidal volumes seem to be detrimental because of the resulting volutrauma or barotrauma. This is compounded in situations in which damaged lung results in a smaller ventilated lung volume, as in ARDS. The lesson from this landmark study is that the tidal volume should be set as low as practical with the goal of keeping the plateau airway pressure less than 30 cm H_2O even at the expense of mild hypercapnia. Thus, the tidal volume should be set between 6 and 10 mL/kg depending on the plateau airway pressure. Conscious nonsedated foals ventilated using a low tidal volume (eg, 6 mL/kg) frequently stack breaths so that the effective tidal volume is higher (eg, 12 mL/kg). The breath stacking can go undetected unless the clinician is quite observant. Sedation, with its associated complications, to achieve a low tidal volume may be more detrimental than a slightly higher tidal volume. Indeed, in human studies, low tidal volumes have been associated with systemic problems, suggesting that although this approach may be beneficial for the lungs, it may be detrimental overall [28,33,36–38].

Respiratory rate is often determined by the patient, because most ventilator modes allow the patient to initiate more breaths than the set machine breath rate. The set rate on the machine is in essence a minimum breath rate. For patients that have poor central sensitivity to CO_2, the respiratory rate should be set in conjunction with the tidal volume to achieve a desired minute volume adequate to maintain $Paco_2$ in the range that results in an acceptable pH. Often, critically ill neonates have an abnormal acid-base balance. Significant metabolic alkalosis is frequently present. The target $Paco_2$ is the one that returns the pH to a normal value. A $Paco_2$ of 60 to 65 mm Hg may be appropriate if that level is required to buffer a significant metabolic alkalosis, keeping the pH less than 7.45. This is not permissive hypercapnia with controlled hypoventilation. Permissive hypercapnia is the practice of allowing a $Paco_2$ higher than what is required to correct an acid pH, avoiding the possible lung trauma that could be caused in pursuit of full correction of the pH and allowing more optimal expiratory time. The goal of permissive hypercapnia is to maintain an arterial pH greater than 7.20 but not necessarily greater than 7.35. The practice of permissive hypercapnia is only needed when ventilating foals with significant underlying lung injury. When placing a foal on a ventilator using a mode other than full pressure support, an initial ventilator rate between 20 and 30 breaths per minute is usually adequate. The rate should be adjusted during the first 30 minutes of ventilation with the aid of capnography, which should be followed up by arterial blood gas measurements. The peak flow, which determines inspiratory time when machine-generated breaths are delivered, should be set in conjunction with the respiratory rate and tidal volume. Other factors that go into selecting and modifying peak flow include pulmonary mechanics, airway resistance, time constants, and airway pressure gradients. There is no clear formula that can be used in setting peak flow, but it is usually initially set so that the inspiratory time is similar to that of the unventilated patient that has an I/E ratio of approximately 1:2; it can then be dynamically adjusted as needed. Improperly set peak flow can be a source of patient-ventilator dyssynchrony when the delivered gas is too rapid or slow for the situation. When airway pressure becomes negative (beyond the trigger point) during inspiration, the patient is demanding gas faster than the ventilator is delivering, which may be because the peak flow is set too low.

The initial Fio_2 setting is dictated by the preventilation Pao_2 and the response observed to intranasal oxygen insufflation. If maintaining an acceptable Pao_2 has not been a problem, beginning with an Fio_2 of 0.3 should be sufficient. If high intranasal flows have been required to maintain blood oxygen, an Fio_2 of 0.5 should be initiated, and if the foal has remained hypoxemic despite high intranasal flows, the initial Fio_2 should be between 0.8 and 1.0. In all cases, the Fio_2 should be titrated as directed arterial blood levels, with the initial measurement within 30 minutes of initiating ventilation with the goal of an Fio_2 less than 0.5. An initial PEEP of 4 to 5 cm H_2O is usually adequate. Once the foal is stable on the ventilator, the PEEP can be further adjusted by the aid of flow loops or a compliance or Pao_2 grid can be constructed to ensure that the PEEP is optimal for the patient.

In cases with low Pao_2 values despite high intranasal oxygen flows, a trial with an Fio_2 of 1.0 can be useful diagnostically in identifying the source of the hypoxemic response. If the Pao_2 is less than 100 mm Hg after 15 to 20 minutes of ventilation with an Fio_2 of 1.0, it is likely that the cause of the hypoxemia is a large cardiac shunt rather than an intrapulmonary problem. In most of these cases, the Pa_{O_2} is often between 20 and 45 mm Hg and only increases to an $F_{I_{O_2}}$ of 2.0 or 3.0. This clinical rule of thumb has been accurate in this author's experience, predicting the presence of persistent fetal circulation with pulmonary hypertension and a large fraction of right-to-left shunting or a significant cardiac malformation resulting in the same. Also, reversion to fetal circulation can easily be detected by this method.

The sensitivity trigger, the patient's inspiratory effort needed to initiate a breath, can be pressure based or flow based. With pressure triggering, the expiratory valve must be closed before the patient generates the preset negative pressure needed to open the flow controller valve. With flow triggering, the inspiratory valve is kept open with a small amount of bias flow and the patient may initiate a breath even if the expiratory valve is still open, allowing for flow-by ventilation. With flow triggering, the patient immediately receives a small amount of flow to satisfy any air hunger, making for a smoother transition to the next breath [3]. Pressure trigger sensitivity is usually set at 2 to 3 cm H_2O. Care should be taken not to set the trigger value so low that any respiratory movement of the foal or bumping of the respiratory circuit triggers a breath. Increasing the trigger point, and thus making the patient use more effort to trigger a breath, is a common way to judge readiness for weaning and to exercise respiratory muscles in preparation for weaning.

The level of pressure support is dependent on the resistance and compliance of the ventilatory circuit, airway resistance, lung compliance, and inspiratory effort of the patient. In the absence of lung disease, such as in an uncomplicated patient that has botulism, 8 to 12 cm H_2O is enough to overcome ventilatory circuit resistance and deliver an adequate tidal volume. In cases of low compliance, pressure support as high as 20 to 25 cm H_2O or higher may be required. Higher pressure support can also be useful in situations in which patient-ventilator dyssynchrony results from a strong patient-derived inspiratory effort that exceeds the rate of gas delivery by the ventilator. Setting the inspiratory time and pressure slope with a rapid peak resulting in a higher peak flow can be helpful in ventilators that allow these adjustments.

All ventilator settings should be adjusted dynamically after initiation of ventilation, because success is highly dependent on tailoring the setting to the individual. A combination of simple pulmonary mechanics, end-tidal CO_2 determination, ventilation pressures, clinical status, and arterial blood gas results should form the basis for the adjustments. Having a feel for which combination of ventilatory adjustments improves successful gas exchange and improves ventilatory synchrony while, at the same time, decreasing ventilator-induced lung trauma only comes with experience and forms the basis of the art of successful ventilatory support.

Preconditioning ventilator gases

With the upper airway bypassed by tracheal intubation, sufficient heat and moisture must be added to the inspired gas mixtures to prevent mucosal injury secondary to drying and cooling. The response of the trachea to such injury is proliferation of goblet cells and production of discharge, which becomes tenacious as it becomes desiccated and can obstruct the airway or endo-tracheal tube. Active humidifiers use external water sources and electrical power to adjust blended gas mixtures to an intratracheal temperature greater than $35\,^{\circ}C$ and a water content greater than 40 mg/L. Passive humidifiers use simple heat-moisture exchange (HME) device filters placed on the ventilator side of the endotracheal tube that use heat and moisture trapped from expired gases (Fig. 3). HME filters trap heat and moisture from the exhaled air and add both to the next breath as it passes through the filter. These disposable units can usually supply adequate heat and moisture (ie, warmer than $30\,^{\circ}C$–$33\,^{\circ}C$ and higher than 28–32 mg H_2O/L) for most foals receiving mechanical ventilation for only short periods [27]. Foals weighing more than 70 kg or those that have large minute volumes for any reason may need more moisture than can be trapped by large HME filters. In these cases, adding a cold active humidifier to a circuit with an HME filter in place may add enough moisture to allow effective ventilator gas preconditioning. In this situation, the humidity must be delivered to the HME filter cold so that it passes through the filter to the patient. Once it is warmed by the patient, the moisture is trapped on the patient side of the filter. In addition to the limitation of high minute volume, HME filter use is not effective in hypothermic patients, and the presence of airway discharge can obstruct the filter, causing a dangerous situation [7]. An advantage of many HME filters is that they act as an efficient antimicrobial filter, excluding nosocomial bacteria and viruses from the patient and confining the patient's pathogens to the endotracheal tube and airway. Thus, with this type of HME filter, sterile ventilator circuit tubing is not needed. Without it, the circuit and active humidifier must be sterile and changed at

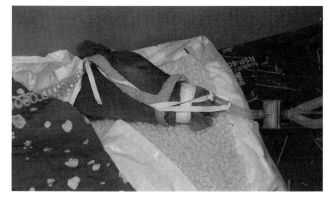

Fig. 3. Foal on ventilator with an HME filter between the endotracheal tube and ventilator circuit wye-piece. Note how the endotracheal tube is secured with ties running from the endotracheal tube and HME tubing to the foal's poll after being laced around the halter cheek pieces to keep the ties away from the eyes.

least every 24 hours. The other practical problem with active humidification is the problem of "rainout" in the circuit as the moist warm gas passes though a cool circuit. This requires the addition of water traps in the circuit that require frequent emptying or the addition of heated circuit tubing. The rainout problem is exacerbated by the cooler environmental temperatures often found in the equine neonatal intensive care unit (NICU) in the winter.

Preparing to place a foal on a ventilator

The time between the decision to use mechanical ventilation as a therapeutic intervention and initiation of ventilation can be minimized by following a routine for ventilator setup. In clinics in which mechanical ventilation of patients is a rare event, having a ventilator setup checklist, dry runs with the staff practicing setting up the equipment, and sessions covering equipment troubleshooting procedures can minimize confusion and uncertainty during the heat of battle. Typical equipment needed includes the ventilator; access to oxygen (with minimal interruption of the patient's oxygen insufflation); access to medical grade compressed air or a compressed air generator; interface lines; a gas blender (often built into the ventilator); a capnograph with lines and an adaptor; a humidifying device (often, an HME filter); a ventilator circuit; an endotracheal tube; sterile gloves; sterile lubrication; a means of securing the endotracheal tube; a stethoscope; a self-inflating bag (in case of an emergency); and, most importantly, adequate trained help to restrain the foal, intubate the foal, secure the endotracheal tube, and begin adjusting the ventilator settings as soon as the foal is intubated (Table 3).

As part of setting up the ventilator, the circuit and other attachments should be inspected to be certain that everything is in proper working order, and the circuit should be checked for leaks. This can be done by attaching an artificial lung to the circuit, occluding the exhalation port, and charging the circuit with a manual breath or checking the ventilator's ability to maintain PEEP. It is convenient to select the initial ventilator setting after checking for leaks. It is also important to check the integrity of the endotracheal tube's cuff before intubation. Leaking endotracheal cuffs are a common problem during ventilation. Sterile endotracheal tubes should be used to minimize introduction of nosocomial bacteria during intubation. While checking the cuff, care should be taken to maintain sterility of the tube beyond the cuff inflation port. During setup, a choice about heating and humidifying the delivered gas should be made and implemented (Fig. 4).

Monitoring during ventilation

The object of monitoring during ventilation is to allow dynamic adjustment of mechanical ventilation parameters, to understand and correct underlying pathophysiology, to prevent damage from the act of mechanical ventilation,

Table 3
Preparation for ventilation

Required equipment resource	Setup
Ventilator	Position in conjunction with foal so that there is easy access to medical gases and there is minimum disruption and danger of extubation when turning the foal from side to side
	Check all attachments, valves, and connections
	Program initial settings, set alarm levels
Oxygen	Access with minimal interruption of the patient's oxygen insufflation until placed on ventilator
Medical grade compressed air	Access to piped compressed air or a compressed air generator
Interface lines	From O_2/air source and compressed air source to ventilator
Gas blender	Often built into the ventilator; set initial F_{IO_2}
Capnograph	Warm up and calibrate; attach sample line to HME filter or endotracheal tube adaptor
Flowmeter	Often built into the ventilator; setup and calibrate; set alarm levels
Humidifying device	New HME filter (keep patient side sterile) or active humidifier with sterile circuit and water traps; place temperature probe at wye-piece; fill with sterile water; set parameters
Ventilator circuit	Circuit tubing, wye-piece, capnograph adaptor, proximal pressure line, HME filter, temperature sensor
	Check that it has been put together properly
	Labeled pictures of the circuit and other parts of the ventilator setup are helpful for inexperienced staff
	Check the assembled circuit for leaks (using an artificial lung and occluding exhalation valve)
Endotracheal tube	Sterile, 55-cm length, at least two sizes (estimated and one size smaller), 2 of each
	Estimate size based on foal's size and relative nasal passage size (IUGR foal often can use a tube larger than estimated by body size)
	Common sizes: STD TB, 9-mm ID; Warmblood, 10-mm ID, Arabian, 8-mm ID
	Sterile gloves, lube; the endotracheal tube should be placed as cleanly as possible to minimize introduction of nosocomial pathogens to the respiratory tract
Securing the endotracheal tube	This can be done with ties running from the endotracheal tube adaptor and HME tubing around the foal's poll; a cloth halter is useful in directing the ties away from the eyes to avoid ocular trauma (see Fig. 3)
Adequate assistance	Help trained to restrain the foal, intubate the foal, secure the endotracheal tube, and begin adjusting the ventilator settings as soon as the foal is intubated
Stethoscope	To ensure proper intubation placement with even gas flow to each lung
Self-inflating bag	In case of ventilator malfunction or other emergency

Abbreviations: ID, inner diameter; STD, standard; TB, Thoroughbred.

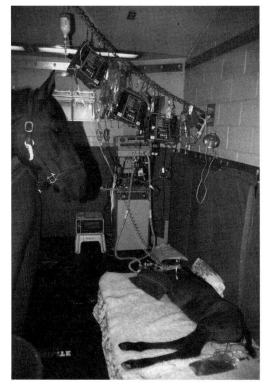

Fig. 4. Typical ventilator setup.

and to decide if it is time to discontinue mechanical ventilation. Monitoring can take many forms, which vary greatly in sophistication. The following are the most useful parameters that can be monitored by the minimum equipment that should be available in support of mechanical ventilation.

Arterial blood gas measurement

Although noninvasive monitoring, such as pulse oximetry and capnography, can be useful, it is not a substitute for an arterial blood gas (ABG) measurement in a critical neonate. If these noninvasive techniques are being used when an ABG measurement is drawn, comparison of the results recorded as the syringe is filling and understanding the underlying pathophysiology causing discrepancies between the two monitoring techniques can be useful in understanding the clinical condition of the patient. Whenever an ABG measurement is drawn, not only should ventilator settings be recorded to help with dynamic adjustments but the capnograph reading should also be noted as the syringe is filling. An ABG measurement should be drawn before beginning ventilation, within 30

minutes of initiation of ventilation and again after 2 to 3 hours of ventilation. Timing of further ABG samples should be undertaken as dictated by
the initial samples and the clinical condition of the patient. Stable patients
that do not have primary pulmonary disease or cardiovascular instability
(eg, botulism) may only require one ABG measurement a day. Others may
require samples every few hours. The goal is to keep the Pao_2 greater than
80 mm Hg and less than 120 mm Hg with an Sao_2 greater than 92% and to
keep the pH greater than 7.340 but less than 7.420.

Capnography

Capnography can be a valuable monitoring technique and should be used
continuously during ventilation. It can be useful for simple but vital matters,
such as detecting loss of endotracheal cuff integrity, an all too common
problem during ventilation. In this situation, the end-tidal CO_2 ($ETCO_2$)
drops to 0 as if the foal is apneic, but the cycling of the ventilator suggests
that apnea is not the problem. Most of the time, this scenario is caused by
a deflated endotracheal cuff with leakage of exhaled gases around the
endotracheal tube. Capnography can also help to diagnose and monitor
complex pathophysiologic conditions.

In patients that have normal hemodynamics and pulmonary function,
the $ETCO_2$ is 2 to 5 mm Hg less than the $Paco_2$, having a strong enough
correlation to safely be relied on as a surrogate for $Paco_2$ [39,40]. In patients
that have severe lung disease or hemodynamic instability, the $ETCO_2$ is not
a good predictor of $Paco_2$ because the difference between the two
measurements varies with changing V/Q relations in the lungs. In these
cases, the emphasis should be on more ABG measurements until the V/Q
mismatch improves (improved hemodynamics and pulmonary function)
and a more consistent relation between $ETCO_2$ and $Paco_2$ is established.
Establishment of a consistent relation implies an improvement in the V/Q
status of the patient [39–41].

$ETCO_2$ is a function of $Paco_2$, cardiac output, alveolar dead space
ventilation (pulmonary perfusion), airway time constants, CO_2 production
(metabolic rate), and bicarbonate therapy. Capnography can be used to
determine the adequacy of alveolar ventilation, the patency and placement
of the endotracheal tube, the relation between alveolar ventilation and
pulmonary perfusion, cardiac output and pulmonary blood flow (especially
useful during cardiopulmonary resuscitation [CPR]), and proper function-
ing of the ventilator (especially if rebreathing of CO_2 is occurring) [42–46].

The $Paco_2$ is determined by the Pco_2 of all perfused alveoli (whether or not
they are ventilated), and the $ETCO_2$ represents the Pco_2 of all ventilated
alveoli (whether or not they are perfused). As a result, the gradient between
$Paco_2$ and $ETCO_2$ reflects alveolar dead space ventilation (V/Q = infinity).
Alveolar dead space is the volume of alveoli that are ventilated but not
perfused. It represents a failure of pulmonary perfusion and is the other end of

the spectrum from shunting or venous admixture in the continuum of V/Q abnormalities. Because the gas leaving alveoli that are ventilated but not perfused does not contain CO_2, it has a diluting effect on the CO_2 leaving other areas of the lung, lowering the $ETCO_2$. The gradient between $PaCO_2$ and $ETCO_2$ reflects the percent of alveolar dead space ventilation and can easily be calculated with the following formula: % alveolar dead space = ($PaCO_2$ − $ETCO_2$/$PaCO_2$) × 100. The two most common reasons for increased alveolar dead space ventilation are decreased perfusion secondary to decreased cardiac output and decreased perfusion secondary increased pulmonary vascular resistance, such as occurs during ventilation with increased alveolar pressure (PEEP level/peak airway pressure/average airway pressure) causing alveolar capillary compression.

Although the $PaCO_2$-$ETCO_2$ gradient usually reflects alveolar dead space ventilation, because there are other factors affecting $ETCO_2$ levels, this is not always true. The $ETCO_2$ is a measure of the CO_2 in the last alveoli to empty. If the lungs have uniform conditions throughout most areas, this reflects the average alveoli. There are often areas of the lungs with different time constants (reflecting how quickly gas enters and leaves these alveoli), however. When there are areas of the lungs with long time constants, these alveoli receive less ventilation. The PCO_2 in these alveoli is higher, and gas from these alveoli is the last to leave the lungs and heavily influences the PCO_2 in the end-tidal gas, thus resulting in an $ETCO_2$ that is higher than that of the average alveoli. In fact, in some cases, the $ETCO_2$ may be higher than the $PaCO_2$. Thus, the $PaCO_2$-$ETCO_2$ gradient underestimates the alveolar dead space ventilation. Inspection of the capnogram readily reveals this situation. This is one of several reasons why, in addition to $ETCO_2$ monitoring, it is important to use capnography, which is the continuous measurement of exhaled CO_2.

Capnography consists of continuous real-time recording of CO_2 as measured from a sample taken at the ventilator end of the endotracheal tube relative to time or to volume of exhaled gases. A volume capnogram is a graph of exhaled CO_2 relative to the volume of gas exhaled. There has been renewed interest in this mode of capnography with the advent of noninvasive cardiac output measurements using CO_2 excretion. Whether or not this technique, which seems to be valuable in patients that have normal physiology, lives up to its promise when applied to critically ill patients remains to be proven. The clinically more common time capnogram graphs CO_2 relative to time throughout the respiratory cycle. In a time capnogram of a normal individual at the initiation of exhalation, the CO_2 is 0, because the first gas to leave the airway exits from anatomic dead space (phase I). As anatomic dead space gas begins to mix with alveolar gas, there is a sudden upstroke of the curve (phase II), which is almost at a right angle to the baseline. The upstroke rapidly reaches a plateau (phase III). The end of the plateau marks the end of exhalation, and that point is the $ETCO_2$. The initial part of inhalation is marked by the downstroke, which rapidly returns to baseline followed by a period with a CO_2 of 0 (phase 0) [47].

Careful observation of the curve for variations from normal can help to characterize abnormalities. An elevated baseline and upstroke (phase II) indicate CO_2 rebreathing if they develop gradually. A sudden increase suggests contamination of the sample cell with water, mucus, or dirt [48]. A prolonged or sloped upstroke that does not meet a clear plateau suggests an obstruction to expiratory gas flow (eg, bronchospasm, obstructive pulmonary disease, kinked endotracheal tube) or leaks in the breathing circuit [47]. Even in normal patients, the plateau, which is alveolar gas, usually has a slight positive slope, indicating a slight rise in CO_2 during expiration. There are two reasons for this increase. First, because CO_2 is being continuously excreted into the alveoli, which are becoming progressively smaller as expiration continues, the last gas emptied from the alveoli has a higher concentration of CO_2. Second, even in normal lungs, there is a wide range of V/Q ratios in different areas of the lungs. Some alveoli have a higher V/Q ratio because they are more readily ventilated (have shorter time constants) and thus have a relatively lower PCO_2. Others have a lower V/Q ratio because of underventilation (longer time constants), resulting in a relatively higher PCO_2. The delayed emptying of these alveoli with a low V/Q (high PCO_2) contributes to the rising slope of the plateau. Factors like changes in cardiac output, CO_2 production, airway resistance, and FRC may further affect the V/Q status of the various areas in the lung, and thus influence the height or the slope of the plateau. The presence of a steep slope of this plateau indicates abnormalities in V/Q mismatch of the lung [40]. The V/Q difference can be great enough that the $ETCO_2$ may be higher than the $PaCO_2$, which reflects the average perfused alveolar CO_2. When there is a significant slope to the plateau phase, the $PaCO_2$-$ETCO_2$ gradient underestimates the amount of alveolar dead space ventilation [49,50].

Fraction of inspired oxygen

It is important to check the accuracy of the FIO_2 setting periodically by measuring the FIO_2 at the endotracheal tube. At times, the gas blender of the ventilator may be inaccurate. Some ventilators have built-in oxygen sensors. Inexpensive handheld oxygen sensors are readily available and convenient for spot monitoring of the FIO_2.

Tidal volume and minute volume

It is important to monitor actual tidal volume and minute volume rather than relying on the intended volumes to monitor for leaks and ventilator malfunction. Also, in ventilator modes like PSV, where the patient sets the tidal volume, which can change at any time, tidal volume monitoring is important. Most modern ventilators have built-in flowmeters, but external flowmeters are available for those that do not. One downfall of common turbine-based flowmeters (where gas moving past the sensor spins a turbine and the volume is measured by counting the revolutions) is that at high respiratory rates, where the expiratory pause is too short to allow the turbine to stop spinning, tidal volume measurements cannot be obtained.

Airway pressure

Many modern ventilators measure airway pressure, volumes, and flows throughout the respiratory cycle and display pressure-volume (compliance) loops and flow-volume (resistance) loops. These graphs can be quite useful in adjusting and monitoring ventilator function. If these displays are not available, the most important airway pressures are peak inspiratory pressure (PIP), plateau pressure (P_{PL}), and PEEP or baseline pressure. The PIP is the highest pressure, usually occurring at the end of inspiration. The P_{PL} is the pressure after the end of inspiration when the gases have arrived at equilibrium and can usually be measured during the inspiratory pause if the ventilator has this capability or by briefly occluding the expiratory port after full inspiration and recording the value once the pressure stabilizes. The PEEP or baseline pressure can be measured between respiratory cycles, again, when no air is moving.

The PIP is the most frequently measured variable of ventilatory function during mechanical ventilation. It depends on lung compliance and airway resistance. Changes in the magnitude of PIP may reflect any of several potentially detrimental problems related to ventilation. In a practical sense, PIP should be considered an additional vital sign for patients on a ventilator. A sudden decrease in PIP suggests a major leak in the circuit but also can be caused by insufficient gas supply to the ventilator, an inadvertent change in settings, unintended extubation, or failure or disconnection of the ventilator. Increases in PIP may indicate endotracheal tube occlusion by secretions or kinking, acute bronchospasm, pneumothorax, or conditions causing decreased lung compliance. High PIP may cause barotrauma and other acute lung injury. PIP is usually monitored by alarms that indicate high values or failure to reach a minimum PIP. The baseline pressure should be 0 or higher if there is a PEEP, except during patient inspiratory efforts. Failure to maintain PEEP usually suggests a small circuit leak.

Compliance and resistance

With measurement of tidal volume, PIP, P_{PL}, and PEEP, effective compliance and airway resistance can be calculated. Effective compliance is the compliance of the lungs and the chest wall. Because chest wall compliance rarely changes acutely and effective compliance does not require pleural pressure measurements, effective compliance is a readily attainable and clinically convenient parameter. Static effective compliance can be calculated by dividing the tidal volume by the difference between the P_{PL} and PEEP. It decreases if there is an abnormality of the chest wall (a flail chest) or a decrease in functional alveolar numbers as with pulmonary edema, pneumonia, or atelectasis as well as for other similar reasons. It may also be used to determine the best PEEP and best tidal volume if serial measurements are obtained at trial settings and a response grid is recorded.

Dynamic effective compliance can be calculated by dividing the tidal volume by the difference between the PIP and PEEP. Dynamic compliance adds the effects of resistance to static compliance. Dynamic compliance decreases with disorders of the airway, lung parenchyma, and chest wall. Dynamic compliance is less than static compliance when there is increased resistance, such as with secretions in the airways or endotracheal tube, bronchospasm, or endotracheal tube kinking.

Changes in airway resistance are most easily detected by monitoring the difference between the PIP and P_{PL}. As the difference increases, so does the airway resistance. PIP and P_{PL} pressures cannot always be accurately measured with spontaneously initiated breaths, especially in PSV. In the pressure support mode, the airway pressure may be variably decreased by the magnitude of the patient's inspiratory effort. As the patient's effort increases and because the ventilator cycles off based on flow rates and not volume or pressure, the PIP may never reach a value close to that if the patient had the breath delivered by a volume or pressure machine breath. In fact, what is traditionally the measure of PIP (at the end of inspiration) may actually be less than the P_{PL}. Therefore, these measurements should only be made during a ventilator-delivered breath that is not pressure supported.

Endotracheal tube

Initially, the endotracheal tube should be changed daily or more often in the face of increased airway resistance. Each time the tube is changed, the amount and quality of the discharge in the tube should be monitored. If the discharge is extremely viscous and difficult to clean from the tube, it suggests inadequate preconditioning of ventilator gases (usually too little humidity), which should be corrected. An increased quantity of clear discharge is also an indication of failure of preconditioning of gases. If the discharge becomes dark or sanguineous (in the absence of traumatic intubation), infection should be suspected. In either case, periodic culturing of the lumen of the endotracheal tube is useful. Generally, several microbes (two to six microbes) can be recovered, even in the absence of significant disease. These isolates should not be viewed as invaders that need to be targeted with antimicrobial treatment but as colonizers that represent the nosocomial population from which the next invader may originate, whether the route is via the respiratory tract, the gastrointestinal tract, or intravenous access. If a secondary infection becomes evident, these culture results give weight to an educated guess of how to modify antimicrobial therapy before definitive culture and sensitivity results are available. Targeting these colonizers with antimicrobials before they invade is likely to select for more resistant nosocomial microbes. It should be remembered that cuffed endotracheal tubes provide a degree of protection from aspiration, but this degree of protection is not complete. Studies in human medicine have found gastric contents in the bronchial secretions of approximately 25% of intubated patients [2,51,52].

Evolving therapies

Newer modes of ventilatory therapy are gaining acceptance in human intensive care, but few have been evaluated by more than small clinical studies. Most of these modes have a firm basis in the theoretic pathophysiology of lung injury and have been added to modern ventilators but largely remain unproven in human medicine and have rarely been tried in foal ventilation. Some of these therapies may have an important role in evolving therapy, but recommendation for widespread adaptation requires further studies [27].

Inverse ratio ventilation (IRV) is mechanical ventilation with an extended inspiratory time greater than expiration. It has been used in infants and adults suffering from ARDS. The purpose is to maintain oxygenation at lower levels of PEEP and airway pressures, thereby minimizing barotrauma. Airway pressure release ventilation (APRV) augments spontaneous breathing with CPAP. The patient's inspiration is aided by CPAP, and expiration is then allowed by periodically releasing the CPAP to a lower level. This modality was designed specifically for patients that have severe restrictive lung disease, who poorly tolerate positive-pressure ventilation because of their susceptibility to barotrauma and cardiac depression. High-frequency ventilation (HFV) is a generic term for any mode of mechanical ventilation that supplies small tidal volumes at rates of more than 60 breaths per minute. HFV is administrated by a jet of gas in the endotracheal tube that entrains additional airway gases, delivering 2- to 5-mL/kg tidal volumes at 60 to 80 breaths per minute. Large studies supporting the use of HFV in clinical critical care are lacking. Proportional assist ventilation (PAV) is an approach to ventilatory support in which the ventilator responds to each spontaneous breath in an independent manner. This modality augments patient effort but leaves the patient completely in control of all aspects of breathing. For a given breath, the pressures, volumes, times, and flows may differ from previous and subsequent breaths. The use of PAV may allow for assisted ventilation with relatively low peak airway pressures and therefore less risk of barotrauma or cardiac depression. Liquid ventilation has also enjoyed some popularity, but reports of successful large scale studies are not yet available [23,53–56].

The use of noninvasive positive-pressure ventilation and noninvasive CPAP has become popular in human medicine. The major stumbling block to this methodology is that successful maintenance is more labor-intensive and requires experienced staff. Adapting this technique requires the development of an effective noninvasive nasal delivery apparatus.

Discontinuing mechanical ventilation

As soon as the foal is begun on mechanical ventilation, the clinician should ask himself if the foal is ready to be weaned. This question should be asked repeatedly until the answer is yes. Because of the threat of secondary nosocomial infections associated with ventilation, it is important to keep the ventilation period as short as possible. Some foals with neonatal encephalopathy can be weaned less than 24 hours after being placed on a ventilator. Some foals with botulism require 10 to 14 days of ventilation, and some foals with significant respiratory injury may require a month or more of ventilatory support.

Before attempting to discontinue mechanical ventilation, patients should show cardiovascular and metabolic stability and sepsis, if present, should be controlled. Also, there should be evidence that the original underlying problem which led to the need for mechanical ventilation has resolved or at least improved. No predictor is reliably able to establish when a foal is ready for weaning.

There are three commonly accepted methods of performing weaning trials [57]. The method I prefer involves having the foal breathe on PSV with a gradual decrease in the level of support as tolerated. When breathing with minimal to no support, the foal is extubated. A second method uses a gradual decrease in the SIMV ventilator rate with constant minimal pressure support until the foal is not receiving any mechanical breaths and instead is maintaining minute ventilation requirements spontaneously. The third method is the spontaneous breathing trial. This involves extubation with constant observation over a period of up to 2 hours. This trial should not be attempted without extubation, because asking a foal that is just ready to wean to breath with the extra resistance posed by the endotracheal tube is a formula for weaning failure. Failure of a weaning trial can be defined by the development of tachypnea, hypoxemia, tachycardia, sustained brady-cardia, hypertension, hypotension, or agitation [2].

Foals that have had prolonged ventilation (>4 days) may benefit from respiratory exercise periods to strengthen respiratory muscles before full weaning. This can most easily be accomplished by decreasing the PSV or SIMV rate or decreasing the trigger sensitivity for periods of 30 to 60 minutes every 4 to 6 hours. During these periods, if the foal shows signs of fatigue, the session should be cut short.

Summary

Critically ill foals often have respiratory failure and benefit from respiratory support. Some only require intranasal oxygen insufflation, whereas others need full respiratory support with mechanical ventilation. Recent developments in chemical adjuncts to ventilatory support allow successful conservative therapy in many foals with neonatal encephalopathy that were previously only saved with mechanical ventilation. Modern mechanical ventilators developed for human medicine are easily adapted to foals and make mechanical ventilation of foals not only possible but frequently successful. Conventional mechanical ventilation using SIMV or PSV along with PEEP is useful in many foals. Initial ventilator settings are based on the underlying cause of respiratory failure and the usual response of similar cases but must be dynamically adjusted from the outset as dictated by the response of the individual. This dynamic process is aided by constant monitoring of parameters, such as pH, Pao_2, $Paco_2$, $ETCO_2$, tidal and minute volume, airway pressures, compliance, and resistance. As soon as the foal is begun on mechanical ventilation, the clinician should ask himself if the foal is ready to be weaned. Early weaning is as important as timely initiation of ventilation. Monitoring also aids in deciding when it is appropriate to wean the foal.

References

[1] Morch E. History of mechanical ventilation. In: Kirby R, Banner M, Downs J, editors. Clinical applications of ventilatory support. New York: Churchill-Livingstone; 1990. p. 1–6.

[2] Gali B, Goyal DG. Positive pressure mechanical ventilation. Emerg Med Clin North Am 2003;21(2):453–73.

[3] Fenstermacher D, Hong D. Mechanical ventilation: what have we learned? Crit Care Nurs Q 2004;27(3):258–94.

[4] MacIntyre NR. Mechanical ventilation: the next 50 years. Respir Care 1998;43:490–3.

[5] Palmer JE. Ventilatory support of the neonatal foal. Vet Clin North Am Equine Pract 1994; 10(2):167–86.

[6] Palmer JE. Respiratory support of critical equine neonates. In: Madewell B, editor. 2003 American College of Veterinary Internal Medicine Forum Proceedings. Lakewood (CO): American College of Internal Medicine; 2003.

[7] Wilkins PA, Palmer JE. Mechanical ventilation in foals with botulism: 9 cases (1989–2002). J Vet Intern Med 2003;17(5):708–12.

[8] Axon JE, Palmer JE, Wilkins PA. Short- and long-term athletic outcome of neonatal intensive care unit survivors. Proc Am Assoc Equine Pract 1999;45:224–5.

[9] Delivoria-Papadopoulos M, McGowan JE. Oxygen transport and delivery. In: Polin RA, Fox WW, Abman SH, editors. Fetal and neonatal physiology. 3rd edition. Philadelphia: WB Saunders; 2004. p. 880–9.

[10] Palmer JE. When fluids are not enough: inopressor therapy. In: Hughes D, editor. Proceedings of the Eighth International Veterinary and Critical Care Symposium. San Antonio (TX): Veterinary Emergency and Critical Care Society; 2002.

[11] Palmer JE. Foal cardiopulmonary resuscitation. In: Orsini JA, Divers TJ, editors. Manual of equine emergencies: treatment and procedures. 2nd edition. Philadelphia: WB Saunders; 2003. p. 581–614.

[12] Chiumello D, Bottino N, Pelosi P. Condition of medical gases during spontaneous breathing. In: Vincent JL, editor. Intensive care medicine annual update 2003. Heidelberg, Germany: Springer-Verlag; 2004. p. 255–63.

[13] Palmer JE. Use of inhaled nitric oxide in improving pulmonary gas exchange in persistent pulmonary hypertension and pulmonary failure secondary to septic shock in the neonatal foal and calf. In: Proceedings of the Dorothy Havemeyer International Workshop on Neonatal Septicemia. Boston (MA): Dorothy Russell Havemayer Foundation; 1998. p. 22–6.

[14] Lester GD, DeMarco VG, Norman WM. Effect of inhaled nitric oxide on experimentally induced pulmonary hypertension in neonatal foals. Am J Vet Res 1999; 60(10):1207–12.

[15] Gross I. Recent advances in respiratory care of the term neonate. Ann NY Acad Sci 2000; 900:151–8.

[16] Nagaya N. Drug therapy of primary pulmonary hypertension. Am J Cardiovasc Drugs 2004; 4(2):75–85.

[17] Wilkins MR, Moller GM, Ren X, et al. Developments in therapeutics for pulmonary arterial hypertension. Minerva Cardioangiol 2002;50(3):175–87.

[18] Slutsky AS. Mechanical ventilation (American College of Chest Physicians' Consensus Conference). Chest 1993;104:1833–59.

[19] Esteban A, Anzueto A, Frutos F, et al. Characteristics and outcomes in adult patients receiving mechanical ventilation: a 28-day international study. JAMA 2002;287:345–55.

[20] Tobin MJ. Medical progress: advances in mechanical ventilation. N Engl J Med 2001;344: 1986–96.

[21] Pollack CV. Mechanical ventilation and noninvasive ventilatory support. In: Marx JA, Hockberger RS, Walls RM, editors. Marx-Rosen's emergency medicine—concepts and clinical practice. 5th edition. St. Louis, MO: Mosby; 2002. p. 21–8.

[22] MacIntyre NR. Respiratory function during pressure support ventilation. Chest 1986;89: 677–83.

[23] MacIntyre N. Recent innovations in mechanical ventilatory support. In: Vincent JL, editor. Intensive care medicine annual update 2003. Heidelberg, Germany: Springer-Verlag; 2004. p. 264–71.

[24] Marini JJ, Crooke PS, Truwit JD. Determinants of pressure-preset ventilation: a mathematical model of pressure control. J Appl Physiol 1989;67:1081–92.

[25] Muscedere JG, Mullen JB, Gan K, et al. Tidal ventilation at low airway pressures can augment lung injury. Am J Respir Crit Care Med 1994;149:1327–34.

[26] Wyszogrodski I, Kyei-Aboagye K, Taeusch HW Jr, et al. Surfactant inactivation by hyperventilation: conservation by end-expiratory pressure. J Appl Physiol 1975;38:461–6.

[27] Macintyre NR. Principles of mechanical ventilation. In: Murray JF, Nadel JA, editors. Textbook of respiratory medicine. 3rd edition. Philadelphia: WB Saunders; 2000. p. 2471–87.

[28] Anonymous. Ventilation with lower tidal volumes as compared with traditional tidal volumes for acute lung injury and the acute respiratory distress syndrome (The ARDS Network). N Engl J Med 2000;342:1301–8.

[29] Dreyfuss D. Acute lung injury and mechanical ventilation: need for quality assurance. Crit Care Med 2004;32(9):1960–1.

[30] Brower RG, Rubenfeld GD. Lung-protective ventilation strategies in acute lung injury. Crit Care Med 2003;31(Suppl):S312–6.

[31] Vincent JL. Evidence-based medicine in the ICU: important advances and limitations. Chest 2004;126:592–600.

[32] Brun-Buisson C, Minelli C, Bertolini G, et al. Epidemiology and outcome of acute lung injury in European intensive care units (Results from the ALIVE study). Intensive Care Med 2004;30:51–61.

[33] Ricard JD. Are we really reducing tidal volume—and should we? Am J Respir Crit Care Med 2003;167:1297–8.

[34] Weinert CR, Gross CR, Marinelli WA. Impact of randomized trial results on acute lung injury ventilator therapy in teaching hospitals. Am J Respir Crit Care Med 2003;167: 1304–9.

[35] Gajic O, Dara SI, Mendez JL, et al. Ventilator-associated lung injury in patients without acute lung injury at the onset of mechanical ventilation. Crit Care Med 2004;32(9):1817–24.

[36] Brochard L, Roudot-Thoraval F, Roupie E, et al. Tidal volume reduction for prevention of ventilator-induced lung injury in the acute respiratory distress syndrome. Am J Respir Crit Care Med 1998;158:1831–8.

[37] Stewart TE, Meade MO, Cook DJ, et al. Evaluation of a ventilation strategy to prevent barotrauma in patients at high risk for acute respiratory distress syndrome. N Engl J Med 1998;338:355–61.

[38] Brower RG, Shanholtz CB, Fessler HE, et al. Prospective randomized, controlled clinical trial comparing traditional vs. reduced tidal volume ventilation in ARDS patients. Crit Care Med 1999;27:1492–8.

[39] Shankar KB, Moseley H, Kumar Y, et al. Arterial to end-tidal carbon dioxide tension difference during Caesarean section anaesthesia. Anaesthesia 1986;41:698–702.

[40] Fletcher R, Jonson B, Cumming G, et al. The concept of dead space with special reference to the single breath test for carbon dioxide. Br J Anaesth 1981;53:77–88.

[41] Phan CQ, Tremper KK, Lee SE, et al. Noninvasive monitoring of carbon dioxide: a comparison of the partial pressure of transcutaneous and end-tidal carbon dioxide with the partial pressure of arterial carbon dioxide. J Clin Monit 1987;3:149–54.

[42] Maslow A, Stearns G, Bert A, et al. Monitoring end-tidal carbon dioxide during weaning from cardiopulmonary bypass in patients without significant lung disease. Anesth Analg 2001;92:306–13.

[43] Weil MH, Bisera J, Trevino RP, et al. Cardiac output and end-tidal carbon dioxide. Crit Care Med 1985;13:907–9.

[44] Ornato JP, Garnett AR, Glauser FL. Relationship between cardiac output and the end-tidal carbon dioxide tension. Ann Emerg Med 1990;19:1104–6.

[45] Jin X, Weil MH, Povoas H, et al. End-tidal carbon dioxide as a noninvasive indicator of cardiac index during circulatory shock. Crit Care Med 2000;28:2415–9.

[46] Isserles SA, Breen PH. Can changes in end-tidal Pco_2 measure changes in cardiac output? Anesth Analg 1991;73:808–14.

[47] Bhavani-Shankar K, Moseley H, Kumar AY, et al. Anaesthesia and capnometry. Can J Anaesth 1992;39:617–32.

[48] Sweadlow DB, Irving SM. Monitoring and patient safety. In: Blitt CD, editor. Monitoring in anesthesia and critical care medicine. 2nd edition. New York: Churchill Livingstone; 1990. p. 64–82.

[49] Nunn JF, Hill DW. Respiratory dead space and arterial to end-tidal CO_2 tension difference in anesthetized man. J Appl Physiol 1960;15:383–9.

[50] Shankar KB, Moseley H, Kumar Y. Negative arterial to end-tidal gradients. Can J Anaesth 1991;38:260–1.

[51] Young P, Basson C, Hamilton D, et al. Prevention of tracheal aspiration using the pressure-limited tracheal cuff tube. Anaesthesia 1999;54:559–63.

[52] Orozco-Levi M, Torres A, Ferrer M, et al. Semirecumbent position protects from pulmonary aspiration but not completely from gastroesophageal reflux in mechanically ventilated patients. Am J Respir Crit Care Med 1995;152:1387–90.

[53] Sydow M, Burchardi H, Ephraim E, et al. Long-term effects of two different ventilatory modes on oxygenation in acute lung injury: comparison of airway pressure release ventilation and volume-controlled inverse ratio ventilation. Am J Respir Crit Care Med 1994;149:1550–6.

[54] Burchardi H. New strategies in mechanical ventilation for acute lung injury. Eur Respir J 1996;9:1063–72.

[55] Herridge MS, Slutsky AS, Colditz GA. Has high-frequency ventilation been inappropriately discarded in adult acute respiratory distress syndrome? Crit Care Med 1998;26:2073–7.

[56] Wrigge H. Proportional assist versus pressure support ventilation: effects on breathing pattern and respiratory work of patients with chronic obstructive pulmonary disease. Intensive Care Med 1999;25:790–8.

[57] Bernard GR, Artigas A, Brigham KL, et al. Report of the American-European Consensus Conference on ARDS: definitions, mechanisms, relevant outcomes and clinical trial coordination (The Consensus Committee). Intensive Care Med 1994;20:225–32.

ELSEVIER
SAUNDERS

VETERINARY
CLINICS
Equine Practice

Vet Clin Equine 21 (2005) 487–510

Nutritional Support for Neonatal Foals

Virginia A. Buechner-Maxwell, DVM, MS

Department of Large Animal Clinical Sciences, Virginia-Maryland Regional College of
Veterinary Medicine, Virginia Tech, Phase II, Duck Pond Drive,
Blacksburg, VA 24061–0442, USA

Energy requirements of the normal foal

The neonatal foal is born with minimal energy stores as compared with the adult horse. The body composition of the newborn foal differs significantly from that of the adult horse, and these differences contribute to the foal's inability to survive periods of nutritional deprivation. The total body water of newborn full-term foals is approximately 79% of body weight as compared with that of adult horses (60%) [1]. Premature mature foals have an even greater percentage of body weight in the form of water (83%) [1]. These differences are attributable to less body fat and greater blood volume in the neonatal foal as compared with the adult. The blood volume of the newborn foal has been reported to be 93 to 150 mL/kg [2]. Over the first 30 days of life, increase in body weight exceeds increase in blood volume, such that by 100 days, the proportion of body weight to blood volume approaches that of the adult [2].

Foals also have minimal energy stores. Glycogen, stored predominantly in liver and muscle, is one source of energy for the neonate. Compared with other species, hepatic glycogen stores in foals are minimal (wet weight <20 mg/g as compared with sheep, rat, and pig neonates [wet weight of 90–120 mg/g]) [3,4]. These stores are adequate to maintain newborn body temperature for less than 1 hour postpartum [5]. After this time, energy is derived from endogenous fat. This source is also limited in newborn foals and is only adequate to maintain body temperature for a maximum of 24 hours. Studies from other mammals also suggest that nearly 50% of fat in newborns is structural and not available as an energy source [6].

Newborn foals also require a great deal of energy to support their rapid growth [7]. Foals increase body weight by approximately 1.3 to 1.5 kg/d during the first 30 days of life [8,9]. Within the first 6 months, Thoroughbred foals

E-mail address: bmax@vt.edu

doi:10.1016/j.cveq.2005.04.003   *vetequine.theclinics.com*

attain 83% of their adult height and 46% of their adult weight [10]. Ultrasonographic evaluation of foals' thoracic and abdominal viscera indicates that the most rapid growth in these organs occurs during the first 30 days of life [11]. Foals also attain adult bone diameter by 12 to 18 months [7,10].

Feeding behavior and milk consumption of the normal foal

The National Research Council's recommended nutrient requirements for the horse do not provide specific information about feeding foals that are less than 3 months of age, and information for this age group is sparse. Some indication of a young foal's requirements have been derived by observation of normal feeding behavior, measurements of milk consumption, and evaluation of milk composition.

Observations of stabled and pastured foals indicate that neonates successfully suckle approximately five times an hour [12]. By 2 weeks of age, foals decrease the frequency of suckling to approximately four times an hour. Normal foals tend to suckle each teat successfully an equal number of times. During the first week of the foal's life, the mare assists her offspring by shifting to positions that make the teat more accessible. For 1 to 2 weeks after this time, the mare becomes more resistant, resulting in early termination of the foal's nursing. After this period, mares once again become more cooperative, terminating foals' nursing less often, until foals are 16 weeks of age. From 16 to 24 weeks, termination of the nursing sessions again becomes increasingly frequent, suggesting that mares begin weaning foals at approximately 16 weeks of age [12].

Studies using a double-isotope dilution or radiolabeled water (^3H_2O) technique have shown that foals consume between 20% and 27% of their body weight in the form of milk [9,13]. Based on this information, a 50-kg foal may consume as much milk as 12.5 L/d. Eleven-day-old foals consume a quantity of milk adequate to provide a daily mean of gross energy of 159 kcal/kg/d and a daily mean of crude protein of 7.2 g/kg/d. This provides the foal a total gross energy of 9830 kcal and crude protein of 422 g on a daily basis [13]. Although these values decreased to a daily mean of gross energy of 98 kcal/kg and a daily mean of crude protein of 3.7 g/kg as the foal approaches the end of the first month of life, they far exceeded the requirements of an adult horse on a body weight basis [14].

The composition of mare's milk has been investigated extensively. A compilation of this research has been previously published and is shown in Table 1 [9,13,15–17]. Each milliliter of early lactation milk (1–4 weeks postpartum) contains 0.48 kcals of digestible energy (DE) [17]. Based on the volume consumed, foals acquire 120 kcal/kg/d of DE from milk. Early lactation milk also contains approximately 2.7% protein, which is equivalent to 27 mg crude protein/mL [17]. Again, based on the foal's

Table 1
Composition of mare's milk over time

Time post partum	Total solids (%)	Digestible energy (kcal/kg)	Protein (%)	Fat (%)	Lactose (%)	Concentration (mg/kg or ppm) in milk as consumed							
						Calcium	Phosphorus	Magnesium	Potassium	Sodium	Copper	Zinc	Selenium
Colostrum	25	1000	19	0.7	5	400	400	100	700	200	0.8	2–3	0.04
1–4 weeks	10.7	480	2.7	1.8	6.2	800–1200	500–750	90	700	225	0.3–0.5	2.5	0.01
5–8 weeks	10.5	460	2.2	1.7	6.4	1000	600	60	500	290	0.25	2.0	0.005
9–21 weeks	10.0	420	1.8	1.4	6.5	800	500	45	400	250	0.2	1.8	

Data from Lewis LD. Growing horse feeding and care. Media (PA): Williams & Wilkins; 1995. p. 341.

milk consumption, daily ingestion is equivalent to 6.75 g of crude protein per kg of body weight. As compared with cow's milk, mare's milk contains less total solids and DE as well as a lower concentration of protein and fat on a per milliliter basis [15,17]. In contrast, the lactose concentration is greater. This information provides insight to the general requirements of the normal neonatal foal. Milk composition changes throughout lactation, however, suggesting that a foal's needs also change during this period (see Table 1) [13,17]. Significant breed and horse-to-horse variations in milk composition have also been observed [13,17]. These findings indicate that measurements of milk composition and consumption are at best rough indicators of the normal foal's nutritional requirements.

Monitoring for adequate nutrition in the nursing foal

In nursing foals, growth is one means of determining if the foal is receiving adequate nutrition. Although there is little direct evidence that supplementing adequately fed mares significantly improves foal growth, restricting a mare's feed during lactation does compromise the foal [18]. To determine if a foal is receiving adequate nutrition, height and body weight should be measured every 2 weeks and plotted over time. Comparison of the growth of an individual foal with breed-specific growth charts may help to identify those foals that do not have access to an adequate diet. These charts are published elsewhere [17]. Growth may not be a sensitive method for detecting dietary imbalances in micronutrients that contribute to congenital lesions like developmental orthopedic disease, however. When these diseases are identified in foals, a more thorough evaluation of the diet is required.

Energy requirements of the sick foal

The relation between diseases and energy requirements has not been well explored in the neonatal foal, and information from the human literature is conflicting. Some studies provide evidence that disease increases the energy requirements of affected people and animals [19,20]. Others suggest that the delivery of caloric amounts normally required for healthy infants is inappropriate for critically ill infants, because sick human infants have lower total energy requirements attributable to inhibited growth, reduced insensible losses, and decreased activity [21]. Results from recent studies of sick foals also indicate that their caloric requirements are far less than their normal counterparts [85].

The consequences of underfeeding or overfeeding can also be significant. In the treatment of human neonates, delivery of adequate support is considered essential, because the impact of catabolism on growing tissue may have profound long-term effects on health. Epidemiologic and animal studies have shown that perinatal growth retardation is associated with increased risk of coronary heart disease, hypertension, and type 2 diabetes

[22–25]. These data are interpreted as evidence that interruptions in the immediate growth pattern of the neonate have a long-term negative effect on programming and development of somatic cells. In contrast, overfeeding occurs when patients are administered calories or a specific substrate that exceeds their requirements or their ability to maintain metabolic homeostasis [21]. The effects of overfeeding include azotemia, hypertonic dehydration, metabolic acidosis, hyperglycemia, sepsis, hypertriglyceridemia, hepatic stenosis, and hypercapnia [26]. Thus, the clinician is presented with the challenge of providing adequate nutritional support without inducing the negative effects of overfeeding.

To achieve a balance, nutritional support of the sick neonate requires a two-step approach:

1. Initially, the nutritional plan should provide a conservative estimate of the foal's energy and protein requirements. This approach is taken to minimize the risk of developing complications like hyperglycemia, hyperlipemia, and azotemia.
2. Once the patient's condition is stabilized, nutritional support should be gradually increased to provide the nutrients required for typical growth and weight gain. The rate at which this can occur depends on the animal's ability to tolerate a change in its diet. Careful monitoring of the patient's response to a reformulated diet is essential to avoid complications associated with overfeeding.

Initiating nutritional support

Before administering nutritional support, every effort should be made to correct the electrolyte, acid-base, and hydration status of the patient. This is not always possible in sick foals because they do not have adequate energy stores to delay institution of support while all deficits are corrected. Close monitoring is essential to prevent hyperglycemia, hyperlipemia, and other complications that can exacerbate the foal's clinical problems.

Enteral nutrition

Nutritional support can be delivered by the enteral or parenteral route. If the foal has a functional gastrointestinal tract, the enteral route is preferred because it is less expensive and permits the safe delivery of a more complex diet. Delayed feeding of sick human neonates has also been associated with a number of negative effects on tissue development. These include the following:

- Reduction in intestinal villi height
- Decreased weight of the stomach, pancreas, and intestine
- Increased mucosal permeability, permitting translocation of bacteria
- Increased risk of necrotizing enterocolitis

• Decreased secretion of gut hormones that stimulate gastrointestinal development [27–30]

For human neonates who cannot tolerate large volumes of enteral nutrition, even small amounts have been shown to improve outcome [29,31].

Enteral products

Mare's milk is the preferred source of enteral nutrition (Table 2). Milk is described as a complex species-specific biologic fluid adapted to satisfy the nutritional and immunologic needs of the offspring perfectly [32–34]. Mare's milk is the most likely source of an inexpensive balanced diet for the foal. Human milk has been shown to contain protectants like secretory IgA, lactoferrin, lysozyme, lactadherin, numerous cytokines, and oligosaccharide analogues for microbial receptors on mucosal membranes [35]. Human milk fat is a primary source of energy for the human infant, and the fatty acid composition supports optimal neural and visual development [36,37]. Human breastfeeding is considered protective against necrotizing enterocolitis, chronic lung disease of prematurity, otitis media, and general infection in infants [35,38–44]. Although less species-specific information is available for the horse, Cymbaluk and Laarveld [45] demonstrated that mare's milk is a source of insulin-like growth factor-1, which stimulates gut and somatic development. Stripping milk from the foal's dam promotes continued

Table 2
Composition of mare's, cow's, and goat's milk and manufacturer milk replacers

Nutrient	Milk			Milk Replacers		
	Mare[a]	Cow	Goat	Mare's[b] Match	Foal-Lac[c]	Mare's Milk Plus[d]
Total solids (DM) (%)	10.7	12.5	13.5	11–13	16	12.5
Crude protein (%)	25	27	25	24	min 19.5	min 21
Crude fat (%)	17	38	31	16	min 14	min 14
Crude fiber (%)	0	0	0	0.15	max 0.1	max 0.15
Calcium (%)	1.1	1.1	1.0	0.65–1.15	0.9–1.2	0.7–1.10
Phosphorus (%)	0.7	0.7	0.8	0.6	min 0.75	min 0.65
Zinc (ppm)	23	40	30	40	min 50	min 110
Copper (ppm)	4	3	2	10	min 18	min 35
Selenium (ppm)	0.04	0.024	—	0.3	0.10	min 0.3

Values for total solids or dry matter are for the milk as fed or milk replacers as diluted as recommended by the manufacturer. All other values are given for the amount in the total solids or dry matter.

Abbreviations: DM, dry matter; max, maximum; min, minimum.

[a] During the first 4 weeks of lactation.

[b] Land O' Lakes, Arden Hills; Minnesota.

[c] Pet-Ag, Inc., Hampshire, Illinois.

[d] Acidified Mare's Milk Replacer; Buckeye Nutrition, Dalton, Ohio.

Data from Lewis LD. Growing horse feeding and care. Media (PA): Williams & Wilkins; 1995. p. 342.

lactation, increasing the chance of reuniting the foal with the mare once it has recovered. Maintaining the foal-mare association is advantageous, because rearing orphan foals requires a considerable amount of labor and can produce an animal with behavioral problems.

If mare's milk is not available, goat's milk or cow's milk may be used as an alternative source of fresh milk products. Cow's milk and goat's milk are less dilute than mare's milk and contain nearly twice as much fat. Cow's milk and goat's milk also contain less lactose or carbohydrates but are similar in protein and mineral content to mare's milk [17]. Although the carbohydrate content is less in cow's milk and goat's milk, the fats are highly digestible, making both acceptable food sources for the foal.

Unmodified cow's milk may cause diarrhea. Cow's milk can be adapted by using low-fat (2%) milk or by diluting two parts of whole milk with one part of saturated lime water [17]. Saturated lime water can be prepared by adding lime (calcium oxide) to water and allowing the mix to sit for several hours. The water that is removed off the remaining sediment is saturated lime water. Low-fat milk and diluted whole milk also require the addition of 20 g of dextrose per liter [17]. Other sugars (eg, table sugar or sucrose) should not be used, because foals do not have the ability to digest these carbohydrates and develop osmotic diarrhea from diets that contain them [46]. The amount of dextrose that should be added is equal to four level teaspoons of dextrose or 40 mL of 50% dextrose per liter of milk. If it is not pasteurized, milk should be heated to 170°F (70°C) for 15 minutes to kill or decrease the number of pathogenic bacteria [47].

Goat's milk is similar to cow's milk, but foals find it more palatable and grow well even when it is fed unmodified [17,48]. Goat's milk may also be modified as previously described for cow's milk. Goat's milk may cause constipation in some foals, which can be avoided by adding 30 to 60 mL of mineral oil to two or three feedings of milk per day during the period that this diet is being introduced [49]. Over 5 to 7 days, reduce the frequency and amount of mineral oil and observe the foal's fecal consistency to be certain that it does not become abnormally dry.

Milk from cows or goats may provide some benefits beyond nutritional support to neonatal foals. Evidence of cross-species protection from ingestion of immunoglobulins indicates that milk from other species provides some of the immunoprotective benefits derived from mare's milk [50].

A number of commercial mare's milk replacers are available (see Table 2; Table 3) that are formulated to match closely the energy, protein, mineral, and vitamin content of mare's milk closely [14,17]. Constipation, dehydration, and hypernatremia have resulted from feeding milk replacers that are not adequately diluted [17]. Milk replacers should have a final concentration of total solids or dry matter between 10% and 17%, because the concentration of mare's milk is 10% to 11% [17]. Some manufacturers' directions for reconstituting milk result in solutions that are nearly twice as concentrated. Water volume should be adjusted to provide a more dilute

Table 3
Sources of additional milk replacers

Product	Species	Source
Foal Mate	Foals	Manna Pro, Chesterfield, Missouri
Unimilk	Multispecies, including foals	Manna Pro, Chesterfield, Missouri
Supreme All Milk Calf Milk Replacer	Calves	Blue Seal Dairy Feed, Londonderry, New Hampshire
Nonmedicated		
Blue Ribbon Nutra-Gro	Calves, lambs, kids, foals, piglets, puppies	Tractor Supply Company distributor

final product, and the total volume of milk replacer offered to the foal should be proportionally increased to be certain that the foal receives an adequate amount of nutrients.

Calf and kid milk replacers have been used to feed foals (see Table 3). These are not as nutritionally matched to meet the foal's requirements as mare's milk replacers [48]. Products that contain milk protein are preferred. The crude fiber content in replacers should not be greater than 0.2%, because products with a crude fiber content of 0.5% to 1% likely contain soy protein, which is difficult for the foal to digest [17]. Calf milk replacers often contain antibiotics, and these should be not be used in foals. If choosing a calf or goat milk replacer, the product's nutritional analysis should be examined to be certain that the mineral and vitamin requirements of the foal will be met [14,17].

Human products have been used for short-term enteral support of foals. Foals have been shown to tolerate a low-residue human liquid diet for 7 days [51]. Long-term use of these diets is impractical because they are expensive and are not formulated for this purpose.

Acidified milk replacers were originally developed for calves but are available in formulas for the foal. Mare's Milk Plus (Buckeye Feeds, Dalton, Ohio) is one example and is designed to be fed free choice and to remain fresh for up to 3 days. Reportedly, foals find this formula palatable, and the use of this replacer reduces labor significantly [48]. Mare's Milk Plus does not contain antibiotics and meets the requirements established by the National Research Council for growing horses. When introducing foals to this product, they should be carefully monitored because some may not find it immediately palatable. This product is probably more useful for feeding foals that are orphaned or require long-term supplementation.

Delivery of enteral nutrition

In examining the sick neonatal foal, some emphasis should be placed on the patient's ability to nurse the mare effectively. Ineffective suckling is a significant problem encountered in the human neonatal intensive care unit (NICU), in part, because this is a highly coordinated activity requiring the input of five cranial nerves (Table 4) [52]. As foals become weak or depressed, their ability to suckle diminishes. This change in suckle efficiency, coupled with the foal's head position while nursing, puts the sick neonate at risk for aspiration pneumonia. Compromised suckle ability should be considered if a foal fails to empty or reduce udder size significantly after completing a nursing bout and may also be suspected if milk appears in the foal's nares after nursing. If aspiration is a concern, auscultation of the trachea while the foal suckles assists in identifying this problem. There are several alternative methods for delivering nutritional support to foals that do not have an adequate ability to suckle.

Bottle feeding is one way to deliver nutrition to normal foals when suckling the mare is not an option. Bottle feeding is not recommended for foals with compromised suckling ability, because the animal's head must be elevated to evacuate the bottle effectively, placing the foal at risk for

Table 4
Cranial nerves involved in human suckle response

Cranial nerve	Sensory function	Motor function
Trigeminal (V)	General sensation Anterior two thirds of tongue Soft palate Nasopharynx Mouth	Innervates muscles of mastication Contributes to oral phase of swallowing
Facial (VII)	Taste Anterior two thirds of tongue Sensation Lips Face	Innervates lip sphincter and face muscles
Glossopharyngeal (IX)	Taste and sensation Posterior two thirds of tongue Sensation Tonsils Pharynx Soft palate	Pharyngeal phase of swallowing
Vagus (X)	Sensation Pharynx Larynx Viscera Tongue base	Pharyngeal phase of swallowing Innervation of extrinsic muscles of the tongue and esophagus
Hypoglossal (XII)	None	Innervation of the intrinsic muscles of the tongue

From Jones MW, Morgan E, Shelton JE. Dysphagia and oral feeding problems in the premature infant. Neonatal Netw 2002;21:51; with permission.

aspiration. Lamb nipples work well for foals because they are similar in shape to the mare's nipple. Even in the normal foal, care must be taken to prevent milk from running out of the nipple at a rate that exceeds the foal's ability to swallow. If milk is observed in the foal's mouth immediately after swallowing or if the foal coughs while suckling, the nipple should be examined to be certain that large volumes of milk do not spontaneously flow from the bottle.

Bucket or pan feeding can be used for foals that have a moderate suckle reflex but are too weak to hold their head in position and evacuate the teat. Pan feeding is beneficial for foals that have pneumonia and are unable to interrupt respiration for prolonged periods to suckle the teat. Suckling from a pan requires less energy and permits the foal's head to remain in a flexed vertical position. This minimizes the likelihood of milk flowing into the trachea by gravity. Bucket feeding is also a less labor-intensive means of rearing an orphan foal as compared with bottle feeding. Foals must be taught to drink from a bucket, and this process can take from several hours to several days.

Feeding tubes permit access to the gastrointestinal tract of foals that can tolerate enteral support but have a poor suckle reflex. A 14- or 16-French stallion catheter can be easily placed in the foal's esophagus when one-time or short-term feeding is required. Milk readily flows through these catheters, but their rigid nature may cause trauma to the foal's larynx if left in place for more than a few days. Feeding tubes made of polyurethane (14-French × 50-inch nasogastric feeding tube; Mila International, Florence, Kentucky) are much less traumatic and may be kept in place for several weeks. These tubes are smaller in diameter and less rigid, making them more difficult to place. Some tubes are available with an internal wire stylet that is removed after the tube is in position. The stylet increases the rigidity of the tube, making it easier to pass. Occasionally, the stylet is difficult to remove once the tube is positioned. Prewetting the inside of the tube with water decreases the drag on the stylet and allows for easier withdrawal. Tube rigidity can also be increased temporarily by storing it in a freezer for 10 to 15 minutes before placement. Rigid tubes, such as the stallion catheter, should be placed in the esophagus rather than the stomach to avoid gastric reflux between feedings. Smaller diameter tubes of softer material may be placed in the stomach to permit the feeder to check for reflux between feedings.

Sick foals should not be fed by syringe dosing. Nutrient requirements cannot be met through this technique. Dosing foals with a compromised suckle reflex places that animal at high risk for aspiration pneumonia.

Initiating enteral nutrition

Normal foals consume as much as 27% of their body weight in the form of milk on a daily basis [9]. Sick foals generally do not tolerate this volume of milk during the acute phase of the disease. The initial volume of enteral support that is provided for the sick neonatal foal is based on the foal's status at the time of presentation and its response to initial therapy. In human infants, gut ischemia occurs with hypoxia, septic shock, and dehydration. A conservative approach to enteral support is applied to patients with these problems, and this tactic should also be used with sick foals [41]. For sick full-term foals, initial daily support is aimed at providing an amount of milk equal to 5% to 10% of the foal's body weight in multiple small feedings. Milk contains DE at a rate of 0.48 kcal/mL, so providing 10% of the foal's body weight on a daily basis is equivalent to providing a total of 48 kcal/kg/d. Initial feedings can be as frequent as every hour and then decreased to every 2 hours (with double the volume) once the foal's condition stabilizes. For premature neonates, even small amounts of milk (25 mL/h for a 50-kg foal) may be beneficial. Necrotizing enterocolitis is a life-threatening that has been observed in sick foals [68]. Early enteral feeding and feeding of breast milk have been shown to decrease the risk associated with this disease in human infants [29,41,43,69]. Enteral support may provide the same benefit to neonatal foals. Most foals tolerate enteral feeding, which can be gradually increased to 25% of their body weight over several days, but they should be carefully monitored during this period for complications associated with nutritional support.

If adequate nutritional support cannot be achieved through the enteral route, a combination of parenteral and enteral nutrition should be attempted. Parenteral nutrition can allow for a more gradual introduction to enteral support, preventing complications associated with feeding a compromised gut. Nutritional plans that use parenteral and enteral nutrition together should be formulated so that the contributions of both nutrient sources add up to the calculated energy requirements for the foal.

Complications associated with enteral feeding

Complications associated with enteral feeding are most commonly attributable to mismanagement of the tube or overfeeding. Aspiration may occur even when the tube is properly placed. Large-bore tubes placed into the stomach permit dilation of the distal esophageal sphincter and regurgitation of stomach contents. Tubes may also become dislodged between feedings, especially as foals become more active. Careful evaluation of tube placement before every feeding can reduce these problems. Also, placement of large-bore tubes in the esophagus or use of small-bore tubes can minimize regurgitation from the stomach and decrease the risk of aspiration.

Foals' gastrointestinal tracts do not tolerate distention well. Intraluminal pressures that exceed 25 cm H_2O cause collapse of the capillary beds in the wall of the gut, resulting in poor tissue perfusion and reperfusion injury [53]. Monitoring for abdominal bloating must be done on a regular basis. This can be accomplished by marking an area on the foal's abdomen and measuring the diameter using a tape or string before each feeding. If diameter size increases over several consecutive feedings, further evaluation is warranted. Ultrasound examination of the foal's gastrointestinal tract permits a better estimate of small intestinal and gastrointestinal distention. If bloating is suspected, an attempt should be made to reflux the foal. Enteral feeding should be discontinued for 4 to 6 hours, or until the distention resolves. Feeding should then be reinstituted at a smaller volume.

Parenteral nutrition

Some sick foals cannot tolerate enteral feeding or have conditions that require gut rest. For these animals, support can bypass the gut and be delivered directly to the blood in the form of parenteral nutrition. Parenteral nutrition has been used in the treatment of sick foals for 20 years or more and no longer represents a "frontier" therapy. Evidence-based information regarding parenteral support for foals is sparse, however, and is predominantly adapted from recommendations for human infants. Current understanding of nutritional requirements of the sick animal has also resulted in some significant changes in the way parenteral nutrition is formulated.

Formulas for parenteral support may be designed to meet part of or all the patient's needs. Most parenteral formulations for foals are designed to provide energy and protein requirements. Multivitamin and electrolyte supplements may also be added. Meeting the foal's full nutritional requirements with parenteral feeding is unlikely, however, because the current understanding of these requirements is limited. In most cases, parenteral feeding serves as a bridge to enteral support by allowing more time for this transition to occur, and whenever possible, some amount of enteral nutrients should be included in the diet of the neonate.

Parenteral products

There any many sources for parenteral nutrition solutions, and some of these are listed in Table 5. The energy nutrient sources in parenteral nutrition are dextrose solutions, lipid emulsions, and protein provided in the form of amino acids.

Dextrose solutions

Dextrose solutions can be obtained in wide range of concentrations, but a 50% concentration is most commonly used to formulate parenteral nutrition for foals (Table 6) [54]. A single gram of dextrose provides 3.4 kcal of energy. Consequently, each milliliter of a 50% dextrose solution provides 1.7 kcal of energy. Fifty-percent solutions are hypertonic and should not be delivered without first being diluted to a 10% or less solution.

Table 5
Sources of parenteral solutions

Company name	Location
Abbott Laboratories, Animal Health	North Chicago, Illinois
Baxter Health Care Corporation	Deerfield, Illinois
B. Braun Medical Inc.	Bethlehem, Pennsylvania

Lipid emulsions

A single gram of lipid provides approximately 10 kcal of energy (based on the specific composition of fats). Parenteral products are 10% or 20% emulsions, which provide 1 kcal/mL or 2 kcal/mL of energy, respectively.

Protein (amino acids)

Amino acids provide approximately 4 kcal/g of protein. Amino acid solutions come in a variety of concentrations, ranging from 3.5% to 15%. Solutions containing 8.5% amino acids are most commonly used in veterinary medicine and provide 85 mg of protein or 0.34 kcal/mL. A summary of product information is provided in Table 7.

Parenteral admixtures may also include multivitamins or B vitamins. Electrolytes, such as potassium, can be added to the parenteral formulation. The addition of 20 mEq/L of potassium is routinely recommended for foals that cannot tolerate any enteral nutrition. This amount should be adjusted for foals that are hypokalemic or hyperkalemic. The initial formulation of parenteral support also does not meet the foal's fluid needs, which must be achieved by supplementing with isotonic crystalloid fluids.

Formulating parenteral nutrition

Calculation of parenteral nutritional requirements is usually achieved in several steps. These include the following:

- Determination of DE to be provided in the form of carbohydrates and fats. This is also considered the non-nitrogen (non-N_2) kilocalories that

Table 6
Characteristics of dextrose solutions

Dextrose concentration (%)	Dextrose (g/L)	Calories (kcal/L)	Osmolality (mOsm/L)
2.5	25	85	126
5	50	170	253
10	100	340	505
20	200	680	1010
25	250	850	1330
50	500	1700	2525
70	700	2380	3535

Data from Plumb DC. Table of parenteral fluids. In: Veterinary drug handbook. 4th edition. St. Paul, IA: Iowa State Press; 2002. p. 804.

Table 7
Caloric values of parenteral solutions

Nutrient	Commonly used concentration	Kcal/mL
Dextrose	50%	1.7
Lipid	20% emulsion	2
Protein (amino acids)	8.5%	0.34

the foal receives, because carbohydrates and fats (as compared with proteins) do not contain nitrogen
• Determination of protein to be provided as a ratio of DE

As a starting point, the amount of DE required to meet the foal's RER based on body weight, BW, is calculated using the following interspecies equation [65]:

$$RER(kcal) = 70 \times [BW\ (kg)]^{0.75}$$

More simply, the foal's RER can be met by providing non-N_2 calories at a rate of 30 kcal/kg/d. Based on this estimate, a 50-kg foal would require non-N_2 calories at a rate of 1500 kcal/kg/d to meet its RER. These calories are derived from dextrose and lipids. In foals, lipids can provide up to 60% of non-N_2 caloric requirements, with the remainder derived from dextrose solutions [66]. The ratio of dextrose to lipids is dependent on the foal's response to these nutrients. As an example, foals that are hyperglycemic may require diets that contain a greater percentage of lipids.

Although there are several methods for calculating protein, a simple approach is to provide non-N_2 energy by administration of protein at a rate of 4 to 6 g per 100 kcal. Foals that are hypoproteinemic or have ongoing protein losses should receive 6 g of protein per 100 kcal non-N_2 energy. Foals that are azotemic or have other evidence of renal disease should be provided less protein (4 g/100 kcal non-N_2 energy). Using this formula, a 50-kg foal receiving 5 g of protein per 100 kcal non-N_2 energy is provided 75 g of protein in the form of amino acids.

The volume of each nutrient is calculated based on the proportion of energy derived from dextrose and lipids as well as on the grams of protein that the foal requires. The dextrose concentration is adjusted to 10% by adding crystalloid fluids to the final admixture. Once the final volume is determined, an hourly infusion rate is calculated by dividing the total volume in milliliters by 24 hours. Parenteral nutrition should be delivered using a volumetric constant-infusion pump. Infusion of parenteral nutrition should not be interrupted once it is initiated unless the foal is unable to tolerate parenteral nutrition. An example of these calculations is provided in Table 8.

Initiating parenteral nutrition should be done gradually, especially in critically compromised foals. In these patients, start the parenteral nutrition infusion at half the calculated infusion rate for the first 4 to 8 hours of administration. If parenteral nutrition is tolerated, increase the infusion rate

Table 8
Calculation of initial parenteral nutrition formulation and example (50-kg foal, 50% energy from dextrose, 50% from lipids, 5 g protein/100 kcal)

	Formula	Example (50-kg foal)
RER	Foal's weight (kg) × 30 kcal/ kg = total kilocalories non-N_2 energy	1500 kcal
Dextrose		
Dextrose (kcal)	(Percent of energy from dextrose)(Total kilocalories non-N_2 energy)	750 kcal
Volume of 50% (mL)	Dextrose (kcal) ÷ 1.7 kcal/mL	441 mL of 50% dextrose
Lipids		
Lipid (kcal)	(Percent of energy from lipids) (Total kilocalories non-N_2 energy)	750 kcal
Volume of 50% (mL)	Lipids (kcal) ÷ 2 kcal/mL	325 mL of 20% lipids
Amino acids		
Grams	[(Total kilocalories non-N_2 energy) ÷ 100] × [desired grams (4–6) of protein per 100 kcal]. For this example, 5g/100 kcal was used.	75 g of amino acids
Kilocalories from amino acids	Grams of protein × 4 kcal/g	300 kcal
Volume of 8.5% (mL)	Grams of protein ÷ 0.85 g/mL	353 mL of 8.5% amino acids
Dextrose concentration		
Actual volume of PN (L)	[Dextrose (mL) + lipids (mL) + protein (amino acids) (mL)]/1000	1119-mL actual volume
Dextrose (g)	(Volume of 50% dextrose) ÷ 2	220.5 g
Desired volume of PN (mL) (for 10% dextrose)	Dextrose (g) × 10	2205-mL desired volume
Volume of additional crystalloid fluid (mL)	Desired volume − actual volume	1086 mL
Final formulation of PN	Volume of 50% (mL) =	441 mL
	Volume of 50% (mL) =	325 mL
	Volume of 8.5% (mL) =	353 mL
	Volume of additional crystalloid fluid (mL) =	1086 mL
	Total volume =	2205 mL
Hourly infusion rate	Total volume ÷ 24	92 mL/h
Total energy (non-N_2 and protein)	Dextrose (kcal) + lipids (kcal) + amino acids (kcal)	1800 kcal

Abbreviation: PN, parenteral nutrition.

by 25% increments every 4 to 8 hours, depending on the patient's response. As an example, if the calculated infusion rate is 100 mL/h, start at 50 mL/h for the first 8 hours and monitor the foal's response. If parenteral nutrition is tolerated well, increase the rate to 75 mL for the next 8 hours and reassess the foal's response. Again, if the diet is well tolerated, increase the rate to 100 mL/h. For some foals, it may take 3 to 4 days to achieve the desired infusion rate, whereas others may achieve it within the first 24 hours of administration.

As the foal's condition stabilizes, the parenteral nutrition solution can be reformulated to provide more calories and protein. Ousey and colleagues [67] reported that normal pony foals, receiving parenteral nutrition at a rate of 75 kcal/kg/d experienced a negative energy balance by the second day on this diet. These findings suggest that the daily DE requirements of the normal neonatal foal are greater than 75 kcal/kg. For foals that require long-term parenteral nutrition, the nutrients in the diet should be gradually increased to exceed this amount of energy. This can be achieved without complication if the patient's response is adequately monitored.

Preparation of parenteral nutrition

The components of a parenteral diet should be mixed in a clean environment, preferably under a laminar hood. Solutions are usually mixed by transferring the calculated amount into a sterile bag. The order in which solutions are transferred is important. Dextrose and amino acids are mixed first, with lipids added after the amino acids. This procedure prevents lipids from becoming unstable and coming out of solution. Although many parenteral nutrition products are available, products from the same source should be selected for formulation so as to minimize incompatibility of solutions.

Delivery of parenteral nutrition

To deliver the diet, an intravenous catheter is placed aseptically in the jugular or peripheral vein. Catheters made of polyurethane or silastic are minimally thrombogenic and are recommended and readily available for veterinary use (Mila International). A double-lumen catheter is preferred, with one lumen dedicated to delivery of parenteral nutrition. This minimizes contamination and eliminates the need to stop and start the solution when delivering additional medications, such as antibiotics. Nutrition should be delivered at a constant rate using an infusion pump to avoid fluctuations in glucose delivery, and the actual volume of parenteral nutrition delivered to the patient should be carefully monitored and recorded.

Complications associated with parenteral nutritional support

Common complications associated with parenteral nutrition in human infants include catheter dysfunction, thrombosis, perivascular leakage, contamination, sepsis, and major organ failure. Similar complications can occur in neonatal foals and can be minimized with proper monitoring and managing of the catheter site as well as cautious handling of the parenteral nutrition solutions. Several times a day, the catheter site and jugular vein should be carefully examined for evidence of infection, thrombosis, or perivascular leakage. If a catheter is wrapped, the wrap should be removed daily to permit close visualization of the site. Before replacing the bandage, the site should be gently cleaned with an antiseptic nonirritating scrub like Nolvasan (Wyeth, Madison, New Jersey) and rinsed with sterile normal saline or water. If it is not bandaged, the site should be cleaned several times a day to minimize infection at the point where the catheter penetrates the skin. Parenteral solutions, once prepared, should be immediately refrigerated or used. Parenteral nutrition can be stored for up to 24 hours in a refrigerator before use. Once in use, any residual parenteral nutrition solution should be discarded after 24 hours. In sick neonates, all fluid transfer lines should be changed every 24 hours, and all injection ports should be cleaned with alcohol and allowed to dry before any substance is injected through them.

Complications common to enteral and parenteral nutrition

In the past, human patients receiving parenteral nutrition were thought to be at greater risk for developing sepsis than patients receiving enteral nutrition. This was in part attributable to gut atrophy and the increased risk of bacterial translocation across the gut wall. Human studies have not documented similar alterations in gut morphology in patients who were restricted to parenteral nutrition for 1 month [55]. A review of human subjects with intestinal obstruction provided evidence that the incidence of bacterial translocation occurred with equal frequency in individuals receiving parenteral or enteral nutrition [56].

Hyperglycemia, hyperlipidemia, hypercapnea, azotemia, and major organ injury are side effects frequently associated with parenteral nutrition, but they can occur when patients are being provided any form of nutritional support. More recently, researchers have discovered that these side effects occur most frequently when human patients are being overfed. In an evaluation of 213 human patients on mechanical ventilators, 66.2% had a measured resting energy requirement (RER) of less than 25 kcal/kg/d. Most of the patients were overfed (58.2%), whereas only 12.2% were underfed [57]. The degree of overfeeding had an inverse impact with minute ventilation and also resulted in a significant increase in azotemia. Overfeeding may also be of concern in patients with respiratory disease if elimination of carbon dioxide (CO_2), by production of glucose metabolism, is impaired. Nutritional needs of sick human infants are reported to be less than those of normal children, and formulating diets based on the needs of normal infants can result in overfeeding by 200% [21]. Effects of overfeeding

include azotemia, hypertonic dehydration, metabolic acidosis, hyperglycemia, sepsis, hypertriglyceridemia, hepatic stenosis, and hypercapnia [26].
Patients receiving parenteral nutrition tend to be provided more energy than
individuals receiving enteral nutrition, and overfeeding rather than
parenteral nutrition may be the cause of the side effects so often associated
with this mode of nutritional delivery [57–60].

Hyperglycemia occurs commonly in sick human infants and has been
reported in foals receiving parenteral support [61]. In most cases,
hyperglycemia can be managed by reducing the initial infusion rate of
parenteral nutrition or the delivery rate of enteral nutrition by 50% for 6 to
12 hours and then gradually increasing the amount of the diet until the
desired rate is reached. Some septic animals may become persistently
hyperglycemic, however, significantly limiting the amount of nutrition that
can be delivered to them. The pathogenesis of this hyperglycemia is not well
understood but may be a result of insufficient pancreatic insulin secretion,
failure of insulin to suppress hepatic gluconeogenesis, or insulin resistance of
peripheral tissues to insulin [62]. Stress-induced elevation in glucagons,
epinephrine, and cortisol may also contribute to a persisting hyperglycemia
[63]. Methods for managing hyperglycemia in sick foals are described briefly
in this article and in greater detail elsewhere [61]. Animals that develop
refractory hyperglycemia may benefit from insulin therapy. Regular insulin
can be delivered as a continuous infusion or may be provided as a single
injection. Continuous infusion can be achieved by adding regular insulin to
the parenteral solutions or by infusing it separately. Regular insulin is added
to parenteral solutions by using 1 to 2 IU per 4 g of glucose [64]. For
separate infusion, the addition of regular insulin (20 IU) to normal saline
(500 mL) produces a final solution with an insulin concentration of regular
insulin of 0.04 IU/L. Therapy is started with an infusion rate of
approximately 0.0133 IU/kg/h. For a 40-kg foal, this equals 13.3 mL of
insulin-saline solution per hour. If the blood glucose concentration does not
decrease, the amount of insulin can be increased by small increments (0.002
IU/kg/h) every 6 hours until blood glucose concentrations return to normal.
The rate of glucose infusion should also be decreased initially until
hyperglycemia resolves. Throughout this period, the blood glucose
concentration should be monitored closely (at least every 3 hours) to be
certain that hypoglycemia does not occur. Insulin may also be administered
as an injection. The recommended dose is 0.1 to 0.5 IU/kg given
subcutaneously or intravenously [64]. Again, blood glucose should be
monitored to prevent hypoglycemia.

Monitoring metabolic response to diet

Acutely sick foals may be metabolically intolerant of nutritional support
and should be monitored closely for evidence of complications. This is most
critical in foals whose clinical condition is not yet stabilized or in foals that

are acutely febrile or during periods of dietary change. Table 9 provides some guidelines for frequency of monitoring. If specific problems are identified (eg, persistent severe hyperglycemia), more frequent monitoring may be required. Identifying metabolic problems rapidly and adjusting nutritional plans in response to these problems is the safest approach to providing support for sick neonatal foals.

Probiotics

The use of probiotics is infrequently discussed in the treatment of neonatal foals. Probiotics have been the focus of human research interest in recent years and are believed to have significant clinical application in the treatment of adult and pediatric gastrointestinal disorders [70–74]. A probiotic is defined as "a live microbial feed supplement which beneficially affects the host by improving its intestinal microbial balance" [75]. Because the major site of action is the colon, a probiotic must be able to survive exposure to bile, gastric pH, and pancreatic secretions [74]. Functionally, probiotics should be able to:

- Adhere to cells
- Exclude or reduce pathogenic adherence
- Persist and multiply
- Produce acids, hydrogen peroxide, and bacteriocins antagonistic to pathogen growth
- Reside as safe, noncarcinogenic, and nonpathogenic organisms
- Coaggregate to form a normal balanced flora [71]

The bacterial population of the human colon consists of mostly strict anaerobes, predominant bacteroides, bifidobacteria, eubacteria, methanogens, gram-positive cocci, sulfate-reducing bacteria, and lactobacillus [76].

Table 9
Monitoring foal's status while receiving nutritional support

	Critical foal, change in diet and sudden fever	Foal in stable condition, diet unchanged
Body weight	Daily	Daily
Urine glucose	Every 2 hours	Every 6 hours
Blood glucose	Every 2 to 4 hours and immediately if urine glucose positive	Every 6 to 8 hours
Serum creatinine	Daily	Daily or every other day
Serum protein	Every 4 to 8 hours	Daily or every other day
Serum electrolytes	Every 12 hours if abnormal	Daily or every other day
Serum triglycerides	Daily	If lipemia is noted
Lipemia	Every 4 to 8 hours	Daily
$P\bar{v}CO_2$	Every 4 hours if respiratory compromise is diagnosed	Daily or every other day if respiratory function is normal

Abbreviation: $P\bar{v}CO_2$, partial pressure of carbon dioxide, mixed venous blood.

The main function of the human colonic microflora is the fermentation of carbohydrates that are not digested in the upper gastrointestinal tract. The products of this activity include production of short-chain fatty acids (acetate, propionate, and butyrate); lactate; and the gases hydrogen, CO_2, and methane gases [76]. Short-chain fatty acids are absorbed and metabolized by colonocytes, liver, muscle, and brain tissue [74]. The presence of normal gut flora also limits overgrowth of enteropathogenic bacteria [74]. Manipulation of the flora through the use of probiotics helps to maintain normal gut function and reduces the risk of enteric disease [74]. Human clinical studies have shown that probiotics prevent antibiotic-associated and traveler's diarrhea, reduce the severity of rotavirus diarrhea, and decrease the incidence of diarrhea associated with enteral tube feeding [74,77,78]. The β-galactosidase activity of lactobacilli may also attenuate the symptoms of lactose intolerance [78]. In human pediatric medicine, probiotics have been shown to prevent colonization of the gut with pathogenic bacteria and to decrease the incidence of viral enteric infections (rotavirus), necrotizing enterocolitis, and recurrent diarrhea caused by *Clostridium difficile* [79–81]. The effects are most evident in preterm infants and infants that are not being fed breast milk [82]. Specific bacterial strains that are likely to serve as probiotics include members of the genera *Lactobacillus*, *Bifidobacterium*, and *Enterococcus* [71]. Colonization of the colon by probiotic bacterial strains is species specific, and the development of an effective probiotic requires identification of bacteria that exhibit the ability to survive in the gut of the specific species of interest [70].

Information about equine probiotics is limited, but the microbial composition and function of the horse's colon have some similarities to those of the human colon. The microbial population of the horse's colon consists of anaerobic bacteria (approximately 50%), gram-negative rods (51%–64%), and gram-positive cocci (8%–33%) [83]. The activity of these bacteria includes fermentation of undigested carbohydrates to short-chain fatty acids and production of methane gas [83]. *Lactobacillus* species have been isolated from equine feces, and a subpopulation of this bacterium is capable of attenuating the growth of pathogenic bacteria in vitro [84].

Although the use of probiotics in the treatment of the neonatal foal has not been systematically explored, the addition of plain low-fat yogurt containing live bacterial cultures may be of benefit. Based on human studies, foals being fed through an enteral feeding tube, receiving parenteral nutrition, or consuming a diet of milk replacer should be considered candidates for probiotic supplementation. The additional of 30 to 60 mL every 2 hours to foal diets is well tolerated and palatable. It is unlikely that the bacteria in human yogurt colonize the equine neonatal gut. However, results from human studies indicate that colonization may not be necessary for patients to benefit from probiotic therapy [70]. Although lactose intolerance is also not documented in neonatal horses, the addition of yogurt to the diet of foals that have persistent gassy diarrhea may assist in milk digestion and resolution of their clinical signs.

Summary

Nutritional support is an important component of neonatal care because foals do not have adequate energy stores to survive for prolonged periods without food. The nutritional needs of the normal foal far exceed those of the adult animal on a per kilogram of body weight basis. The impact of disease on the nutritional requirements is not known, but severe complications can results from underfeeding and overfeeding. Methods for delivering nutrients by the enteral or parenteral route are described for the foal. A conservative approach is recommended when initiating nutritional support, accompanied by careful monitoring of the patient's response. As the patient's condition improves, the amount of nutrition can be increased. Complications associated with the method of delivery, formulation, and handling of nutrients can occur. Sick foals may also develop metabolic derangements and tissue injury if they are not monitored carefully while receiving support. A balance between meeting the foal's requirements while avoiding complications is the key to successful nutritional support.

Acknowledgments

The author thanks Dr. Craig Thatcher for his knowledgeable insight regarding normal and sick foal nutrition and Maureen Perry for her assistance with information on enteral and parenteral nutrition products.

References

[1] Spurlock SL, Furr M. Fluid therapy. In: Koterba AM, Drummond WH, Kosch PC, editors. Equine clinical neonatology. Philadelphia: Lea & Febiger; 1990. p. 671–700.
[2] Persson SG, Ullberg LE. Blood volume and rate of growth in Standardbred foals. Equine Vet J 1981;13:254–8.
[3] Fowden AL, Ellis L, Rossdale PD. Pancreatic beta cell function in the neonatal foal. J Reprod Fertil Suppl 1982;32:529–35.
[4] Fowden AL, Mundy L, Ousey JC, et al. Tissue glycogen and glucose 6-phosphatase levels in fetal and newborn foals. J Reprod Fertil Suppl 1991;44:537–42.
[5] Ousey JC, McArthur AJ, Rossdale PD. Metabolic changes in Thoroughbred and pony foals during the first 24 h post partum. J Reprod Fertil Suppl 1991;44:561–70.
[6] Mellor DJ, Cockburn F. A comparison of energy metabolism in the new-born infant, piglet and lamb. Q J Exp Physiol 1986;71:361–79.
[7] Green DA. A study of growth rate in thoroughbred foals. Br Vet J 1969;125:539–46.
[8] Hintz HF. Growth rate of horses. Proc Am Assoc Equine Pract 1978;24:455–9.
[9] Martin RG, McMeniman NP, Dowsett KF. Milk and water intakes of foals sucking grazing mares. Equine Vet J 1992;24:295–9.
[10] Hintz HF, Hintz RL, Van Vleck LD. Growth rate of thoroughbreds, effect of age of dam, year and month of birth, and sex of foal. J Anim Sci 1979;48:480–7.
[11] Aleman M, Gillis CL, Nieto JE, et al. Ultrasonographic anatomy and biometric analysis of the thoracic and abdominal organs in healthy foals from birth to age 6 months. Equine Vet J 2002;34:649–55.

[12] Carson K, Wood-Gush DG. Behaviour of thoroughbred foals during nursing. Equine Vet J 1983;15:257–62.

[13] Oftedal OT, Hintz HF, Schryver HF. Lactation in the horse: milk composition and intake by foals. J Nutr 1983;113:2096–106.

[14] NRC Nutrient requirements of horses. 5th edition. Washington, DC: National Academy of Sciences; 1989.

[15] Koterba AM. Nutritional support: enteral feeding. In: Koterba AM, Drummond WH, Kosch PC, editors. Equine clinical neonatology. Philadelphia: Lea & Febiger; 1990. p. 728–46.

[16] Koterba AM, Drummond WH. Nutritional support of the foal during intensive care. Vet Clin North Am Equine Pract 1985;1:35–40.

[17] Lewis LD. Growing horse feeding and care. Media, PA: Williams & Wilkins; 1995. p. 334–49.

[18] Banach MA, Evans JW. Effects of inadequate energy during gestation and lactation on the estrous cycle and conception rates of mares and on their foal weights. Proc Equine Nutr Physiol Soc Symp 1981;7:97–100.

[19] Neu J, Huang Y. Nutrition of premature and critically ill neonates. In: Nestle Nutrition Workshop Series Clinical & Performance Programme. Volume 8. Basel, Switzerland: Karger AG; 2003. p. 171–85.

[20] Scrimshaw NS. Rhoades Lecture. Effect of infection on nutrient requirements. Journal of Parenteral and Enteral Nutrition 1991;15:589–600.

[21] Chwals WJ. Overfeeding the critically ill child: fact or fantasy? New Horiz 1994;2: 147–55.

[22] Barker DJ. Fetal origins of coronary heart disease. BMJ 1995;311:171–4.

[23] Dusick AM, Poindexter BB, Ehrenkranz RA, et al. Growth failure in the preterm infant: can we catch up? Semin Perinatol 2003;27:302–10.

[24] Osmond C, Barker DJ. Fetal, infant, and childhood growth are predictors of coronary heart disease, diabetes, and hypertension in adult men and women. Environ Health Perspect 2000; 108(Suppl 3):545–53.

[25] Schwarzenberg SJ, Kovacs A. Metabolic effects of infection and postnatal steroids. Clin Perinatol 2002;29:295–312.

[26] Klein CJ, Stanek GS, Wiles CE III. Overfeeding macronutrients to critically ill adults: metabolic complications. J Am Diet Assoc 1998;98:795–806.

[27] Lucas A, Bloom SR, Aynsley-Green A. Gut hormones and 'minimal enteral feeding.' Acta Paediatr Scand 1986;75:719–23.

[28] Lucas A, Bloom SR, Aynsley-Green A. Metabolic and endocrine consequences of depriving preterm infants of enteral nutrition. Acta Paediatr Scand 1983;72:245–9.

[29] Premji SS, Paes B, Jacobson K, et al. Evidence-based feeding guidelines for very low-birth-weight infants. Adv Neonatal Care 2002;2:5–18.

[30] Rothman D, Udall JN, Pang KY, et al. The effect of short-term starvation on mucosal barrier function in the newborn rabbit. Pediatr Res 1985;19:727–31.

[31] Evans RA, Thureen P. Early feeding strategies in preterm and critically ill neonates. Neonatal Netw 2001;20:7–18.

[32] do Nascimento MB, Issler H. Breastfeeding: making the difference in the development, health and nutrition of term and preterm newborns. Rev Hosp Clin Fac Med Sao Paulo 2003;58:49–60.

[33] Picciano MF. Human milk: nutritional aspects of a dynamic food. Biol Neonate 1998;74: 84–93.

[34] Riordan J. The biological specificity of breastmilk. In: Riordan J, Auerbach K, editors. Breastfeed and human lactation. 2nd edition. Boston: Jones and Bartlett Publishers; 1998. p. 121–61.

[35] Hanson LA, Korotkova M. The role of breastfeeding in prevention of neonatal infection. Semin Neonatol 2002;7:275–81.

[36] Jewell VC, Northrop-Clewes CA, Tubman R, et al. Nutritional factors and visual function in premature infants. Proc Nutr Soc 2001;60:171–8.

[37] Morley R, Lucas A. Influence of early diet on outcome in preterm infants. Acta Paediatr Suppl 1994;405:123–6.

[38] Bancalari E. Changes in the pathogenesis and prevention of chronic lung disease of prematurity. Am J Perinatol 2001;18:1–9.

[39] Chandra R, Bhat BV, Puri RK. Why breast feed? Indian Pediatr 1993;30:841–51.

[40] Connor WE, Neuringer M, Reisbick S. Essential fatty acids: the importance of n-3 fatty acids in the retina and brain. Nutr Rev 1992;50:21–9.

[41] Kosloske AM. Breast milk decreases the risk of neonatal necrotizing enterocolitis. Adv Nutr Res 2001;10:123–37.

[42] Neuringer M. Cerebral cortex docosahexaenoic acid is lower in formula-fed than in breast-fed infants. Nutr Rev 1993;51:238–41.

[43] Pellegrini M, Lagrasta N, Garcia Garcia C, et al. Neonatal necrotizing enterocolitis: a focus on. Eur Rev Med Pharmacol Sci 2002;6:19–25.

[44] Sheard NF. Breast-feeding protects against otitis media. Nutr Rev 1993;51:275–7.

[45] Cymbaluk NF, Laarveld B. The ontogeny of serum insulin-like growth factor-I concentration in foals: effects of dam parity, diet, and age at weaning. Domest Anim Endocrinol 1996;13:197–209.

[46] Roberts MC. The development and distribution of mucosal enzymes in the small intestine of the fetus and young foal. J Reprod Fertil Suppl 1975;717–23.

[47] Pugh DG, Williams MA. Feeding foals from birth to weaning. Compend Contin Educ Pract Vet 1992;14:526–33.

[48] Wilson JH. Feeding considerations for neonatal foals. Proc Am Assoc Equine Pract 1988;34: 823–9.

[49] Madigan JE. Some practical aspects of feeding sick and convalescing foals. Ved Med 1987;924–8.

[50] Mitra AK, Mahalanabis D, Ashraf H, et al. Hyperimmune cow colostrum reduces diarrhoea due to rotavirus: a double-blind, controlled clinical trial. Acta Paediatr 1995;84: 996–1001.

[51] Kohn CW, Knight DA, Yvorchyk-St Jean KE, et al. A preliminary study of the tolerance of healthy foals to a low residue enteral feeding solution. Equine Vet J 1991;23:374–9.

[52] Jones MW, Morgan E, Shelton JE. Dysphagia and oral feeding problems in the premature infant. Neonatal Netw 2002;21:51–7.

[53] Lundin C, Sullins KE, White NA, et al. Induction of peritoneal adhesions with small intestinal ischaemia and distention in the foal. Equine Vet J 1989;21:451–8.

[54] Plumb DC. Table of parenteral fluids. In: Veterinary drug handbook. 4th edition. St. Paul, IA: Iowa State Press; 2002. p. 804.

[55] Guedon C, Schmitz J, Lerebours E, et al. Decreased brush border hydrolase activities without gross morphologic changes in human intestinal mucosa after prolonged total parenteral nutrition of adults. Gastroenterology 1986;90:373–8.

[56] Sedman PC, Macfie J, Sagar P, et al. The prevalence of gut translocation in humans. Gastroenterology 1994;107:643–9.

[57] McClave SA, Lowen CC, Kleber MJ, et al. Are patients fed appropriately according to their caloric requirements? Journal of Parenteral and Enteral Nutrition 1998;22:375–81.

[58] Jeejeebhoy KN. Enteral and parenteral nutrition: evidence-based approach. Proc Nutr Soc 2001;60:399–402.

[59] Jeejeebhoy KN. Total parenteral nutrition: potion or poison? Am J Clin Nutr 2001;74: 160–3.

[60] Moore FA, Moore EE, Jones TN, et al. TEN versus TPN following major abdominal trauma–reduced septic morbidity. J Trauma 1989;29:916–22.

[61] Buechner-Maxwell VA. Hyperglycemia in a neonatal foal: management with continuous insulin infusion. Equine Pract 1994;16:13–6.

[62] Kanarek KS, Santeiro ML, Malone JI. Continuous infusion of insulin in hyperglycemic low-birth weight infants receiving parenteral nutrition with and without lipid emulsion. Journal of Parenteral and Enteral Nutrition 1991;15:417–20.

[63] Chan S, McCowen KC, Blackburn GL. Nutrition management in the ICU. Chest 1999; 115(Suppl):S145–8.

[64] Koterba AM. Appendix 1. In: Koterba AM, Drummond WH, Kosch PC, editors. Clinical equine neonatology. Philadelphia: Lea & Febiger; 1990. p. 785.

[65] Kleiber M. Energy metabolism. In: The fire of life: an introduction to animal energetics. 2nd edition. New York: Robert E. Krieger Publishing Company; 1975. p. 40–55.

[66] Hansen TH. Nutritional support: parenteral feeding. In: Koterba AM, Drummond WH, Kosch PC, editors. Equine clinical neonatology. Philadelphia: Lea & Febiger; 1990. p. 747–62.

[67] Ousey JC, Prandi S, Zimmer J, et al. Effects of various feeding regimens on the energy balance of equine neonates. Am J Vet Res 1997;58:1243–51.

[68] Wilson JH, Cudd TA. Gastrointestinal system disorders: common gastrointestinal diseases. In: Koterba AM, Drummond WH, Kosch PC, editors. Equine clinical neonatology. Philadelphia: Lea & Febiger; 1990. p. 412–30.

[69] Diehl-Jones WL, Askin DF. Nutritional modulation of neonatal outcomes. AACN Clin Issues 2004;15:83–96.

[70] Bezkorovainy A. Probiotics: determinants of survival and growth in the gut. Am J Clin Nutr 2001;73(Suppl):S399–405.

[71] Kaur IP, Chopra K, Saini A. Probiotics: potential pharmaceutical applications. Eur J Pharm Sci 2002;15:1–9.

[72] Reid G. The scientific basis for probiotic strains of Lactobacillus. Appl Environ Microbiol 1999;65:3763–6.

[73] Roberfroid MB. Prebiotics: preferential substrates for specific germs? Am J Clin Nutr 2001; 73(Suppl):S406–9.

[74] Whelan K, Gibson GR, Judd PA, et al. The role of probiotics and prebiotics in the management of diarrhoea associated with enteral tube feeding. J Hum Nutr Diet 2001;14: 423–33.

[75] Fuller R. Probiotics in man and animals. J Appl Bacteriol 1989;66:365–78.

[76] Gibson GR, Roberfroid MB. Dietary modulation of the human colonic microbiota: introducing the concept of prebiotics. J Nutr 1995;125:1401–12.

[77] de Roos NM, Katan MB. Effects of probiotic bacteria on diarrhea, lipid metabolism, and carcinogenesis: a review of papers published between 1988 and 1998. Am J Clin Nutr 2000; 71:405–11.

[78] de Vrese M, Stegelmann A, Richter B, et al. Probiotics—compensation for lactase insufficiency. Am J Clin Nutr 2001;73:S421–9.

[79] Dai D, Walker WA. Role of bacterial colonization in neonatal necrotizing enterocolitis and its prevention. Zhonghua Min Guo Xiao Er Ke Yi Xue Hui Za Zhi 1998;39:357–65.

[80] Davidson GP, Butler RN. Probiotics in pediatric gastrointestinal disorders. Curr Opin Pediatr 2000;12:477–81.

[81] Friedrich MJ. A bit of culture for children: probiotics may improve health and fight disease. JAMA 2000;284:1365–6.

[82] Dai D, Walker WA. Protective nutrients and bacterial colonization in the immature human gut. Adv Pediatr 1999;46:353–82.

[83] Hintz HF, Cymbaluk NF. Nutrition of the horse. Annu Rev Nutr 1994;14:243.

[84] Weese JS, Anderson ME, Lowe A, et al. Screening of the equine intestinal microflora for potential probiotic organisms. Equine Vet J 2004;36:351–5.

[85] Paradis MR. Nutrition and indirect calorimetry in neonatal foals. Proceedings of 15th American College of Veterinary Internal Medicine Forum 2001;19:245–7.

VETERINARY
CLINICS
Equine Practice

Vet Clin Equine 21 (2005) 511–535

ELSEVIER
SAUNDERS

Abdominal Surgery in Neonatal Foals

James E. Bryant, DVM[a],*, Earl M. Gaughan, DVM[b]

[a]Pilchuck Veterinary Hospital, 11308 92nd Street SE, Snohomish, WA, 98290, USA
[b]J.T. Vaughan Large Animal Hospital, College of Veterinary Medicine, Auburn University,
Auburn, AL 36849, USA

Abdominal surgery in foals under the age of 30 days has become more common with improved neonatal care [1–9]. Early recognition of a foal at risk and better nursing care have increased the survival rates of foals that require neonatal care [1–11]. The success of improved neonatal care also has increased the need for accurate diagnosis and treatment of gastrointestinal, umbilical, and bladder disorders in these foals. Abdominal surgery can be successful; however, the surgeon must be mindful of the complex nature of the medical conditions of foals and maintain adequate supportive and treatment measures slightly different than in the adult horse or older foal undergoing abdominal surgery [1,3]. The primary indications for abdominal procedures in foals include those presenting for acute or chronic colic, ruptured bladder, or umbilical remnant infection [1–16]. This article focuses on the early and accurate diagnosis of specific disorders that require abdominal exploratory surgery and the specific treatment considerations and prognosis for these disorders in foals under 30 days of age.

Diagnostics

Physical examination and history

Very young foals present unique considerations in the evaluation and diagnosis of disorders that require abdominal surgery. Examination through the rectum, other than a digital examination, is not possible, therefore a physical examination and the results of diagnostic procedures are relied on more heavily in foals [1,3,10]. In the neonatal foal under 7 days of age, an abdominal disorder may be related directly or indirectly to other disease

---

* Corresponding author.
E-mail address: jbryant@pilchuckvet.com (J.E. Bryant).

0749-0739/05/$ - see front matter © 2005 Elsevier Inc. All rights reserved.
doi:10.1016/j.cveq.2005.04.011

processes such as septicemia, hypoxic ischemic encephalopathy, or prematurity [1,11]. The abdominal crisis may be secondary, and therefore,
a thorough physical examination and history are paramount in making an
accurate treatment plan [1,9,10].

The certainty of a foal's age is helpful in sorting out historical
information. Disorders in foals less than 7 days of age can be different
than typical diseases found in 2- to 4-week-old foals. Uroperitoneum
typically occurs in foals under 7 days old and is less likely to be
a consideration in an older foal [11]. Information gained from the history
should include the gestational age, events associated with parturition, fecal
production (ie, meconium), urine output, physical signs, severity and
duration of pain, and any history of previous treatment or medications
[1,10]. A medical history is especially important for foals in the 2- to 4-week
age group, in which previous treatment could increase the possibility of
gastric outflow obstruction secondary to gastric ulceration [2,3,10,17].

Physical examination parameters should include but not be limited to
temperature, heart rate, respiratory rate, gastrointestinal sounds, abdominal
distention, digital examination of the rectum, palpation of the umbilicus,
palpation of the inguinal area, severity of abdominal pain, and ballottement
of the abdomen [1,10]. Fever may be present with generalized sepsis, bowel
ischemia, endotoxemia, or a specific focus of infection, either within the
abdomen (enteritis, colitis, peritonitis, omphalophlebitis, umbilical abscessation, and other conditions) or in the case of many extra-abdominal
conditions (pneumonia, septic arthritis, osteomyelitis, meningitis, and
others). Tachycardia can be present with pain, gastrointestinal obstruction,
endotoxemia, cardiovascular collapse, and dehydration. Tachypnea may be
associated with pain of varying degrees and a variety of respiratory tract
disorders. Foals may exhibit variable clinical signs of abdominal discomfort.
The degree of abdominal pain does not always correlate specifically with the
severity of the disease in foals. Signs of abdominal pain in foals include
stretching to urinate, flagging of the tail, depression, and anorexia.
Moderate signs of pain include pawing, persistent standing and laying
down, lying in recumbency, and possibly, rolling up on their backs. More
severe signs of pain include violent rolling or frequent up and down or
persistent recumbency or both. Neonatal foals that are recumbent or
nonresponsive should be evaluated for septicemia, hypoxic encephalopathy,
gastrointestinal disorders, and uroperitoneum [1,3,11,16]. It has been
reported that foals rolling up on their backs may have gastric ulceration
[1,10]. This clinical sign should still be interpreted as abdominal pain in
general and not simply specific to gastric ulceration, until the definitive
diagnosis has been reached.

Repeated measurement of the abdomen at a location approximating the
level of the second lumbar vertebrae and just caudal to the last rib in the
flank can be helpful to determine progressive distention [1]. If the decision to
perform surgery is delayed because of the need for appropriate medical

treatment or continued monitoring, a measurement of the abdomen obtained every 2 to 4 hours can be important in determining whether continued distention is occurring. The area for measurement can be marked by clipping the hair or placing pieces of tape, which can be placed on the dorsal and ventral aspects of the abdomen. This will help to ensure that each measurement is made in the same area and, therefore, accurately interpreted. Neonatal disorders that increase these measurements include meconium impactions with gas distention in the colon, other physical or functional intestinal obstruction, and uroperitoneum, in which the abdomen continues to fill with fluid. The information obtained from this parameter should be interpreted along with all others and used accordingly. For foals with uroperitoneum, the electrolyte abnormalities should be monitored and evaluated along with the measurement of abdominal distention [1,11, 13–15,18].

Ancillary diagnostic procedures

Nasogastric intubation and evaluation of potential gastric reflux should be performed during the initial evaluation of any foal presenting with abdominal pain. The volume of reflux, the consistency of the ingesta, the pH level of the fluid, and the frequency of accumulation should be evaluated to determine whether a pyloric outflow obstruction, a small intestinal obstruction, or a small intestinal ileus are present [1,3,10,19]. In the neonatal foal, volumes above 500 mL should be considered clinically significant [1,19]. Volumes of 500 to 2000 mL may be supportive evidence of a gastric outflow obstruction. Foals with a pyloric outflow obstruction typically have small volumes of reflux especially if food is withheld. Volumes above 2 L may be supportive of a functional or mechanical obstruction of the small intestine. The pH level of the reflux fluid can be evaluated with a pH strip; a pH level of 6.0 or greater indicates a reverse flow from the small intestine, which is associated with a functional or mechanical outflow obstruction of the small intestine [17]. If feeding by nasogastric tube has been instituted in foals with a suspected outflow obstruction, the stomach should be evaluated for reflux before each feeding. If an obstruction is present, it is likely that a majority of the last volume fed will be retrieved. In the neonatal foal, the consistency of the reflux is important. The presence of milk allows for the assessment of nursing status, and the time since the last observed nursing should be considered to assess gastric emptying; normal gastric emptying of fluid should be 30 minutes [20]. In foals older than 1 week the type of feed material retrieved (such as grass, hay, dirt, or sand) can aid in assessing the intake of inappropriate feed material and the possibility of a foreign body obstruction or impaction. If reflux is present once, continued reevaluation (every 2 hours) and attention to the volume of reflux obtained in repeated attempts are important. If an excessive volume persists, a functional or mechanical obstruction may be present. A repeated evaluation of pain, heart rate, mucous membrane color, and abdominal ultrasonography and radiography is essential to determine whether a surgical lesion is present.

Clinicopathologic findings may be beneficial in the assessment of various surgical disorders. Foals presenting with nonsurgical conditions such as sepsis or hypoxic encephalopathy may have several clinicopathologic changes. Many of the abdominal surgical disorders often are accompanied by values within normal reference ranges. However, certain conditions may be associated with specific changes. The peripheral white blood cell (WBC) count could be elevated in inflammatory bowel conditions and infectious processes of the umbilical remnant structures [1,3,9]. Leukopenia may occur with endotoxemia associated with severe compromise to the bowel from an inflammatory condition such as enterocolitis or a compromised intestine caused by a strangulating lesion. Electrolyte abnormalities present with uroperitoneum can include hyperkalemia, hyponatremia, and hypochloremia [1,11,13–15,18]. However, these abnormalities may not be present in all cases of uroperitoneum, especially in foals already receiving intravenous fluids for the treatment of another disorder [11].

Abdominocentesis is suggested for foals with colic. However, severe distention can increase the risk of lacerating or puncturing the bowel. Ultrasonographic examination of the abdomen is highly encouraged before performing abdominocentesis, to determine the volume, character, and location of free fluid. Ultrasonography also can allow for the evaluation of intestinal distention and therefore the associated risk of intestinal perforation [21,22]. After aseptic preparation of the area, abdominocentesis may be performed with the patient standing or in lateral recumbency. Sedation is typically indicated. Abdominocentesis typically is performed to the right of midline along the ventral abdomen, approximately 5 to 8 cm caudal to the xyphoid. Ultrasonographic examination should be used to identify free fluid and the best site for abdominocentesis. Abdominocentesis can be performed with a teat cannula or a 20-gauge × 1–1.5-in hypodermic needle. The authors' prefer to use a teat cannula inserted through a stab incision made in the skin after applying a local anesthetic in the skin and subcutaneous tissue. The advantages of a teat cannula include a decreased risk of perforating the bowel and accidental laceration of the bowel by a needle [1]. If a large amount of free fluid is evident on ultrasonography, a 20-gauge × 1–1.5-in needle may be used. One advantage of a needle is that it avoids a stab incision in the skin and abdominal musculature, which can lead to herniation of the omentum [19]. Normal abdominal fluid is clear and yellow in appearance [19]. The WBC count should be less than 5000/μL and the total protein less than 2.5 g/dL. Inflammatory diseases such as enteritis are associated typically with elevated total protein and a WBC count within normal limits [1]. In diseases with vascular compromise to the bowel wall and resultant peritonitis, elevations in both WBC count and total protein are expected [1,3]. A normal abdominocentesis does not rule out intestinal disease or ischemic compromise. Foals with uroperitoneum typically have a large volume of free fluid with a creatinine in the peritoneal fluid at least two times higher than the serum creatinine concentration [1,11, 13–15,18].

Abdominal radiography is recommended routinely for neonatal foals with abdominal discomfort [1,3,5,10,20,22,23]. Adequate radiographs can be obtained with most portable radiograph machines and rare earth screens, with the patient standing or in lateral recumbency. Positioning of the patient should be taken into consideration when interpreting gas and fluid interfaces [1,3,20,23]. Radiographs should be evaluated for the distention of bowel with gas or fluid, normal positioning of the intestines, excessive abdominal fluid, or free air within the abdomen [20,23]. The small intestine is considered abnormally distended when the diameter of the lumen is slightly greater than the length of the body of the first lumbar vertebrae [23]. The alignment of the small bowel also is important in determining disease processes. With obstructive small bowel disease, the distended loops tend to become vertical in alignment, over time [1,20]. Pyloric outflow obstructions may be suspected based on the distention of the stomach with fluid and gas but can only be confirmed with contrast radiography [1,3,20,23]. Barium is expected to exit the stomach into the pylorus within 10 minutes and be in the cecum within 4 hours. Delayed emptying of the stomach may be assessed within 4 hours of the administration of contrast material [20,23]. In foals with suspected uroperitoneum, the bladder may not be radiographically visible. If abdominocentesis is not supportive of a ruptured bladder and clinical suspicion is high, double contrast radiography of the bladder may be performed [12,20]. If contrast material is present in the abdomen then uroperitoneum is confirmed (Fig. 1).

The use of abdominal ultrasonography has become more prevalent and is an extremely helpful diagnostic tool in the young foal [1,3,9,21,22]. Ultrasonography can be used to evaluate the abdominal viscera, umbilical remnants, and the bladder. In foals presenting with colic, a thorough systematic ultrasonographic examination should be performed [21,22]. Viscera should be evaluated for the degree and nature of distention (fluid, gas, or feed), motility (normal, absent, or increased), intestinal wall thickness, and the presence or absence of visualization of viscera (ie, large intestinal distention that obstructs the visualization of the small bowel). The volume of abdominal fluid can be evaluated, and an appropriate site for abdominocentesis can be determined. The umbilical remnant structures and bladder should be part of a routine ultrasonographic examination of a foal under 7 days of age [11,12,22]. The presence of a bladder that appears distended does not rule out rupture but does decrease the likelihood. The absence of a distended bladder does not indicate rupture, but with the presence of a large volume of abdominal fluid, the index of suspicion should be increased [1,11,13–15,18,21,22].

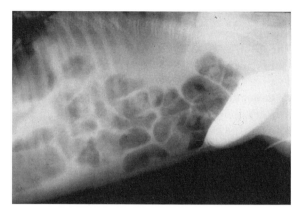

Fig. 1. Positive contrast cystogram of a 24-hour-old Quarter Horse foal presenting for straining to defecate and decreased urine production. Note the outline of the contrast material entering the urachal remnant. The bladder was intact, and no contrast entered the abdomen.

Surgical considerations

In formulating the treatment plan for a foal with abdominal discomfort, all physical examination parameters and results of diagnostic tests should be considered [1]. Together, these data should be used in the decision for immediate surgical intervention or for continued medical therapy. A decision for surgical intervention should be made as rapidly as possible, with consideration of all pertinent data. Foals less than 1 month of age, and more specifically those under 1 week of age, present challenges when making decisions for abdominal surgery. Early intervention is likely to result in a positive outcome for foals with compromised bowel. However, other medical problems, including septicemia and hypoxic encephalopathy, can pose substantial difficulty in interpretation.

The severity of pain and abdominal distention are often used as primary indicators for abdominal exploratory surgery (Fig. 2). In foals with strangulating intestinal lesions, pain control becomes difficult with analgesic drugs, and abdominal distention may be increasing. Nonstrangulating obstructions may be readily treatable with analgesic drugs. If the heart rate, dehydration, and electrolyte disturbances are corrected and controlled, continued medical management is indicated.

The presence of continued gastric reflux should be interpreted in light of pain control and cardiovascular status. A mechanical obstruction of bowel associated with strangulating lesions can result in a heart rate that remains elevated after gastric decompression [1,3,9–11]. Pain also will be persistent between reflux attempts because gastric distention alone is not responsible for the pain. At this point, surgical intervention is indicated. In potentially nonsurgical disorders of functional ileus or enteritis with gastric reflux, the signs of abdominal pain are controlled unless overdistention of the stomach occurs without frequent refluxing.

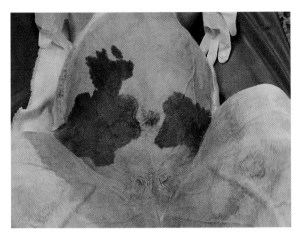

Fig. 2. Severe abdominal distention in a 7-day-old Quarter Horse foal presenting for acute onset of colic.

The results of abdominocentesis should be interpreted in light of other diagnostic results. In cases of small intestinal strangulation, an abnormal white cell count and elevated total protein indicate intestinal compromise. The results of abdominocentesis and ultrasonography examination can be very helpful in determining the need for surgical intervention in foals with small intestinal disease. The presence of numerous loops of distended small intestine with a thickened wall and no motility is likely associated with a strangulating lesion. Enteritis or small intestinal ileus can make the decision for surgery more difficult. An elevation in the peritoneal fluid total protein with a normal white cell count is expected with these disorders; however elevations of the peritoneal white cell count can be present. When pain is not controllable or the patient's condition is deteriorating then surgical intervention is indicated.

Supportive therapy, especially in the form of intravenous fluids to correct various electrolyte, fluid, or acid–base derangements, should not be overlooked before the induction of anesthesia. In the case of foals with uroperitoneum, the serum potassium concentration should be measured before surgery, and correction with intravenous fluids (0.9% saline) should be instituted [24,25]. Broad-spectrum antibiotics and anti-inflammatory agents should be administered before induction of general anesthesia.

After anesthetic induction, a foal should be positioned in dorsal recumbency, and the table should be well padded. A heating pad or other form of external temperature regulation is recommended to maintain acceptable body temperature during anesthesia. If a heating pad is used, adequate protection must be provided to prevent direct contact of the pad to prevent skin burns. The ventral abdomen should be clipped and the skin aseptically prepared. A ventral midline incision is made and, if caudal exposure of the abdomen is required in foals under 1 month of age, the umbilical remnants are resected. For exposure of the caudal abdomen, and specifically in cases of omphallitis and uroperitoneum, an elliptical skin incision is made at the umbilicus. The peritoneum is entered at the cranial edge of the incision, and the umbilical vein is isolated and ligated at the proximal extent of normal tissue. The peritoneum is incised caudally, and the urachus and umbilical arteries are isolated to the level of the bladder, exposing all abnormal tissue. Each umbilical artery is ligated and transected, and the urachus is excised at the bladder, which is closed in two layers. The linea alba is closed with an absorbable suture material of sufficient size (eg, 0-1 polyglactin 910 or polydiaxone), the subcutaneous tissue is closed with 2-0 polyglactin 910 or polydiaxone, and the skin is apposed with 2-0 monocryl. The authors prefer to use an absorbable suture material in the skin so that nonabsorbable sutures or stainless steel staples do not need to be removed from the young foal. Postoperatively, foals may be recumbent or spend a lot of time lying down. Therefore, the authors prefer to cover the incision with either a sterile iodine-impregnated drape or a stent bandage for the recovery and immediate postoperative period. The drape or stent is removed in 1 to 2 days, depending on the length of time the foal has spent in recumbency. After surgery, antibiotics and anti-inflammatory agents should be administered for at least 3 days [3,26]. In cases of septicemia, umbilical remnant infections, or intestinal resection, antibiotic therapy will be continued for a minimum of 5 to 7 days after surgery or 7 to 10 days beyond resolution of clinical signs.

After surgery, foals are typically confined to a stall for 3 weeks, with periods of short walks, and are then allowed small paddock turnout for several hours a day for an additional 4 to 5 weeks. At 7 to 8 weeks after surgery, foals can resume a normal turnout routine [2,3,26]. These recommendations for aftercare are made assuming a foal has no other concurrent diseases or problems. If a foal is recumbent or requires special care, then the postoperative recommendations should be made according to those conditions.

Specific disorders

Small intestinal strangulation

Similar to older horses, a variety of small intestinal strangulations can occur in foals. Entrapments within a body orifice, umbilical or inguinal hernias, small intestinal volvulus, intestinal intussceptions, and mesenteric rents have all been reported in foals (Figs. 3 and 4) [2–9,27,28]. Foals with strangulating lesions typically present with acute abdominal pain charac- terized by increasing intensity followed by cardiovascular compromise resulting in the elevation of heart rate, dehydration, and electrolyte abnormalities associated with strangulated bowel and endotoxemia [1,3].

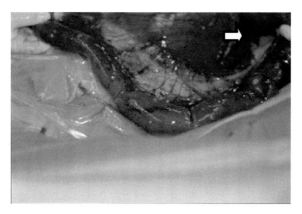

Fig. 3. A tear in the mesentery of the jejunum in a 2-day-old Thoroughbred foal. The vasculature was involved in the tear, resulting in compromised jejunum.

With protracted duration of clinical signs, some foals may present in recumbency or be nonresponsive. In this situation, other causes of recumbency should be investigated, including septicemia, uroperitoneum, and neurologic diseases. Ultrasonographic examination usually reveals dilated loops of small intestine with potentially thickened bowel wall. Peritoneal fluid obtained through abdominocentesis can range from yellow to serosanguinous, with total protein elevated from 2.5 to 5.0 g/dL or greater. The peritoneal WBC count may be normal or elevated. The duration of clinical signs often dictates the severity of the peritonitis and whether there is an elevation in the peritoneal WBC count [1,3,19].

Volvulus of the small intestine is a frequent occurrence in foals that require exploratory celiotomy [4]. Small intestinal volvulus is rotation around the mesenteric origin or root and is believed to occur because of

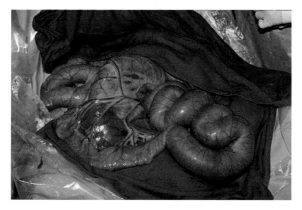

Fig. 4. Jejunojejunal intussusception in a 2-month-old Thoroughbred foal. Approximately 1 foot of jejunum was affected, and a hand-sewn end-to-end jejunojejunostomy was performed.

a hyperactive peristalsis adjacent to an area of temporary or permanent ileus [20,29]. Small intestinal volvulus may occur as a secondary complication in foals being treated for a primary disease process such as neonatal septicemia. This is believed to occur because of the potential for segmental ileus associated with recumbency or changes in feeding patterns. Initial clinical signs are consistent with the acute onset of severe abdominal pain. As the intestinal distention increases so does abdominal distention. Pain associated with strangulating lesions can push and then decline because of ischemia and subsequent necrosis. Abdominal ultrasonography will reveal distended loops of small intestine with little or no motility and potentially thickened walls. Abdominocentesis may reveal normal cell count and protein early in the disease process, because as the bowel becomes compromised the protein level and white cell count will rise. Early surgical intervention increases the likelihood of reducing the volvulus, with healthy bowel still present, and avoiding resection. At the time of surgical intervention and after the volvulus is reduced, the bowel should be assessed for viability. Distinguishing between healthy and compromised bowel can be difficult if the evidence of a complete loss of blood supply is not present. Hemorrhagic, discolored bowel is determined to be nonviable, whereas bowel that assumes normal color may appear viable. If the demarcation of viable and nonviable bowel is not readily apparent, several techniques are available to assess viability, including the use of fluorescein dye, surface oximetry, Doppler ultrasonography, luminal pressure, and histopathology [30].

Intussusception of the small intestine is often considered common in foals; however, retrospective studies [4–8,28,31] have not determined this to occur as frequently as suggested. The small intestine can invaginate, usually at the jejunojejunal or the cecum. In older foals and adults, ileocecal, cecocecal, and cecocolic intussusceptions have been associated with tapeworm infestation [3,32,33]. Clinical signs of an intussusception may begin as those of a simple obstruction and progress to those seen with vascular compromise and strangulation of bowel [1,19]. Depending on the volume and type of bowel involved, foals may show signs of acute or chronic colic. Jejunojejunal intussceptions often are associated with an acute onset of pain similar to other strangulating small intestinal lesions. In those cases that present with subacute or chronic clinical signs, anorexia, mild to moderate pain, and diarrhea may be associated. If the intussusception can be visualized ultrasonographically, immediate surgical intervention is recommended [22,31,34]. The intussusception may be visualized by the characteristic "bull's-eye" sign created by the difference between the edematous inner wall of the intussusceptum and the thinner outer wall of the intussuscipiens [22]. Ultrasonographic examination may reveal only distended small intestine with some motility present or no other visible abnormalities. For these cases, careful assessment and evaluation lead to exploratory celiotomy and discovery of the lesion. In cases with low grade chronic abdominal signs, early surgical intervention may be warranted to identify intussusceptions that are not otherwise visible. Intussusceptions can be reduced manually, and the bowel can be assessed for viability. In acute cases, the bowel may be edematous and inflamed but otherwise viable. In these cases, the bowel is returned to the abdomen, and the foal is monitored for signs of postoperative intestinal compromise. Typically, the affected portion of bowel is hemorrhagic, has lost the mesenteric supply of blood, and is considered nonviable. The nonviable section is then resected [3].

The surgical treatment of a strangulating lesion, regardless of the cause, involves identifying the affected segment followed by resection and anastomosis. Several anastomotic techniques are available for small intestinal resection; a hand-sewn jejunojejunostomy, stapled side-to-side, or a functional end-to-end anastomosis can be performed. In cases in which the distal ileum is involved, a jejunocecostomy may be required. Hand-sewn jejunojejunostomies are preferred in foals with lesions involving the jejunum because of the small lumen size of the bowel and maintenance of the normal flow of ingesta. For end-to-end jejunojejunostomies, the authors prefer a two-layer closure using 2-0 absorbable suture material (eg, polyglactin 910). The first layer apposes the mucosa of the jejunum in two segments of a simple continuous suture pattern set at 90 degrees, and the second layer is two segments of a continuous Lembert suture pattern at 90° in the serosubmucosal layer. This closure results in a good seal of the lumen, a limited decrease in lumen size, and maintenance of normal anatomic flow for ingesta.

With involvement of the distal ileum, either a jejunoileostomy or a jejunocecostomy can be performed. The exposure of a viable segment of distal ileum above the incision line is the deciding factor for the choice of anastomosis technique [29]. Jejunocecostomies result in a new anatomic flow of ingesta and can be associated with more postoperative complications [29]. In young foals, a hand-sewn side-to-side jejunocecostomy is preferred. The size of the intestine allows for accurate apposition with a hand-sewn anastomosis, and conventional staple lengths may be excessive for foals under 1 month of age. Stapled side-to-side jejunocecostomies are appropriate.

Inguinal-scrotal hernias

An inguinal-scrotal hernia may be seen in a foal at birth or within the first few days of life. Typically, soft swellings on one side of the scrotal area and, rarely, bilateral occurrence are noted [1,3,35]. Affected foals are frequently asymptomatic except for the obvious swelling (Fig. 5). The hernia can be easily reduced and may be related to a delayed closure of the internal inguinal ring.

Initial management is directed at repeated manual reduction of the scrotal contents or the application of a truss bandage [3,35]. A truss bandage

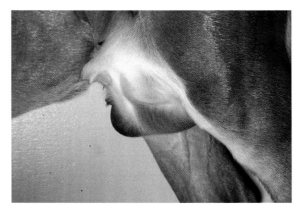

Fig. 5. A 2-day-old Quarter Horse foal with a large inguinal-scrotal hernia.

consisting of a figure-eight of elastikon and cotton can be useful in reducing the hernia [3]. Care is taken not to include the penis or anus in the bandage. Permanent reduction should be achieved by 3 to 6 months of age [3]. Successful manual reduction is achieved typically in the first month. If permanent reduction is not accomplished with manual reduction or a truss bandage, surgical closure of the inguinal ring is recommended [3,35]. The external inguinal ring can be closed through an inguinal approach with castration, laparoscopic repair with castration, an inguinal approach without castration, or through a midline celiotomy with closure of the vaginal ring [28,35,36].

Foals also may present with a nonreducible direct inguinal hernia. A direct inguinal hernia occurs when the vaginal tunic ruptures and bowel passes through the tunic into the subcutaneous tissue [3,35]. Often, foals present with signs consistent with a strangulating intestinal lesion (ie, abdominal pain, elevated heart rate, dehydration, and other typical signs). Typically, there is scrotal and preputial swelling and edema, with skin excoriation and occasionally ulceration. Immediate surgical intervention is recommended [3,35]. The bowel is evaluated, and if it is not compromised, it is returned to the abdomen, and the vaginal tunic and inguinal rings are closed. If necrotic bowel is present then resection and anastomosis is performed as for strangulating lesions.

Meconium impactions

Meconium impactions occur when a foal has been unable to pass all or a sufficient quantity of meconium after birth [1,3,23,37]. Meconium is the mucilaginous material present in the terminal intestine of the term fetus. Meconium is made up of cellular debris, secretions from the intestinal glands, bile, and amniotic fluid [37]. Clinical signs include failure to pass

sepsis, septic arthritis, or other sites of disseminated infection affect the prognosis negatively. Infections that involve the umbilical vein up to and including the liver are more difficult to manage and will carry a poorer prognosis [44].

Diaphragmatic hernia

Diaphragmatic hernias are reported to occur in young foals [3,45–48]. In the neonate with signs of respiratory distress, the integrity of the rib cage should be assessed. In the presence of fractured ribs or a flail chest, thorough evaluation of the diaphragm is indicated [1,3,47,48]. Radiographs may demonstrate abdominal contents within the chest cavity or the presence of pleural fluid. Ultrasonography of the thorax may reveal free pleural fluid, intestinal viscera within the thoracic cavity, or a defect in the diaphragm [13,47]. Foals older than 2 weeks may present with signs of abdominal pain or respiratory distress or both. In older foals, diaphragmatic hernia may be the result of undetected rib fractures, trauma, or congenital diaphragmatic defects [47,48].

Exploratory celiotomy may be elected to assess for the presence of a diaphragmatic hernia and the potential for surgical repair. Depending on the size of a diaphragmatic tear, the abdominal viscera should be removed from the thoracic cavity and assessed for viability. Often a combination of the stomach, small intestine, large intestine, and small colon can be found within the thorax. Small tears in the diaphragm can result in the strangulation of a segment of intestine, and resection and anastomosis will be required. The repair of a diaphragmatic tear in young horses can be accomplished with direct suturing of the edges with appropriately sized absorbable or nonabsorbable suture material [49]. In one case series [49] of three young horses, of which 2 were under 80 days of age, all three recovered and eventually raced after the surgical repair of a diaphragmatic hernia and small intestinal resection and anastomosis.

Intestinal atresia

Intestinal atresia is a rare condition in foals. Atresia of the colon, rectum, and anus have been reported [3,50–52]. This condition is often fatal, and early recognition is important. Possible causes consist of imperfect re-canalization, vascular accidents, anomalies, possible genetic factors, and persistent anal membrane [50–52].

The clinical signs are consistent with failure to pass meconium, but there is usually a complete lack of passage of fecal material. Other forms of abdominal discomfort should be considered and ruled out. Repeated enemas do not produce any fecal material. To confirm a diagnosis of atresia, abdominal radiographs and a barium enema can be used to prove a disruption of the intestinal tract. If the area of disruption is more proximal in the colon, barium can be administered in the stomach, and demonstration of the obstruction can be seen.

Exploratory celiotomy is required to confirm the diagnosis in some cases. If the disease process involves the large or small colon, anastomotic bypass techniques may be used to establish normal intestinal flow (Fig. 10). In one case report [51] of four foals with colonic atresia, only one foal survived. Careful consideration should be exercised before initiating surgical treatment. If surgery is successful, sterilization should be considered because of the possible genetic components of this disorder.

In cases of anal atresia, the imperforate membrane can be resected. Care should be taken to ensure that a rectovaginal or rectourethral atresia is not present as well [3,50].

Adhesions

Foals are considered to be more prone to intra-abdominal adhesion formation [2,7,53]. Adhesions occur as a result of fibrin adhering to areas of serosal injury [16]. Over several days, fibroblasts appear at a traumatic site, and the fibrin scaffold results in mature fibrous adhesions. Adhesions can result in the obstruction of the gastrointestinal tract, causing acute or chronic clinical signs (Fig. 11) [26]. Acute, severe colic episodes often require a second celiotomy or euthanasia [3–9].

Second celiotomies and adhesion formation have been associated with a decrease in long-term survival in one study [6] of foals undergoing abdominal surgery. There are several strategies used to decrease adhesion formation, and these techniques are often used together. Good surgical technique is imperative to decrease adhesions. Inflammation can be minimized by keeping bowel moist with saline, limiting handling, gentle

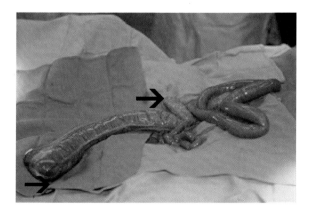

Fig. 10. Atresia coli in a 36-hour-old Quarter Horse foal. The agenesis in this case was located between the ventral and dorsal colons. The blind sac of the ventral colon can be seen, and the right dorsal colon is visualized close to the incision at the top of the picture.

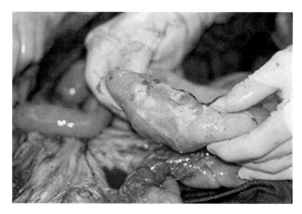

Fig. 11. Fibrous-to-fibrous adhesions on the bowel of a 1-month-old Thoroughbred foal presenting for repeat colic signs after exploratory abdominal surgery 3 weeks earlier for a small intestinal volvulus without resection of bowel.

manipulation of the bowel, good sterile technique, abdominal lavage, and omental resection [3,26,32–34,54]. Broad-spectrum antibiotics seem to be helpful in preventing or minimizing peritonitis. Systemic anti-inflammatory drugs in the form of nonsteroidal anti-inflammatory agents and dimethyl sulfoxide (DMSO) have been recommended to limit inflammation on the serosal surfaces of bowel [26,54]. In a model of ischemia reperfusion in 6-week-old foals, adhesions were not found in four foals that received flunixin meglumine, procaine penicillin G, and gentamicin or in four foals that received DMSO [54].

Additional therapies have been advocated for preventing adhesion formation, including systemic heparin administration, hyaluronate membranes, intra-abdominal sodium carboxymethylcellulose, and omentectomy. The administration of sodium heparin, 40 IU/kg subcutaneously (SQ), twice or three times daily, may aid in the prevention of adhesions. Heparin binds to antithrombin (AT) III, thereby enhancing the effect of AT III and, therefore, inhibiting thrombin-mediated conversion of fibrinogen to fibrin [26]. A recent study, however, found adhesion formation in three of four foals that received heparin (80 IU/kg SQ, twice daily) in a ischemia reperfusion model. [54] The use of hyaluronate membranes or intravenous sodium hylauronate also has been advocated. Receptors for hyaluronan (CD44) have been identified on the serosal surface of intestine, omentum, and peritoneum [55]. The administration of sodium hyaluronate may potentially add to adhesion-prevention strategies. Sodium carboxymethylcellulose has experimentally decreased the rate of adhesion formation in horses undergoing exploratory celiotomy [56]. Carboxymethylcellulose acts as a mechanical lubricating barrier between adjacent serosal surfaces. Removal of the omentum at the end of surgery has been advocated by some to prevent adhesion formation in foals [2,57]. The omentum can be a part of adhesions forming within the abdomen and may be associated with bowel-to-bowel and bowel-to-omentum adhesions. Omentectomy markedly reduces this risk [57].

A combination of the above strategies is recommended to reduce the incidence of adhesions in foals. Decreasing the incidence of adhesions may decrease the incidence of postoperative morbidity and mortality associated with abdominal surgery in foals.

Prognosis

Abdominal surgery in young foals has been associated with high mortality rates [3–9]. It is important to remember that the prognosis for survival after abdominal surgery in foals also depends on the presence of concurrent neonatal diseases. Foals with sepsis, concurrent joint infections, or recumbency resulting from neurologic disorders may not survive, based on the primary disease process [11]. Therefore, an accurate prognostic assessment can only be made in the context of the foal's overall health.

A study [11] evaluating 31 cases of foals with uroperitoneum undergoing surgical correction revealed a survival rate of 100% for 17 foals that had negative sepsis scores and 57% (8/14) for foals that had a positive sepsis score. In another study [15], 11 of 18 foals undergoing surgical correction survived. Surgical correction of septic umbilical structures had a postoperative survival rate of 21 of 23 in one study [12].

In a report [8] of 67 foals less than 150 days of age undergoing surgical therapy for colic, the short-term survival was 63%. The long-term survival (greater than 1–2 years' postoperative) rates of 45% to 58% have been reported for foals undergoing abdominal procedures between birth to 6 months [5–9]. Surgery for nonstrangulating lesions of the large colon had higher survival rates than rates for foals with primary small intestinal or strangulating lesions by 70% to 85% versus 20% to 34%, respectively [5–9]. These rates are consistent with adults, in which nonstrangulating lesions carry a more favorable prognosis. A recent study [9] evaluating long-term survival and racing performance documented a similar short-term survival of 85%, with lesion type and location having a significant effect on long-term survival. This study also reported 63% starters in those foals surviving to racing age, compared with 82% in unaffected siblings. Foals that were able to race were as likely to make the same number of starts, race as often, and make as much money as their sibling counterparts [9].

Postoperative complications associated with adhesions have been recognized in recent retrospective studies. In one study, eight of 51 (17%) foals had clinically influential adhesions that were associated with either a second celiotomy or colic episodes, resulting in euthanasia [6]. In another study, 19 of 90 (33%) foals were found to have adhesions, and 9 of the 19 were believed to be clinically important [6].

Overall, the prognosis for foals with an abdominal accident should be made based on the type of lesion (strangulating versus nonstrangulating), duration of illness, concurrent disease processes, and at the time of surgery the likelihood of postoperative complications such as adhesions. For thoroughbred foals, if the foal survives to racing age, the ability to successfully race is not affected negatively by abdominal surgery [9].

Summary

Neonatal foals requiring an evaluation for gastrointestinal or urinary disorders present different considerations than in older foals and adults. The surgeon must consider these differences in the evaluation of a foal when making a diagnosis, a decision for surgery, the postoperative treatment plan, and in formulating a prognosis for the owner. Nonstrangulating conditions of the intestinal tract and disorders of the urinary tract can be managed successfully in foals. Strangulating intestinal lesions may decrease the long-term survival of an affected foal, and client education is important in any surgical plan for these individuals.

References

[1] Bernard WV, Reimer JM. Examination of the foal. Vet Clin North Am Equine Pract 1994; 10(1):37–66.
[2] Embertson RE. Abdominal surgery in foals: an update. In: Proceedings of the 28th Annual Surgical Forum of the American College of Veterinary Surgeons. Arlington, VA, 2000. p. 31–33.
[3] Orsini JA. Abdominal Surgery in foals. Vet Clin North Am Equine Pract 1997;13(2): 393–413.
[4] Crowhurst RC, Simpson DJ, McEnery RJ, et al. Intestinal surgery in foals. J S Afr Vet Assoc 1975;46(1):59–67.
[5] Adams R, Koterba AM, Brown MP. Exploratory celiotomy for gastrointestinal disease in neonatal foals: a review of 20 cases. Equine Vet J 1988;20(1):9–12.
[6] Cable CS, Fubini SL, Erb HN, et al. Abdominal surgery in foals: a review of 119 cases (1877–1994). Equine Vet J 1997;29(4):257–61.
[7] Singer ER, Livesey MA. Evaluation of exploratory laparotomy in young horses: 102 cases (1987–1992). J Am Vet Med Assoc 1997;211(9):1158–62.
[8] Vatistas NJ, Synder JR, Wilson WD, et al. Surgical treatment for colic in the foal (67 cases): 1980–1992. Equine Vet J 1996;28(2):139–45.
[9] Santschi EM, Slone DE, Embertson RM, et al. Colic surgery in 206 juvenile thoroughbreds: survival and racing results. Equine Vet J Suppl 2000;32:32–6.
[10] Cohen ND, Chaffin MK. Assessment and initial management of colic in foals. Compendium of Continuing Education 1995;17(1):93–103.
[11] Kablack KA, Embertson RM, Bernard WV, et al. Uroperitoneum in the hospitalized equine neonate: retrospective study of 31 cases, 1988–1997. Equine Vet J 2000;32(6):505–8.
[12] Reef VB, Collatos C, Spencer PA, et al. Clinical, ultrasonographic, and surgical findings in foals with umbilical remnant infections. J Am Vet Med Assoc 1989;195(1):69–72.
[13] Robertson JT, Embertson RM. Surgical management of congenital and perinatal abnormalities of the urogenital tract. Vet Clin North Am Equine Pract 1988;4(3):359–79.
[14] Hackett RP. Rupture of the urinary bladder in neonatal foals. Compendium of Continuing Education for the Practicing Veterinarian 1984;6:S488–92.
[15] Richardson DW, Kohn CW. Uroperitoneum in the foal. J Am Vet Med Assoc 1983;182(3): 267–71.

[16] Adams SB, Fessler JF. Umbilical cord remnant infections in foals: 16 cases 9 (1975–1985). J Am Vet Med Assoc 1987;190(3):316–8.

[17] Orsini JA, Donawick WJ. Surgical treatment of gastroduodenal obstruction in foals. Vet Surg 1986;15:205–8.

[18] Lillich JD, Debowes RM. Bladder. In: Auer JA, Stick JA, editors. Equine surgery. 2nd edition. Philadelphia: WB Saunders; 1999. p. 596–8.

[19] Steckel RR. Diagnosis and management of acute abdominal pain (colic). In: Auer JA, editor. Equine surgery. 1st edition. Philadelphia: WB Saunders; 1992. p. 348–60.

[20] Lester GD, Lester NV. Abdominal and thoracic radiography in the neonate. Vet Clin North Am Equine Pract 2001;17(1):19–46.

[21] Lavan RP, Craychee T, Madigan JE. Practical method of umbilical ultrasonographic examination of one-week-old foals: the procedure and the interpretation of age-correlated size range of umbilical structures. Journal of Equine Veterinary Science 1997;17(2):96–101.

[22] Reef VB. Pediatric abdominal ultrasonography. In: Reef VB, editor. Equine diagnotic ultrasound. Philadelphia: WB Saunders; 1998. p. 364–403.

[23] Cornick-Seahorn J. Anesthesia of the critically ill equine patient. Vet Clin North Am Equine Pract 2004;20(1):127–49.

[24] Butler JA, Colles CM, Dyson SJ, et al. Alimentary system. In: Butler JA, Colles CM, Dyson SJ, et al, editors. Clinical radiology of the horse. 2nd edition. Oxford: Blackwell Science Ltd; 2000. p. 529–63.

[25] Fisher AT, Yarborough TB. Retrograde contrast radiography of the distal portions of the intestinal tract in foals. J Am Vet Med Assoc 1995;207:734–7.

[26] Hardy J, Rakestraw PC. Postoperative care and complications associated with abdominal surgery. In: Auer JA, Stick JA, editors. Equine surgery. 2nd edition. Philadelphia: WB Saunders; 1999. p. 294–306.

[27] Stephen JO, Corley KT, Johnston JK, et al. Small intestinal volvulus in 115 horses: 1988–2000. Vet Surg 2004;33(4):333–9.

[28] Greet TR. Ileal intussusception in 16 young thoroughbreds. Equine Vet J 1992;24(2):81–3.

[29] Freeman DE. Small intestine. In: Auer JA, Stick JA, editors. Equine surgery. 2nd edition. Philadelphia: WB Saunders; 1999. p. 232–56.

[30] Moore RM. Principles of intestinal injury and determining intestinal viability. In: Auer JA, Stick JA, editors. Equine surgery. 2nd edition. Philadelphia: WB Saunders; 1999. p. 216–24.

[31] Bernard WV, Reef VB, Reimer JM, et al. Ultrasonographic diagnosis of small intestinal intussusception in three foals. J AM Vet Med Assoc 1989;194:424–6.

[32] Little SE. Adult tapeworms in horses: clinical significance. Compendium of Continuing Education 1999;21(4):356–60.

[33] Martin BB, Freeman DE, Ross MW, et al. Cecocolic and cecocecal intussusception in horses: 30 cases (1976–1996). J Am Vet Med Assoc 1999;214(1):80–4.

[34] Fontaine-Rodgerson G, Rodgerson DH. Diagnosis of small intestinal intussusception by transabdominal ultrasonography in 2 adult horses. Can Vet J 2001;42(5):378–80.

[35] Gaughan EM. Inguinal hernias in horses. Compendium of Continuing Education 1998; 20(9):1057–9.

[36] Klohen A, Wilson DG. Laparoscopic repair of scrotal hernia in two foals. Vet Surg 1996; 25(5):414–6.

[37] Pusterla N, Magdesian KG, Maleski K, et al. Retrospective evaluation of the use of acetylcysteine enemas in the treatment of meconium retention in foals: 44 cases (1987–2002). Equine Veterinary Education 2004;6(3):170–4.

[38] Marr CM. Cardiac emergencies and problems of the critical care patient. Vet Clin North Am Equine Pract 2004;20(1):217–30.

[39] Morisset S, Hawkins JF, Frank N, et al. Surgical management of a ureteral defect with ureterorrhaphy and of ureteritis with ureteroneocystostomy in a foal. J Am Vet Med Assoc 2002;220(3):354–8.

[40] Robertson JT, Spurlock GH, Bramlage LL, et al. Repair of ureteral defect in a foal. J Am Vet Med Assoc 1983;183(7):799–800.
[41] Divers TJ, Byars TD, Spirito M. Correction of bilateral ureteral defects in a foal. J Am Vet Med Assoc 1992;192(3):384–6.
[42] Adams R, Koterba AM, Cudd TC, et al. Exploratory celiotomy for suspected urinary tract disruption in neonatal foals: a review of 18 cases. Equine Vet J 1988;20(1):13–7.
[43] Voss ED, Taylor DS, Slovis NM. Use of a temporary indwelling ureteral stent catheter in a mare with a traumatic ureteral tear. J Am Vet Med Assoc 1999;214:1523–6.
[44] Edwards RB, Fubini SL. A one stage marsupialization procedure for management of infected umbilical vein remnants in calves and foals. Vet Surg 1995;20(1):32–5.
[45] Santschi EM, Juzwiak JS, Moll HD, et al. Diaphragmatic hernia repair in three young horses. Vet Surg 1997;26:242–5.
[46] Jean D, Laverty S. Thoracic trauma in foals. In: Proceedings of the American College of Veterinary Internal Medicine Forum, Charlotte, NC, May 24–28, 2003.
[47] Sprayberry KA, Bain FT, Seahorn TL, et al. 56 cases of rib fractures in neonatal foals hospitalized in a referral center intensive care unit from 1997–2001. In: Proceedings of the 47th Annual American Association of Equine Practitioners, 2001.
[48] Bellezzo F, Hunt RJ, Provost P, et al. Surgical repair of rib fractures in 14 neonatal foals: case selection, surgical technique and results. Equine Vet J 2004;36(7):557–62.
[49] Fischer AT. Laparoscopically assisted resection of umbilical structures in foals. J Am Vet Med Assoc 1998;214(12):1813–6.
[50] Benamou AE, Blikslager AT, Sellon DC. Intestinal atresia in foals. Compendium of Continuing Education 1995;17(12):1510–7.
[51] Estes R, Lyall W. Congenital atresia of the colon: a review and report of four cases in the horse. Journal of Equine Medicine and Surgery 1979;3:495–8.
[52] Young RL, Linford Rl, Olander HJ. Atresia coli in the foal: a review of 6 cases. Equine Vet J 1992;24(1):60–2.
[53] Southwood LL, Baxter GM, Hutchinson JM, et al. Survey of diplomats of the American College of Veterinary Surgeons regarding postoperative intra-abdominal adhesion formation in horses undergoing abdominal surgery. J Am Vet Med Assoc 1997;211(12):1573–6.
[54] Sullins KE, White NA, Lundin CS, et al. Prevention of ischaemia-induced small intestinal adhesions in foals. Equine Vet J 2004;36(5):370–5.
[55] Frees K, Gaughan E, Lillich J, et al. Identification of the hyaluron receptor CD44 on equine peritoneum, serosa and omentum [master's thesis]. Manhattan (KS): University of Kansas; 2002.
[56] Mueller PO, Hunt RJ, Allen D, et al. Intraperitoneal use of sodium carboxymethylcellulose in horses undergoing exploratory celiotomy. Vet Surg 1995;24:112–7.
[57] Kuebelbeck KL, Slone DE, May KA. Effect of omentectomy on adhesion formation in horses. Vet Surg 1998;27:132–7.

VETERINARY
CLINICS
Equine Practice

Vet Clin Equine 21 (2005) 537–545

Index

Note: Page numbers of article titles are in **boldface** type.

A

Abdominal surgery
    in neonatal foals, **511–535**. See also
        *Neonatal foals, abdominal
        surgery in.*

Abdominal ultrasonography
    equine neonatal, **407–429**
        of gastrointestinal tract,
            408–414
        of kidneys, 419–421
        of liver, 422–423
        of spleen, 423–424
        of urogenital tract, 415–418
        technique for, 407–408

ABG measurement. See *Arterial blood gas
    (ABG) measurement.*

Abiotrophy
    cerebellar
        in neonatal foals, 399–400

Acid–base balance
    in diarrhea management in neonatal
        foals, 307

Adaptive immunity
    in neonatal foals, 245–246

Adhesion(s)
    abdominal surgery for
        in neonatal foals, 530–532

Agammaglobulinemia
    in neonatal foals, 256–257

Aganglionosis
    in neonatal foals, 327

Airway pressure
    monitoring of
        during ventilatory support for
            critically ill foals, 480

Allogenic incompatibilities
    in neonatal foals, 259–266

Anemia, immunodeficiency, and peripheral
    ganglionopathy
        in Fell pony foals, 257–258

Angular limb deformities
    in neonatal foals, 372–376

Antacid(s)
    for equine neonatal sepsis, 284

Antiendotoxin(s)
    for equine neonatal sepsis, 283
    in diarrhea management in neonatal
        foals, 309

Antifungal agents
    for equine neonatal sepsis, 283

Antimicrobial agents
    for equine neonatal sepsis, 281–283
    systemic
        in diarrhea management in
            neonatal foals, 310

Anus
    disorders of
        in neonatal foals, 323–327

Arterial blood gas (ABG) measurement
    monitoring of
        during ventilatory support for
            critically ill foals, 476–477

Arthritis
    septic
        equine neonatal sepsis and, 286
        in neonatal foals, 359–368

Asphyxia-associated gastroenteropathies
    in neonatal foals, 296

Atresia
    intestinal
        abdominal surgery for
            in neonatal foals, 529–530
        in neonatal foals, 326–327

B

Bacterial meningitis
    in neonatal foals, 394–395

Botulism
    in neonatal foals, 401–402

Breathing
    in cardiopulmonary cerebral
        resuscitation
        in neonatal foals, 435–437

C

Candidiasis
    oral
        in neonatal foals, 316–317

Capnography
    monitoring of
        during ventilatory support for
            critically ill foals, 477–479

Cardiac arrest
    in neonatal foals
        recognition of, 432

Cardiopulmonary cerebral resuscitation
    in neonatal foals, **431–455**
        airway in, 434–435
        breathing in, 435–437
        care after, 442
        cessation of, 441–442
        circulation in, 437–438
        drugs in, 438–441
        effectiveness of
            monitoring of, 441
        equipment for, 432–433
        new directions in, 442–443
        plan for
            outline of, 433–441
        preparation for, 433

Cataplexy
    in neonatal foals, 398–399

Central nervous system (CNS) trauma
    in neonatal foals, 395–396

Cerebellar abiotrophy
    in neonatal foals, 399–400

Chemical adjuncts
    for critically ill foals, 461–462

Chyloabdomen
    in neonatal foals, 327

Circulation
    in cardiopulmonary cerebral
        resuscitation
        in neonatal foals, 437–438

Cleft palate
    in neonatal foals, 314–315

Clostridial enteritis
    in neonatal foals, 299–302

CNS trauma. See *Central nervous system
    (CNS) trauma.*

Coagulopathy
    equine neonatal sepsis and, 287

Colon
    disorders of
        in neonatal foals, 323–327

Complement
    immune system in neonatal
        foals and, 244

Compliance
    monitoring of
        during ventilatory support for
            critically ill foals, 480–481

Congenital anomalies
    in neonatal foals, 357–359

Contractural deformities
    in neonatal foals, 369–372

Critically ill foals
    ventilatory support for, **457–486**
        chemical adjuncts, 461–462
        evolving therapies, 482
        mechanical ventilation, 462–463
            discontinuation of, 483
        monitoring during, 474–482
            ABG measurement,
                476–477
            airway pressure, 480
            capnography, 477–479
            compliance, 480–481
            endotracheal tube, 481–482
            fraction of inspired
                oxygen, 479
            resistance, 480–481
            tidal volume and minute
                volume, 479–480
        oxygen therapy, 458–461
        preconditioning ventilator gases
            in, 472–474
        preparation for, 474, 475
        ventilator modes in, 463–469
        ventilator settings in, 469–472

D

Dermatitis
    ulcerative
        neonatal alloimmune
            thrombocytopenia with
            or without
            in neonatal foals, 265–266

Dextrose solutions
    for neonatal foals, 498

Diaphragmatic hernia
    abdominal surgery for
        in neonatal foals, 529

Diarrhea
    foal heat, 295–296
    in neonatal foals, **295–312.** See also
        Neonatal foals, diarrhea in.

Drug(s)
    in cardiopulmonary cerebral
        resuscitation
        in neonatal foals, 438–441

Dysmature foals
    treatment of, 344–352

Dysphagia
    in neonatal foals, 315–316

E

EDM. See *Equine degenerative
    myeloencephalopathy (EDM).*

Electrolyte(s)
    in diarrhea management in neonatal
        foals, 307–308

Emergency fluid resuscitation
    in neonatal foals, 443–446

Emergency glucose support
    in neonatal foals, 449–450

Emergency oxygen therapy
    in neonatal foals, 450–452

Endotracheal tube
    changing of
        during ventilatory support for
            critically ill foals, 481–482

Enteral nutrition
    for neonatal foals, 491–498
        complications of, 497–498,
            503–504
        delivery of, 494–496
        initiation of, 496–497
        products, 492–494

Enteritis
    clostridial
        in neonatal foals, 299–302
    viral
        in neonatal foals, 303–304

Enterocolitis
    mechanical
        in neonatal foals, 298–299
    necrotizing
        in neonatal foals, 296–298

Equine degenerative myeloencephalopathy
    (EDM)
    in neonatal foals, 398

Equine neonatal abdominal
    ultrasonography, **407–429.** See also

*Abdominal ultrasonography, equine
    neonatal.*

Equine neonatal sepsis, **273–293**
    causative organisms, 279–281
    clinical signs of, 276–279
    coagulopathy and, 287
    definitions associated with, 273–274
    diagnosis of, 276–279
    focal infection, 285–287
    gastrointestinal involvement in, 285
    meningitis and, 286–287
    ocular involvement in, 287
    osteomyelitis and, 286
    pathophysiology of, 273–274
    predisposing factors for, 273–275
    prevention of, 288–289
    prognosis of, 287–288
    respiratory involvement in, 285
    routes of infection, 273–275
    septic arthritis and, 286
    sequelae of, 285–287
    treatment of, 281–284
        antacids in, 284
        antiendotoxin therapy in, 283
        antifungal agents in, 283
        antimicrobial agents in, 281–283
        cardiovascular support in,
            283–284
        experimental therapy in, 284
    umbilical involvement in, 285–286

Equine neonatal thoracic ultrasonography,
    407–429. See also *Thoracic
    ultrasonography, equine neonatal.*
    technique for, 407–408

Esophagus
    disorders of
        in neonatal foals, 317–318

Experimental therapy
    for equine neonatal sepsis, 284

F

Failure of passive transfer (FPT) of
    immunoglobulins
    in neonatal foals, 249–253

Fell pony foals
    anemia, immunodeficiency, and
        peripheral ganglionopathy in,
        257–258

Fetal hypothalamic-pituitary-adrenal axis
    maturation of
        accelerated, 341–342
        in neonatal foals, 339–341

Fluid balance
    in diarrhea management in neonatal
        foals, 305–307

Fluid therapy
  for hypovolemia
    in neonatal foals, 446–449
Foal(s)
  critically ill. See *Critically ill foals.*
  dysmature
    treatment of, 344–352
  Fell pony
    anemia, immunodeficiency, and
      peripheral ganglionopathy
      in, 257–258
  mule
    neonatal isoerythrolysis in,
      264–265
  neonatal. See *Neonatal foals.*
  normal
    energy requirements of,
      487–488
    feeding behavior of, 488–490
    milk consumption of, 488–490
  premature
    treatment of, 344–352. See also
      *Premature foals, treatment
      of.*

Foal heat diarrhea, 295–296

FPT. See *Failure of passive transfer (FPT)
  of immunoglobulins.*

Fraction of inspired oxygen
  monitoring of
    during ventilatory support for
      critically ill foals, 479

G

Gas(es)
  ventilator
    preconditioning
      for critically ill foals,
        472–474

Gastric ulcer medications
  in diarrhea management in neonatal
    foals, 308–309

Gastric ulceration
  in neonatal foals, 318–321

Gastroduodenal ulceration
  diarrhea in neonatal foals and, 298

Gastroenteropathy(ies)
  asphyxia-associated
    in neonatal foals, 296

Gastrointestinal protectants
  in diarrhea management in neonatal
    foals, 308

Gastrointestinal tract
  in neonatal foals
    nondiarrheal disorders of,

313–332. See also *Neonatal
  foals, nondiarrheal disorders
  of gastrointestinal tract in.*
  neonatal
    ultrasonography of, 408–414

Glucocorticoid(s)
  for premature foals, 349–350

H

Hernia(s)
  diaphragmatic
    abdominal surgery for
      in neonatal foals, 529
  inguinal-scrotal
    abdominal surgery for
      in neonatal foals, 521–522

HIE. See *Hypoxic-ischemic encephalopathy
  (HIE).*

Hydrocephalus
  in neonatal foals, 403–404

Hyperextension
  in neonatal foals, 368–369

Hypovolemia
  fluid therapy for
    in neonatal foals, 446–449

Hypoxic-ischemic encephalopathy (HIE)
  in neonatal foals, 391–394

I

Ileus
  disorders of
    in neonatal foals, 322–323

Immune system
  in neonatal foals, 241–247. See also
    Neonatal foals, immune system in.

Immunity
  adaptive
    in neonatal foals, 245–246
  treatment of premature foals
    and, 350–352

Immunodeficiency disorders
  in Fell pony foals
    anemia, immunodeficiency, and
      peripheral ganglionopathy,
      257–258
  in neonatal foals, 248–259
    agammaglobulinemia, 256–257
    described, 248–249
    FPT, 249–253
    SCID, 253–255
    selective IgM deficiency,
      255–256

Immunoglobulin(s)
    FPT of
        in neonatal foals, 249–253
Immunologic disorders
    in neonatal foals, **241–272**. See also
        Immunodeficiency disorders, in
        neonatal foals.
        allogenic incompatibilities,
            259–266
        immunodeficiencies, 248–259
        neonatal alloimmune
            thrombocytopenia with or
            without ulcerative
            dermatitis, 265–266
        neonatal isoerythrolysis,
            259–264
Impaction
    meconium
        in neonatal foals, 323–326
            abdominal surgery for,
                522–523
Infection(s)
    in premature foals
        treatment-related, 350–352
Inguinal-scrotal hernias
    abdominal surgery for
        in neonatal foals, 521–522
Intestinal atresia
    abdominal surgery for
        in neonatal foals, 529–530
    in neonatal foals, 326–327
Isoerythrolysis
    neonatal
        in foals, 259–264
        in mule foals, 264–265

K

Kidney(s)
    abdominal ultrasonography of,
        419–421

L

Lipid emulsions
    for neonatal foals, 499
Liver
    abdominal ultrasonography of,
        422–423

M

Mare(s)
    pregnant
        late

at-risk
    treatment of, 342–343
Mechanical enterocolitis
    in neonatal foals, 298–299
Mechanical ventilation
    for critically ill foals, 462–463
        discontinuation of, 483
Meconium impaction
    in neonatal foals, 323–326
        abdominal surgery for, 522–523
Meningitis
    bacterial
        in neonatal foals, 394–395
    equine neonatal sepsis and, 286–287
Minute volume
    monitoring of
        during ventilatory support for
            critically ill foals, 479–480
MODS. See *Multiple organ dysfunction*
    syndrome (MODS).
Mule foals
    neonatal isoerythrolysis in,
        264–265
Multiple organ dysfunction syndrome
    (MODS)
    described, 274
Musculoskeletal system
    in treatment of premature foals, 350

N

Narcolepsy
    in neonatal foals, 398–399
Necrotizing enterocolitis
    in neonatal foals, 296–298
Neonatal alloimmune thrombocytopenia
    with or without ulcerative dermatitis
    in neonatal foals, 265–266
Neonatal foals
    abdominal surgery in, **511–535**
        considerations related to,
            516–518
        disorders requiring
            diagnostics for, 511–516
        for adhesions, 530–532
        for diaphragmatic hernia, 529
        for inguinal-scrotal hernias,
            521–522
        for intestinal atresia, 529–530
        for meconium impaction,
            522–523
        for small intestinal strangulation,
            518–521

Neonatal foals (*continued*)
  for umbilical remnant infections
    and patent urachus,
    527–529
  for uroperitoneum, 523–527
  prognosis after, 532–533
  adaptive immunity in, 245–246
  aganglionosis in, 327
  anus disorders in, 323–327
  cardiac arrest in
    recognition of, 432
  chyloabdomen in, 327
  cleft palate in, 314–315
  colon disorders in, 323–327
  congenital anomalies in, 357–359
  diarrhea in, **295–312**
    asphyxia-associated
      gastroenteropathies, 296
    causes of
      dietary, 299
      nutritional, 299
    clostridial enteritis, 299–302
    foal heat diarrhea, 295–296
    gastroduodenal ulceration
      and, 298
    infectious, 299–305
    management of, 305–310
      acid–base balance in, 307
      antiendotoxin modalities
        in, 309
      electrolytes in, 307–308
      fluid balance in, 305–307
      gastric ulcer medications in,
        308–309
      gastrointestinal protectants
        in, 308
      nutrition in, 309–310
      systemic antimicrobial
        agents in, 310
    mechanical enterocolitis, 298–299
    necrotizing enterocolitis, 296–298
    noninfectious, 295–299
    parasitic agents of, 305
    protozoal agents of, 305
    viral enteritis, 303–304
  dysphagia in, 315–316
  emergency fluid resuscitation in,
    443–446
  emergency glucose support for,
    449–450
  emergency management for, **431–455**
  emergency oxygen therapy for,
    450–452
  esophageal disorders in, 317–318
  fluid therapy for hypovolemia in,
    446–449
  gastric ulceration in, 318–321
  ileus disorders in, 322–323
  immune system in, 244–246

assessment of, 247–248
complement and, 244
development of, 241–242
immunodeficiencies in, 248–259
neutrophils and, 244–245
immunologic disorders in, **241–272.**
  See also *Immunologic disorders,
  in neonatal foals.*
intestinal atresia in, 326–327
maturity of, **333–355**
  causes of, 336–338
  clinical progression of, 344
  definitions associated with,
    334–335
  laboratory assessment of,
    343–344
  maturation of fetal hypothalamic-
    pituitary-adrenal axis and,
    339–341
    accelerated, 341–342
  physical characteristics of,
    335–336
  prognosis for, 352
meconium impaction in, 323–326
neurologic development in
  normal, 387–388
neurologic disorders in, **387–406.** See
  also *Neurologic disorders, in
  neonatal foals.*
neurologic examination in, 388–391
nondiarrheal disorders of
  gastrointestinal tract in, **313–332**
  monitoring of
    routine, 313–314
  physical examination of, 313–314
normal gestational period, 333–334
nursing
  adequate nutrition in
    monitoring for, 490
  nutritional support for, **487–510**
    enteral nutrition, 491–498.
      See also *Enteral nutrition,
      for neonatal foals.*
    in diarrheal management,
      309–310
    initiation of, 491
    monitoring response to diet,
      504–505
    parenteral nutrition, 498–503.
      See also *Parenteral nutri-
      tion, for neonatal foals.*
    probiotics, 505–506
oral cavity–related disorders in,
  314–317
orthopedic disorders in, **357–385.**
  See also *Orthopedic disorders, in
  neonatal foals.*
passive immunity in
  transfer of, 242–244

peritoneal disorders in, 327–328
rectal disorders in, 323–327
respiratory arrest in
recognition of, 432
respiratory system in
host defense mechanisms of,
246–247
resuscitation in, **431–455**
sepsis in, **273–293**. See also *Equine
neonatal sepsis.*
septic peritonitis in, 327–328
sick
energy requirements of, 490–491
small intestine–related disorders in,
322–323
stomach disorders in, 318–321
terminology associated with, 334–335
thrush in, 316–317

Neonatal isoerythrolysis
in mule foals, 264–265
in neonatal foals, 259–264

Neonatal sepsis
equine, **273–293**. See also *Equine
neonatal sepsis.*

Neurologic development
in neonatal foals
normal, 387–388

Neurologic disorders
in neonatal foals, **387–406**
bacterial meningitis, 394–395
botulism, 401–402
cataplexy, 398–399
cerebellar abiotrophy, 399–400
CNS trauma, 395–396
EDM, 398
HIE, 391–394
hydrocephalus, 403–404
narcolepsy, 398–399
neuroanatomic localization of,
391
occipitoatlantoaxial malformation, 400
peripheral nerve injury, 397–398
tetanus, 402–403

Neurologic examination
in neonatal foals, 388–391

Neutrophil(s)
and immune system in neonatal foals,
244–245

Nondiarrheal disorders of gastrointestinal
tract
in neonatal foals, **313–332**. See also
*Neonatal foals, nondiarrheal
disorders of gastrointestinal
tract in.*

Nursing
of neonatal foals
adequate nutrition in
monitoring for, 490

Nutrition
enteral
for neonatal foals, 491–498. See
also *Enteral nutrition, for
neonatal foals.*
parenteral
for neonatal foals, 498–503. See
also *Parenteral nutrition,
for neonatal foals.*

Nutritional support
for neonatal foals, **487–510**. See also
*Neonatal foals, nutritional
support for.*
in diarrhea management in neonatal
foals, 309–310

O

Occipitoatlantoaxial malformation
in neonatal foals, 400

Oral candidiasis
in neonatal foals, 316–317

Oral cavity
disorders of
in neonatal foals, 314–317

Orthopedic disorders
in neonatal foals, **357–385**
angular limb deformities,
372–376
congenital anomalies, 357–359
contractural deformities,
369–372
hyperextension, 368–369
osteomyelitis, 286, 359–368
physitis, 376–377
septic arthritis, 359–368

Osteomyelitis
equine neonatal sepsis and, 286
in neonatal foals, 359–368

Oxygen
inspired
fraction of
monitoring of
during ventilatory
support for critically
ill foals, 479

Oxygen therapy
emergency
in neonatal foals, 450–452
for critically ill foals, 458–461

P

Palate(s)
  cleft
    in neonatal foals, 314–315

Parasite(s)
  diarrhea in neonatal foals due to, 305

Parenteral nutrition
  for neonatal foals, 498–503
    complications of, 502–504
    delivery of, 502
    dextrose solutions, 498
    formulation of, 499–502
    lipid emulsions, 499
    preparation of, 502
    products, 498
    protein, 499

Patent urachus
  umbilical remnant infections and abdominal surgery for
    in neonatal foals, 527–529

Peripheral nerve injury
  in neonatal foals, 397–398

Peritoneal disorders
  in neonatal foals, 327–328

Peritonitis
  septic
    in neonatal foals, 327–328

Physitis
  in neonatal foals, 376–377

Pregnancy
  steroidogenesis during, 338–339

Pregnant mare
  late
    at-risk
      treatment of, 342–343

Premature foals
  prognosis for, 352
  treatment of, 344–352
    body temperature regulation and, 349
    gastrointestinal function and, 348–349
    glucocorticoids in, 349–350
    hypoglycemia and, 349
    immunity and, 350–352
    infections and, 350–352
    musculoskeletal system and, 350
    perfusion failure in, 347–348
    respiratory system in, 346–347

Probiotics
  for neonatal foals, 505–506

Protein
  for neonatal foals, 499

Protozoa
  diarrhea in neonatal foals due to, 305

R

Rectum
  disorders of
    in neonatal foals, 323–327

Resistance
  monitoring of
    during ventilatory support for critically ill foals, 480–481

Respiratory arrest
  in neonatal foals
    recognition of, 432

Resuscitation
  cardiopulmonary cerebral
    in neonatal foals, **431–455.** See also *Cardiopulmonary cerebral resuscitation, in neonatal foals.*
  emergency fluid
    in neonatal foals, 443–446

S

SCID. See *Severe combined immunodeficiency (SCID).*

Selective IgM deficiency
  in neonatal foals, 255–256

Sepsis
  equine neonatal, **273–293.** See also *Equine neonatal sepsis.*

Septic arthritis
  equine neonatal sepsis and, 286
  in neonatal foals, 359–368

Septic peritonitis
  in neonatal foals, 327–328

Severe combined immunodeficiency (SCID)
  in neonatal foals, 253–255

SIRS. See *Systemic inflammatory response syndrome (SIRS).*

Small intestinal strangulation
  abdominal surgery for
    in neonatal foals, 518–521

Small intestine
  disorders of
    in neonatal foals, 322–323

Spleen
  abdominal ultrasonography of, 423–424

Steroidogenesis
    during pregnancy, 338–339

Stomach
    disorders of
        in neonatal foals, 318–321

Systemic inflammatory response syndrome (SIRS)
    described, 273–274

T

Tetanus
    in neonatal foals, 402–403

Thoracic ultrasonography
    equine neonatal
        of abnormal structures, 426–429
        of normal structures, 424–425
        techniques for, 407–408
            scanning, 424

Thrush
    in neonatal foals, 316–317

Tidal volume
    monitoring of
        during ventilatory support for critically ill foals, 479–480

Trauma
    CNS
        in neonatal foals, 395–396

U

Ulceration
    gastric
        in neonatal foals, 318–321
    gastroduodenal
        diarrhea in neonatal foals and, 298

Ulcerative dermatitis
    neonatal alloimmune thrombocytopenia with or without
        in neonatal foals, 265–266

Ultrasonography
    abdominal, **407–429**
        equine neonatal. See *Abdominal ultrasonography, equine neonatal.*
    thoracic
        equine neonatal, **407–429**. See also *Thoracic ultrasonography, equine neonatal.*

Umbilical remnant infections and patent urachus
    abdominal surgery for
        in neonatal foals, 527–529

Urogenital tract
    neonatal
        ultrasonography of, 415–418

Uroperitoneum
    abdominal surgery for
        in neonatal foals, 523–527

V

Ventilation
    mechanical
        for critically ill foals, 462–463
            discontinuation of, 483

Ventilator gases
    preconditioning
        for critically ill foals, 472–474

Ventilator modes
    for critically ill foals, 463–469

Ventilator settings
    for critically ill foals, 469–472

Ventilatory support
    for critically ill foals, **457–486.** See also *Critically ill foals, ventilatory support for.*

Viral enteritis
    in neonatal foals, 303–304

Changing Your Address?

Make sure your subscription changes too! When you notify us of your new address, you can help make our job easier by including an exact copy of your Clinics label number with your old address (see illustration below.) This number identifies you to our computer system and will speed the processing of your address change. Please be sure this label number accompanies your old address and your corrected address—you can send an old Clinics label with your number on it or just copy it exactly and send it to the address listed below.

We appreciate your help in our attempt to give you continuous coverage. Thank you.

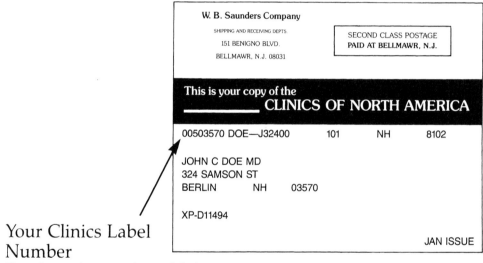

W. B. Saunders Company
SHIPPING AND RECEIVING DEPTS.
151 BENIGNO BLVD.
BELLMAWR, N.J. 08031

SECOND CLASS POSTAGE
PAID AT BELLMAWR, N.J.

This is your copy of the
_____ CLINICS OF NORTH AMERICA

00503570 DOE—J32400   101   NH   8102

JOHN C DOE MD
324 SAMSON ST
BERLIN   NH   03570

XP-D11494

JAN ISSUE

Your Clinics Label Number

Copy it exactly or send your label along with your address to:
W.B. Saunders Company, Customer Service
Orlando, FL 32887-4800
Call Toll Free 1-800-654-2452

Please allow four to six weeks for delivery of new subscriptions and for processing address changes.

8 Ways To Expand Your Practice
Step 1: Return this card.

Elsevier Clinics and Journals offer you that rare combination of up-to-date scholarly data, step-by-step techniques and authoritative insights...information you can easily apply to the situations you encounter in daily practice. You'll be better able to diagnose and treat a wider range of veterinary problems and broaden your client base.

Just indicate your choice(s) on the card below, fill out the rest of the card and drop it in the mail.

Your satisfaction is guaranteed. If you do not find that the periodical meets your expectations, write *cancel* on the invoice and return it within 30 days. You are under no further obligation.

SUBSCRIBE TODAY!
DETACH AND MAIL THIS NO-RISK CARD TODAY!

YES! Please start my subscription to the periodicals checked below with the ❑ first issue of the calendar year or ❑ current issues. If not completely satisfied with my first issue, I may write "cancel" on the invoice and return it within 30 days at no further obligation

Please Print:

Name _____

Address _____

_____

City _____ State _____

ZIP _____

Method of Payment

❑ Check (payable to **Elsevier**; add the applicable sales tax for your area)

❑ VISA ❑ MasterCard ❑ AmEx ❑ Bill me

Card number _____

Exp. date _____

Signature _____

Staple this to your purchase order to expedite delivery

*To receive in-training rate, orders must be accompanied by the name of affiliated institution, dates of residency and signature of coordinator on institution letterhead. Orders will be billed at the individual rate until proof of resident status is received.

This is not a renewal notice. Professional references may be tax-deductible.
© **Elsevier 2005.** Offer valid in U.S. only. Prices subject to change without notice. **MO 10806 DF4169**

❑ **Clinical Techniques in Equine Practice**
Volume 4 (4 issues)
Individuals $124; Institutions $209; In-training $62*

❑ **Clinical Techniques in Small Animal Practice**
Volume 10 (4 issues)
Individuals $134; Institutions $220; In-training $67*

❑ **Journal of Equine Veterinary Science**
Volume 22 (12 issues)
Individuals $171; Institutions $242; In-training $54*

❑ **Seminars in Avian and Exotic Pet Medicine**
Volume 4 (4 issues)
Individuals $116; Institutions $220; In-training $54*

❑ **Veterinary Clinics-Equine Practice**
Volume 21 (3 issues)
Individuals $145; Institutions $230

❑ **Veterinary Clinics-Exotic Animal Practice**
Volume 8 (3 issues)
Individuals $130; Institutions $215

❑ **Veterinary Clinics-Food Animal Practice**
Volume 21 (3 issues)
Individuals $115; Institutions $182

❑ **Veterinary Clinics-Small Animal Practice**
Volume 35 (6 issues)
Individuals $170; Institutions $260

Elsevier, the premier publisher in veterinary medicine, keeps you current with the latest developments in your field to help you achieve optimal patient care. Subscribe today to any of the publications listed below and save considerably over the single issue price.

Clinical Techniques in Equine Practice

Clinical Techniques in Small Animal Practice

Journal of Equine Veterinary Science

Seminars in Avian and Exotic Pet Medicine

Veterinary Clinics – Equine Practice

Veterinary Clinics – Exotic Animal Practice

Veterinary Clinics – Food Animal Practice

Veterinary Clinics – Small Animal Practice

Just fill out the card on the reverse and drop it in the mail.
YOUR SATISFACTION IS GUARANTEED.

NO POSTAGE
NECESSARY
IF MAILED
IN THE
UNITED STATES

BUSINESS REPLY MAIL
FIRST-CLASS MAIL   PERMIT NO 7135   ORLANDO FL

POSTAGE WILL BE PAID BY ADDRESSEE

PERIODICALS ORDER FULFILLMENT DEPT
ELSEVIER
6277 SEA HARBOR DR
ORLANDO FL 32821-9816

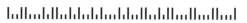